T0383126

Chronic Myeloproliferative Disorders

Chronic Myeloproliferative Disorders

Edited by

Tariq I Mughal MD FRCP FACP
Professor of Medicine and Hematology – Oncology
University of Texas Southwestern Medical School
Dallas, TX, USA
and Consultant Haematologist
Guy's, Kings', & St. Thomas' NHS Hospitals
London, UK

and

John M Goldman DM FRCP FMedSci
Emeritus Professor of Haematology
Department of Haematology
Imperial College London
London, UK

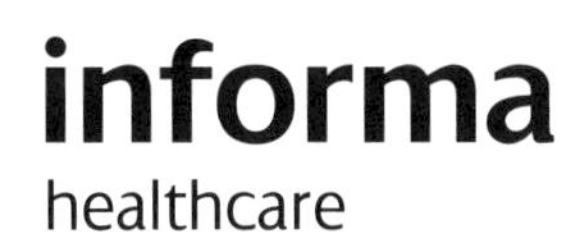

First published in the United Kingdom in 2008 by Informa Healthcare, Telephone House, 69–77 Paul Street, London EC2A 4LQ. Informa Healthcare is a trading division of Informa UK Ltd. Registered Office: 37/41 Mortimer Street, London W1T 3JH. Registered in England and Wales number 1072954.

Tel: +44 (0)20 7017 5000
Fax: +44 (0)20 7017 6699
Website: www.informahealthcare.com

Library of Congress Cataloging-in-Publication Data

Chronic myeloproliferative disorders/edited by Tariq I. Mughal and John M. Goldman.
p. ; cm.
Includes bibliographical references and index.
ISBN-13: 978-0-415-41598-9 (hb : alk. paper)
ISBN-10: 0-415-41598-5 (hb : alk. paper) 1. Myeloproliferative disorders. 2. Chronic diseases. I. Mughal, Tariq I. II. Goldman, J.M. (John Michael)
[DNLM: 1. Leukemia, Myeloid. 2. Myeloproliferative Disorders. WH 250 C5578 2008]
RC645.75.C45 2008
616′.044–dc22

2008028733

ISBN-10: 0 415 41598 5
ISBN-13: 978 0 415 41598 9

Distributed in North and South America by
Taylor & Francis
6000 Broken Sound Parkway, NW, (Suite 300)
Boca Raton, FL 33487, USA

Within Continental USA
Tel: 1 (800) 272 7737; Fax: 1 (800) 374 3401
Outside Continental USA
Tel: (561) 994 0555; Fax: (561) 361 6018
Email: orders@crcpress.com

Book orders in the rest of the world
Paul Abrahams
Tel: +44 207 017 4036
Email: bookorders@informa.com

Composition by Exeter Premedia Services Pvt Ltd., Chennai, India
Printed in the United States of America.

Contents

Part II Philadelphia-negative chronic myeloproliferative disorders

Contributors

Michele Baccarani MD
Department of Hematology-Oncology
'L. and A. Seràgnoli'
Bologna University
Bologna
Italy

Tiziano Barbui MD
Department of Hematology and Oncology
Ospedali Riuniti di Bergamo
Bergamo
Italy

Sonja Burgstaller MD
Wessex Regional Genetics Laboratory
University of Southampton
Salisbury District Hospital
Salisbury
UK

Peter J Campbell MD
Department of Hematology
Cambridge Institute for Medical Research
University of Cambridge
Cambridge
UK

Fausto Castagnetti MD
Department of Hematology – Oncology
'L. and A. Seràgnoli'
University of Bologna
Bologna
Italy

Richard E Clark MA MD FRCP FRCPath
Department of Hematology
Royal Liverpool University Hospital
Liverpool
UK

Jorge Cortes MD
Department of Leukemia
MD Anderson Cancer Center
University of Texas
Houston, TX
USA

Nicholas CP Cross PhD FRCPath MA
Wessex Regional Genetics Laboratory
University of Southampton
Salisbury District Hospital
Salisbury
UK

Michael W Deininger MD PhD
Oregon Health and Science University
Center for Hematologic Malignancies
Portland, OR
USA

Guido Finazzi MD
Department of Trasfusion Medicine
Ospedali Riuniti di Bergamo
Bergamo
Italy

Sergio Giralt MD
Department of Stem Cell Transplantation and
Cellular Therapy
MD Anderson Cancer Center
University of Texas
Houston, TX
USA

John M Goldman DM FRCP FMedSci
Department of Haematology
Imperial College London
London
UK

Anthony R Green PhD FRCP FMedSci
Department of Hematology
Cambridge Institute for Medical Research
University of Cambridge
Cambridge
UK

Devendra K Hiwase MD FRACP FRCPA
Division of Hematology
Institute of Medical and Veterinary Science
Adelaide, SA
Australia

Timothy Hughes MD FRACP FRCPA
Division of Hematology
Institute of Medical and Veterinary Science
Adelaide, SA
Australia

Ilaria Iacobucci MD
Department of Hematology–Oncology
'L. and A. Seràgnoli'
University of Bologna
Bologna
Italy

Elias Jabbour MD
Department of Leukemia
MD Anderson Cancer Center
University of Texas
Houston, TX
USA

Hagop M Kantarjian MD
Department of Leukemia
MD Anderson Cancer Center
University of Texas
Houston, TX
USA

Nicolaus Kröger MD PhD
Department of Stem Cell Transplantation
University Hospital Hamburg-Eppendorf
Hamburg
Germany

Paul La Rosée MD
Faculty of Medicine
III. med. Universitsklinik
Mannheim
Germany

Tariq I Mughal MD FRCP FACP
Department of Hematology–Oncology
University of Texas Southwestern Medical School
Dallas, TX
USA

Francesca Palandri MD
Department of Hematology–Oncology
'L. and A. Seràgnoli'
University of Bologna
Bologna
Italy

Animesh Pardanani MBBS PhD
Division of Hematology
College of Medicine
Mayo Clinic
Rochester, MN
USA

Uday Popat MD
Department of Stem Cell Transplantation and Cellular Therapy
MD Anderson Cancer Center
University of Texas
Houston, TX
USA

Anna Pusiol MD
Department of Pathology and Experimental and Clinical Medicine
Pediatric Section
University of Udine
Italy

Andreas Reiter MD
Faculty of Medicine
III. Medizinische Universitätsklinik
Mannheim
Germany

Jürg Schwaller MD
Division of Childhood Leukemia
Department of Research
University Hospital Basel
Basel
Switzerland

Radek Skoda MD
Division of Experimental Hematology
Department of Research
University Hospital Basel
Basel
Switzerland

Ayalew Tefferi MD
Division of Hematology
College of Medicine
Mayo Clinic
Rochester, MN
USA

Srdan Verstovsek MD PhD
Department of Leukemia
MD Anderson Cancer Center
University of Texas
Houston, TX
USA

Preface

Claims of priority can almost always be challenged but it is generally agreed that John Hughes Bennett in Edinburgh and Rudolph Virchow in Berlin were the first to publish accurate case reports of what must surely have been chronic myeloid leukaemia. Both published in 1845 and probably neither was aware of the other's publication until later. In 1879 a German surgeon, Gustav Heuck, described two young patients with massive splenomegaly and abnormal leukocytes and nucleated red cells in the blood – a condition we would accept today as primary myelofibrosis. Louis Vaquez can legitimately claim credit for the first description of polycythemia vera in 1892, though of course the disease was for many years known as Osler-Vaquez disease in recognition of Osler's description in 1903 of four cases of what today we accept as polycythemia vera. Epstein and Goedel were the first to describe the condition known to as essential thrombocythemia. These four conditions were generally regarded as distinct though various haematologists in the first half of the 20th century had noted trilineage involvement in each. In the editorial he wrote in Blood in 1951 William Dameshek's contribution unquestionably was to group these three disorders together with others under the general heading of myeloproliferative disorders and to draw attention to their common features. He did not specifically refer to essential thrombocythemia.

"....*To put together such apparently dissimilar diseases as chronic granulocytic leukemia, polycythemia, myeloid metaplasia and diGuglielmos's syndrome may conceivably be without foundation, but for the moment at least, this may prove useful and even productive. What more can one ask of a theory?" (Dameshek, 1951)*

He speculated that they might all be due to some ill-defined exogenous factor stimulating excessive haemopoiesis but of course the emphasis has shifted in recent years to the notion that molecular defects acquired in single haemopoietic stem cells may be the primary cause of these different but related disorders. This then is the justification for attempting to cover in a single book the various chronic myeloproliferative disorders. The only major distinction that we have adopted, conveniently but perhaps somewhat artificially, is to divide them into Ph-positive and Ph-negative MPDs, but the two categories do resemble each other almost as much as they differ individually.

If progress in understanding the biology of the MPDs was rather slow in the first half of the 20th century, the MPD student has been richly rewarded in the subsequent 60 years. Obviously important landmarks, to mention only a few, were the discovery of the Ph chromosome, the characterisation of the (9;22) translocation, the identification of the breakpoint cluster region and of the BCR-ABL fusion gene. These major developments were followed much more recently by the identification of the V617F mutation in JAK2 exon 14 and other mutations in JAK2 exon 12, which seem to play a key role in the Ph-negative MPDs. One may well ask whether this remarkable progress in understanding the molecular biology of the MPDs will presage similar advances in understanding other malignant conditions with ensuing implications for therapy - the so-called paradigm shift in the overall orientation of research. Early indications suggests that the answer may well be 'yes'.

For this edition we have asked a number of experts to contribute individual chapters summarising the state of play for 2008. We recognize that each chapter necessarily relies heavily on published work but we believe that to bring the various topics together in one easily readable book will be a real benefit for scientists, clinical haematologists and students who are not already working in the field and do not have time to read all the original literature – at last search Google produced 12 million references to leukaemia and PubMed more than 200 000 for myeloproliferative diseases.

So we must express our thanks to the authors who all contributed their excellent chapters. Actually writing for a book of this kind always takes much longer than one imagines when one accepts the original invitation so we appreciate their efforts. We hope the reader will too.

Tariq Mughal
John Goldman
London, 2008

Acknowledgments

We would like to thank all the authors who contributed to this book, as well as Kelly Cornish and Georgina Adams of Informa Healthcare for their help (and patience) in collating the work. T.M. wishes to thank Sabena and Alpa for the loving attention, support and some comments expressed during preparation, and dedicates the book to the memory of his father, Imdad Ali.

Chronic myeloid leukemia: a historical perspective

1

Tariq I Mughal, John M Goldman

INTRODUCTION

The story of what we now know as chronic myeloid leukemia (CML) began in the early 19th century as a result of astute clinical observations. Thereafter, with the dawn of the era of medical microscopy and the use of aniline-based dyes to stain human tissues, leukemias were recognized as a distinct nosological entity. Many of the initial efforts focused on therapy and led to the introduction of arsenicals in the later part of the 19th century for symptomatic relief. This was largely supplanted by the introduction of ionizing radiation at the beginning of the 20th century and later by the alkylating agent, busulfan, though many hematologists were suspicious that this agent might, in some cases, expedite transformation of the initial chronic phase to the more advanced phases of CML. Major progress in both the therapy and, indeed, the understanding of the disease did not occur until 1960 when advances in the technology of cytogenetics led to the discovery of a consistent chromosomal abnormality in bone marrow cells of patients with CML. This was later termed the 'Philadelphia' or Ph^1 chromosome to acknowledge the city where the discovery took place. The era of molecular biology unfolded in the early 1980s, and led to the molecular unraveling of the 'pathogenetic' or apparent 'initiating' event for the chronic phase of CML. This, in turn, paved the way to the successful introduction of the original ABL kinase inhibitor, imatinib mesylate, as initial treatment for the majority of, if not all, newly diagnosed patients in chronic phase. In this chapter we address the principal historical events leading to the current treatment algorithms for the various phases of CML. The chronology of events is summarized in Table 1.1 and Figure 1.1.

THE 17th AND 18th CENTURIES

Microscopy was first introduced by Robert Hooke in England in 1665 and Anton van Leeuwenhoek in The Netherlands in 1674.[1,2] Many efforts were undertaken thereafter to study blood cells. Initial descriptions of red blood cells appear to have been made by Jan Swammerdam in 1668 and Leeuwenhoek in The Netherlands in 1674, and of white blood cells by Joseph Lieutaud in France in 1749 and William Hewson in England around 1765.[3–5] The description of platelets, however, did not occur until the 19th century, just ahead of the efforts led by Paul Ehrlich in Germany in the

Table 1.1 Milestones in the study of chronic myeloid leukemia

1960	'Philadelphia' chromosome
1973	Philadelphia chromosome is t(9;22)
1982	ABL involved in t(9:22)
1984	Discovery of BCR on chromosome 22
1985	*BCR-ABL* chimeric mRNA
1985	$p210^{BCR\text{-}ABL}$ has enhanced tyrosine kinase activity
1987	$p190^{BCR\text{-}ABL}$ Ph-positive ALL
1990	$p210^{BCR\text{-}ABL}$ murine model simulating the human disease
1997	$p230^{BCR\text{-}ABL}$ in CNL

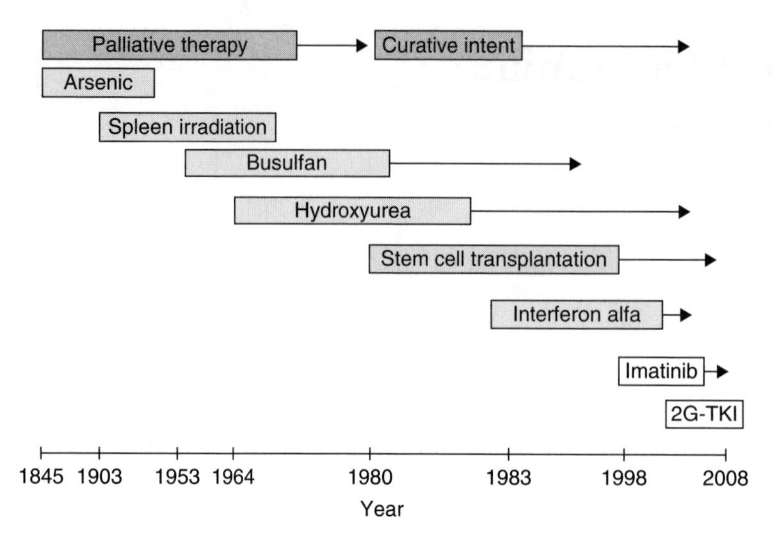

Figure 1.1 Milestones in the treatment of chronic myeloid leukemia. 2G-TKI, second generation tyrosine kinase inhibitors.

use of chemical dyes for better morphological assessment of the various blood cells.[6,7]

It is, of course, likely that one of the first people to publicize the potential role of bone marrow and blood might have been William Shakespeare, who at the end of the 16th century wrote 'Thy bones are marrowless, thy blood is cold' (*Macbeth*).

THE 19th CENTURY

Though the initial descriptions of human leukemias probably began early in the 1800s, Alfred Velpeau in France is credited with the first detailed description of what must have been leukemia in 1827.[8,9] He described a 63-year-old florist and lemonade salesman who presented with gross hepatosplenomegaly and was noted to have 'globules of pus' in his blood. The precise diagnosis, however, remained elusive. The first plausible references to the entity now known as CML were probably made in 1845, almost simultaneously, by John Bennett in Edinburgh, who reported a 28-year-old slater, and Rudolf Virchow in Berlin, who reported a 50-year-old cook.[10,11] They both described autopsy reports in their respective patients who appeared to have been unwell for about 2 years before their deaths and were noted to have very large spleens and an unusual consistency of the blood, which Virchow described as 'weisses blut' and for which Bennett proposed the term 'leucocythaemia'[12] (Figure 1.2). Such was the interest in these initial clinical descriptions, that by 1846, a further nine cases were documented by Virchow. Thereafter cases were described by Craigie, Fuller, and others with increasing frequency.[13–15] Wood in 1850 is credited with the initial description of CML in USA, coincidentally as it turns out in the city of Philadelphia.[16]

Gustav Heuck in Germany in 1879 recognized what he thought was a variant of leukemia when he described two cases of young patients presenting with massive splenomegaly, circulating 'nucleated red cells', and 'abnormal leukocytes', and termed this 'splenic-medullary leukemia', an entity subsequently known by a number of names, including Heuck–Assmann syndrome (1902), agnogenic myeloid metaplasia (1940), chronic idiopathic myelofibrosis (2001), and most recently in 2006 termed primary myelofibrosis by the International Working Group for Myelofibrosis Research and Treatment.[17–23]

Though Alfred Donne in France is credited with the initial description of platelets in 1842, both Max Schultze in Germany and Giulio Bizzozero made significant contributions.[24,25] In 1868 Ernst Neumann in Germany introduced the concept of blood cells being formed in the bone marrow and the notion of

Bennett

LEUCOCYTHEMIA,

WHITE CELL BLOOD,

PHYSIOLOGY AND PATHOLOGY OF THE LYMPHATIC GLANDULAR SYSTEM.

BY JOHN HUGHES BENNETT, M.D., F.R.S.E.,

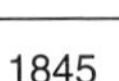

EDINBURGH: SUTHERLAND AND KNOX.
LONDON: SIMPKIN, MARSHALL, & CO.

MDCCCLII.

1845

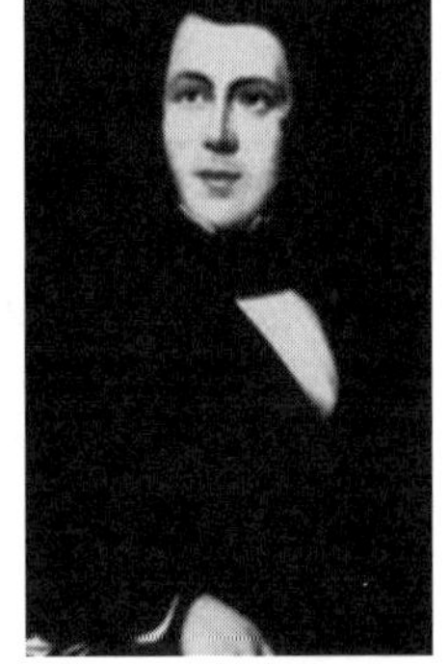

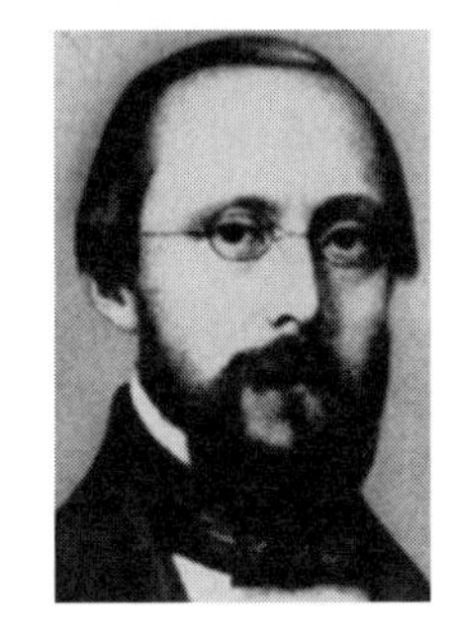

Virchow

Weißes Blut.

Außer sehr wenig rothen Blutkörperchen bestand der ungleich größere Theil aus denselben farblosen oder weißen Körpern, die auch im normalen Blut vorkommen, nämlich kleinen, nicht ganz regelmäßigen Proteinmolecülen, größeren, körnigen, fetthaltigen, kernlosen Körperchen und granulirten Zellen mit einem rundlichen, hufeisenförmigen oder kleeblattartigen oder mit mehreren napfförmigen, distincten Kernen. Die größeren dieser Zellen hatten ein leicht gelbliches Aussehen. Das Verhältniß zwischen den farbigen und farblosen Blutkörperchen stellte sich hier ungefähr umgekehrt, wie im normalen Blut, indem die farblosen die Regel, die farbigen eine Art von Ausnahme zu bilden schienen. Wenn ich daher von weißem Blute spreche, so meine ich in der That ein Blut, in welchem die Proportion zwischen den rothen und farblosen (in Masse weißen) Blutkörperchen eine umgekehrte ist, ohne daß eine Beimischung fremdartiger chemischer oder morphologischer Elemente zu bemerken wäre.

ich würde mich glücklich schätzen, der Wissenschaft dadurch zu einer neuen und, wie es mir scheint, nicht unwichtigen Thatsache verholfen zu haben. —

Dr. Virchow.

Figure 1.2 Virchow and Bennett.

'leucocythemia' arising in the marrow rather than the spleen, as Virchow and others had thought.[26] The 'modern' era of medical microscopy began in the 1880s with the introduction of panoptic staining methods by Paul Ehrlich in Germany[6,27] (Figure 1.3). By this time Neumann was already working on a remarkably detailed description of the cellular components of the bone marrow and probably introduced the notion of an 'ancestral cell' that resulted in the production of circulating red cells.[28] In 1891 Ehrlich compiled the first classification of 'leukemias' with the description of not only 'myeloid' and 'lymphoid' types, but also the various major subtypes of leukemias, including a better microscopic description of CML. Remarkably he also speculated that the 'ancestral cell' proposed by Neumann might actually represent a cell which gave rise to not only circulating red cells, but also white cells and platelets.

From a therapeutic perspective, efforts to improve the symptoms of CML probably began with the use of arsenicals by Thomas Fowler.

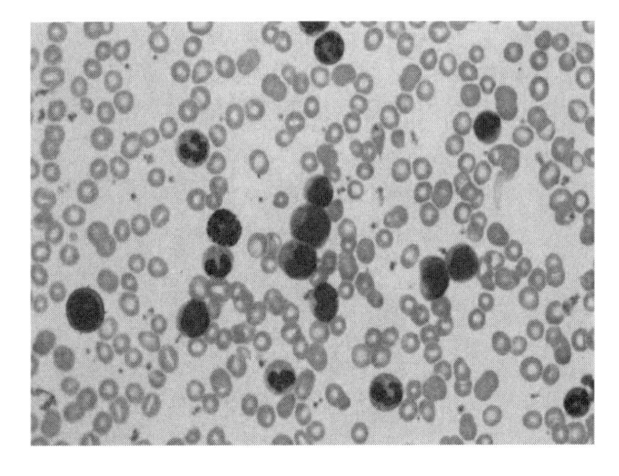

Figure 1.3 Peripheral blood film depicting chronic myeloid leukemia.

He described a 1% solution of potassium arsenite as a general 'tonic' for humans and animals, and its first documented use was by Lissauer in Germany in 1865.[29] The first report of arsenic to treat a patient with the probable diagnosis of CML was published in *The Lancet* by Arthur Conan Doyle from Birmingham, England, in 1882; there is some ambiguity about the letter since the author's name appears as Arthur 'Cowan' Doyle and not Arthur Conan Doyle, but this is probably merely a printer's error. Conan Doyle is, of course, rather more famous for his stories of Sherlock Holmes[30] (Figure 1.4). Blood transfusion was performed, but largely without success, and did not become a safe procedure until the discovery of the human blood groups by Landsteiner in 1935. Splenectomy was also used but often resulted in the death of the patient.

Towards the end of the 19th century, an increasing number of cases were described in different parts of the world characterized by an increase in the number of the different blood cells and often accompanied by an enlarged spleen. Louis Vaquez in France in 1892 described the case of a middle-aged man with marked erythrocytosis, hepatosplenomegaly, and a 'ruddy' complexion.[31] Though it was initially thought that the underlying disease was 'congenital heart disease', an autopsy revealed a normal heart; in view of the enormous hepatosplenomegaly, it was speculated that the underlying disease was probably hematological and it was given the term 'maladie de Vaquez' or 'Vaquez's disease'. In 1899, Richard Cabot in America described additional cases and the disease was later named polycythemia vera by William Osler in England in 1903.[32,33]

THE 20th CENTURY

At the turn of the 20th century, Osler, Turk, and Parkes-Weber provided detailed descriptions of polycythemia vera and its features which overlapped with the leukemias in general.[34,35] Remarkably, Turk, Weber, and Watson also described bilineage proliferation in polycythemia vera.[36] In 1917, a further entity was added to this list of blood disorders, when Giovanni Di Guglielmo in Italy coined the phrase 'eritroleuco-piastrinaemia' to describe a patient with circulating erythroid progenitors, myeloblasts, and megakaryoblasts.[37] The clinical features of CML were well characterized in a classical paper by Minot and colleagues in 1924.[38] This paper also recognized that age was an important prognostic factor. In 1934 Emil Epstein and Alfred Goedel in Austria described a patient with 'extreme' thrombocytosis, absence of 'panmyelosis', and an enlarged spleen, and termed this 'hemorrhagic thrombocythemia' (later termed 'essential thrombocythemia').[20]

The notion of trilineage hematopoietic proliferation was introduced by Vaughan and

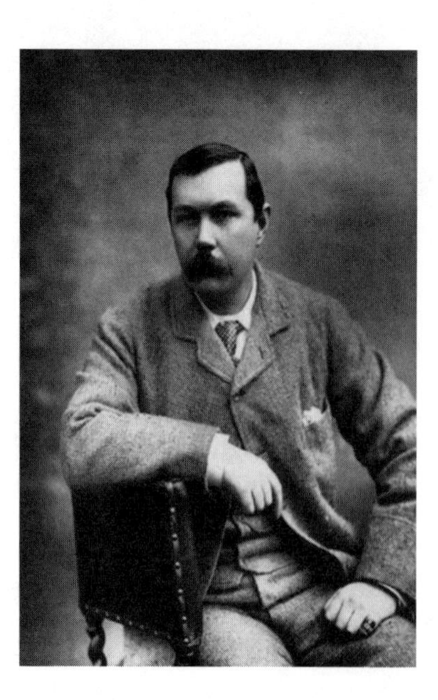

Figure 1.4 Sir Arthur Conan Doyle (1892).

- Dr Arthur Conan Doyle, the author, then in medical practice in Birmingham, UK, described the use of arsenic (Fowler's solution) to treat a case of leuco-cythaemia (CML) in a letter to *The Lancet* (1882).
- Picture of Sir Arthur Conan Doyle in 1892 by which time he was becoming famous as the author of the Sherlock Holmes detective stories.

Harrison in 1939 when they described two cases of 'leucoerythroblastic anemia and myelosclerosis' and suggested that the trilineage proliferation arose from a 'common primitive reticulum cell'.[39] By now efforts were in place to recognize 'myeloproliferative diseases' as a separate entity from 'acute leukemias'. In 1951, William Dameshek, a distinguished American hematologist who started the journal *Blood*, grouped CML with polycythemia vera, essential thrombocythemia, and myelosclerosis, and called the diseases collectively 'chronic myeloproliferative diseases' in a seminal *Blood* editorial[40] (Figure 1.5).

In 1960 Peter Nowell and David Hungerford, in Philadelphia, described the presence of an abnormally small acrocentric chromosome, which resembled a Y chromosome, in two male patients with what was then called chronic granulocytic leukemia[41] (Figure 1.6(a) and (b)). They subsequently described the presence of this chromosomal abnormality in a further seven patients, including two females, with CML. They then speculated that the abnormal chromosomal abnormality was probably not constitutive and may well be causally associated to CML. This abnormality was heralded as the first consistent cytogenetic abnormality in a human cancer at the First International Conference on Chromosomal Nomenclature in 1960 in Denver. It was at this conference that the abnormal chromosome described by Nowell and Hungerford was named Philadelphia (Ph^1) chromosome, after the city of its discovery. The superscript '1' was added on the premise that additional abnormalities originating from Nowell and Hungerford's work, would be discovered in Philadelphia. This, of course, did not occur and the superscript had been dropped by most hematologists by 1990. The formal recognition that a human cancer might be caused by an acquired chromosomal aberration, of course, vindicated to some degree the hypothesis postulated by Theodore Boveri in Germany in 1914 that cancer may be caused by acquired chromosomal abnormalities.[42]

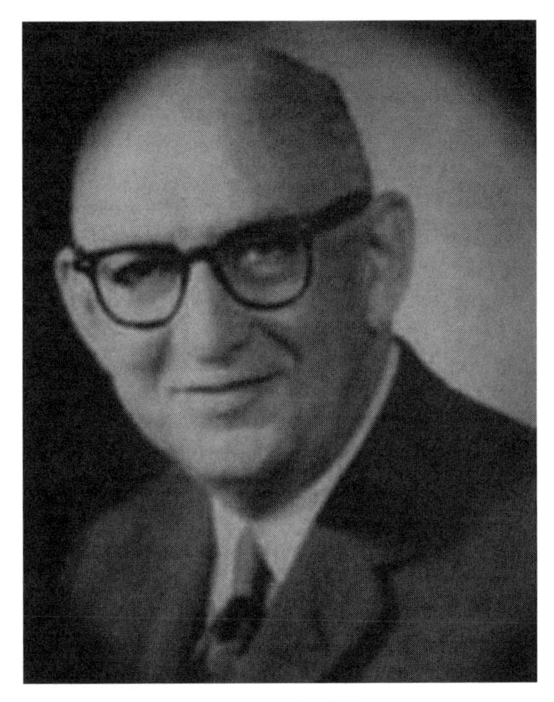

Figure 1.5 William Dameshek (1951).

The next important observations which established that CML was a stem cell-derived clonal disease came from Phillip Fialkow and colleagues in 1967.[43] They applied a genetic technique developed by Susumu Ohno, Ernest Beutler, and Mary Lyon, based on X chromosome mosaicism in females, and by exploiting the polymorphism in the X-linked glucose-6-phosphatase dehydrogenase locus in female patients, they established the clonal nature of not only CML, but also polycythemia vera, essential thrombocythemia, and primary myelofibrosis (albeit in later papers published in 1976, 1978, and 1981, respectively).[44,45]

In 1972, Janet Rowley in Chicago described the morphological aspects of the Ph chromosome in some detail and confirmed that it arose as a consequence of a reciprocal translocation of genetic material between the long arms of chromosomes 9 and 22, t(9;22)(q34;q11) (Figure 1.7).[46] She deserves credit for making an observation that strongly supported the notion that cytogenetic changes play an important role in leukemogenesis.

The molecular events underlying the genesis of the Ph chromosome began to unfold in 1982, when Heisterkamp and colleagues in Rotterdam mapped to chromosome 9 the

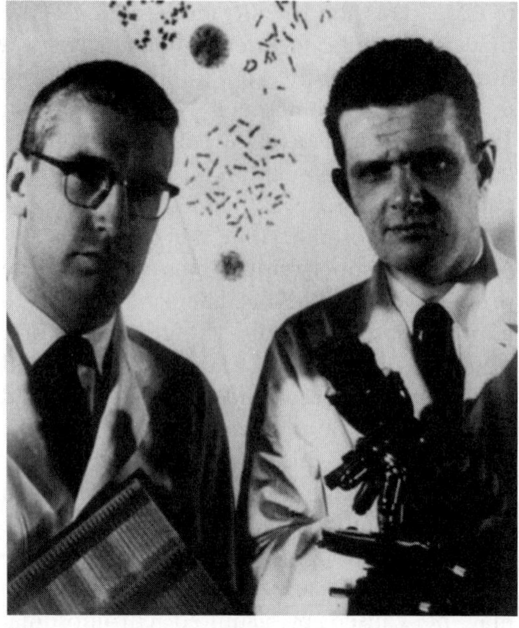

(a)

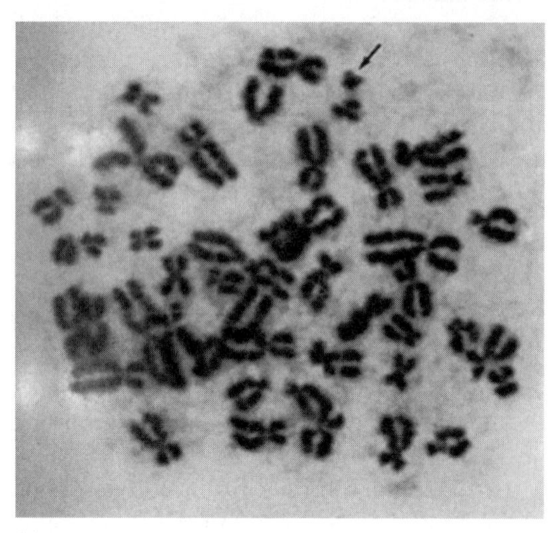

(b)

Figure 1.6 (a) Nowell and Hungerford (1960). (b) Imatinib and a schematic representation of how it might work in CML.

human homolog of the recently described Abelson murine leukemia virus.[47,48] In 1984, the same group, led by John Groffen, Gerard Grosveld, and others, described the so-called 'breakpoint cluster region' (*bcr*).[49] Subsequently, Canaani, Collins, and colleagues described an 8.5-kb *ABL* transcript and, in 1985, the *BCR-ABL* fusion gene that expressed a p210 oncoprotein was identified by Shtivelman, Stam, Ben-Neriah, and colleagues.[50–52] Three separate breakpoint locations on the *BCR* gene on chromosome 22 are now recognized (Figure 1.8). The break in the major breakpoint cluster region (M-BCR) occurs nearly always in the intron between exon e13 and e14 or in the intron between exon e14 and e15 (toward the telomere). By contrast, the position of the breakpoint in the *ABL1* gene on chromosome 9 is highly variable and may occur at almost any position upstream of exon a2. This translocation results in the generation of the chimeric *BCR-ABL* fusion gene transcribed as an 8.5-kb mRNA which encodes a protein of 210 kDa ($p210^{BCR\text{-}ABL1}$) that has a greater tyrosine kinase activity compared with the normal ABL protein. The different breakpoints in the M-BCR result in two slightly different chimeric *BCR-ABL1* genes, resulting in either an e13a2 or e14a2 transcript. The type of BCR-ABL transcript has no important prognostic significance. The second breakpoint location on the *BCR* gene was noted to occur between exons e1 and e2 in an area designated the minor breakpoint cluster region (m-bcr) and forms a BCR-ABL transcript that is transcribed as an e1a2 mRNA which encodes for $p190^{BCR\text{-}ABL1}$. This is found in about two-thirds of patients with Ph-positive acute lymphoblastic leukemia (ALL).

The presence of the $p190^{BCR\text{-}ABL1}$ fusion protein in patients with Ph-positive ALL was described by Erickson, Chan, Hermans, and colleagues between 1985 and 1987.[53] In 1988, Kurzrock and colleagues described the presence of the Ph chromosome in all leukemic cells of the myeloid lineage, and in some B cells and in a very small proportion of T cells in CML patients.[54] The transforming ability of these BCR-ABL fusion proteins was demonstrated convincingly by George Daley and David Baltimore, in Boston, in 1988.[55] The precise nature of the transforming property of the *BCR-ABL1* fusion gene was attributed to the enhanced tyrosine kinase activity. Daley and Baltimore also showed, in 1990, the induction

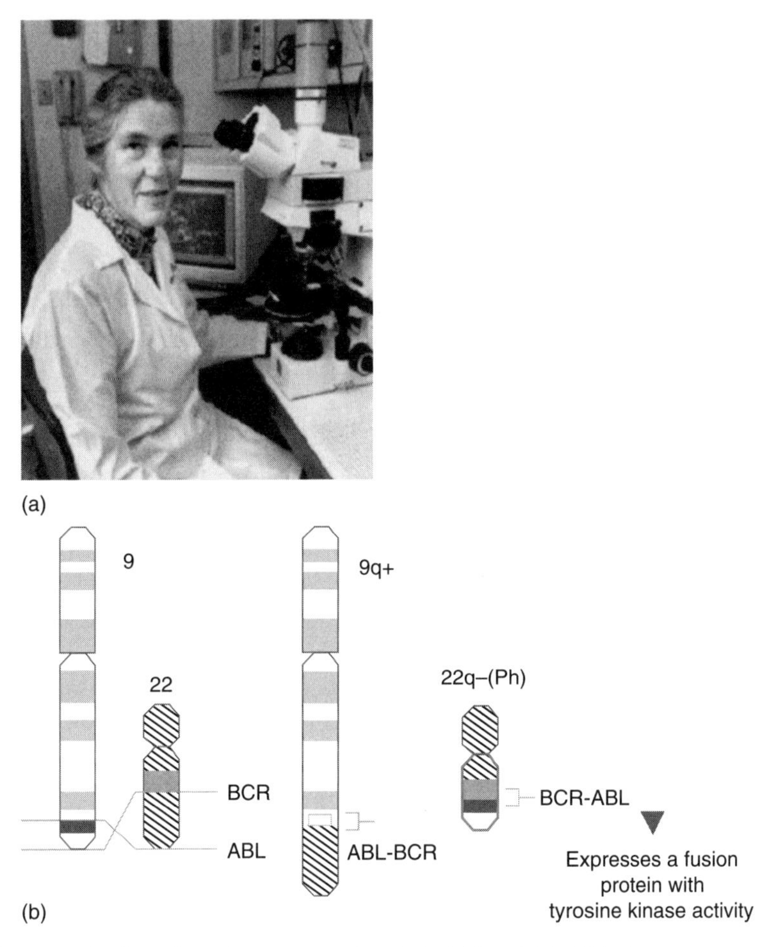

Figure 1.7 (a) Janet Rowley (b) Schematic representation of the Philadelphia (Ph) chromosome.

of a CML-like disease in mice, following the transduction of a retroviral infection of hematopoietic stem cells with p210$^{BCR\text{-}ABL1}$.[56] This was confirmed by work done by Elephanty and colleagues, in Australia and Kelliher and colleagues in Los Angeles. The notion of the *BCR-ABL1* fusion gene having a central role in CML was then generally accepted.[57]

With a general improvement in cytogenetic and molecular technology, the 'classical' Ph chromosome was easily identified in 80% of CML patients; in a further 10% of patients, variant translocations which may be 'simple' involving chromosome 22 and a chromosome other than chromosome 9, or 'complex', where chromosome 9, 22, and other additional chromosomes are involved. About 8% of patients with classical clinical and hematological features of CML lack the Ph chromosome and are referred to as cases of Ph-negative CML. About half of such patients have a *BCR-ABL* fusion gene and are referred to as Ph-negative, *BCR-ABL*-positive cases; the remainder are *BCR-ABL* negative and some of these have mutations in the *RAS* gene. It is probable that these latter patients have a more aggressive clinical course. Some patients acquire additional clonal cytogenetic abnormalities as their disease progresses. The emergence of such clones often heralds development of blastic transformation.

In 1996 a third breakpoint location was found by Pane and colleagues in Italy.[58] Patients with the very rare Ph-positive chronic neutrophilic

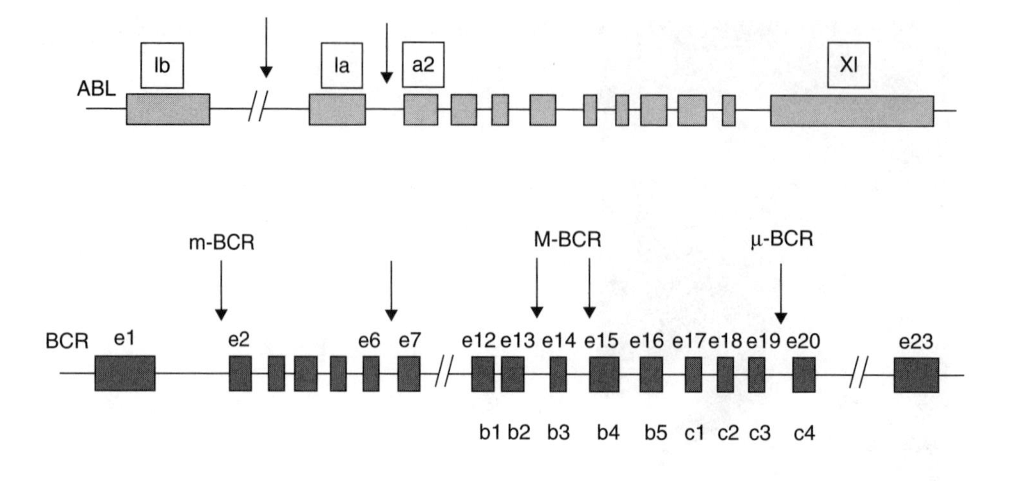

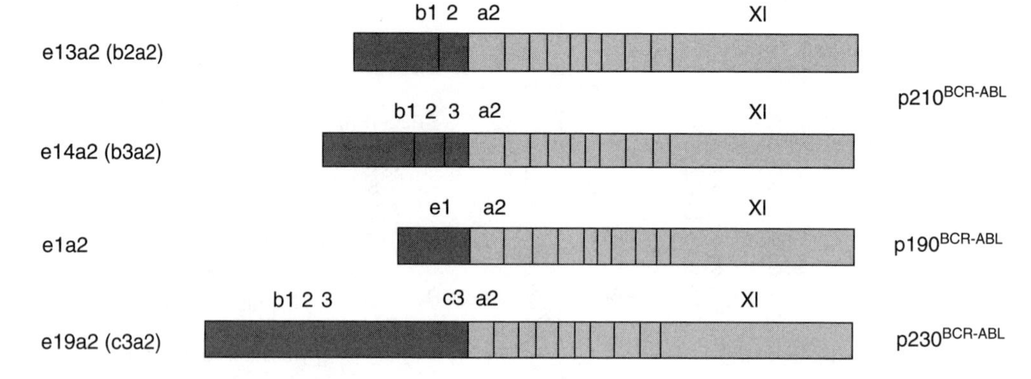

Figure 1.8 The various BCR-ABL transcripts.

leukemia had a much larger BCR-ABL fusion protein, $p230^{BCR\text{-}ABL1}$. This was designated the micro breakpoint cluster region (μ-bcr) and results in e19a2 mRNA, which encodes a larger protein of 230 kDa. The remarkable consistency of these breakpoint locations paved the way to use of the polymerase chain reaction (PCR) technology to amplify small quantities of residual disease which might persist after effective treatment. This technique is now the preferred method for molecular monitoring of individual patients with CML.

Over the past decade much attention has focused on determining the precise role played by the various BCR-ABL proteins in the pathogenesis of CML. A number of possible mechanisms of BCR-ABL mediated malignant transformation have been implicated, not necessarily mutually exclusive. These include constitutive activation of mitogenic signaling, reduced apoptosis, impaired adhesion of cells to the stroma and extracellular matrix, and proteasome-mediated degradation of ABL inhibitory proteins. The deregulation of the ABL tyrosine kinase facilitates autophosphorylation, resulting in a marked increase of phosphotyrosine on BCR-ABL itself, which creates binding sites for the SH2 domains of other proteins. A variety of such substrates, which can be tyrosine phosphorylated, have now been identified. Although much is known of the abnormal interactions between the BCR-ABL oncoprotein and other cytoplasmic molecules, the finer details of the pathways through which the 'rogue' proliferative signal is mediated, such as the RAS-MAP kinase, JAK-STAT, and the PI3 kinase pathways, are incomplete and the relative contributions to the leukemic 'phenotype' are still unknown. Moreover, the multiple signals initiated by the BCR-ABL have both proliferative and anti-apoptotic qualities, which are often difficult to separate. Much remains to be learned about the significance of tyrosine phosphatases in the transformation process.

Work done by Epstein, Melo, and others supported the notion that the Ph-positive cell was prone to acquire additional chromosomal changes, putatively as a result of increasing 'genetic instability', and this presumably underlies progression to advanced phases of the disease.[59] At the cytokinetic level, the mechanism by which the *BCR-ABL1* gene results in the preferential proliferation and differentiation of myeloid progenitors remains an enigma. There is evidence from the work of Holyoake and others, suggesting the presence of normal progenitors cells maintained in G_0 as a result of proliferation of leukemic cells which can, under certain circumstances, be induced to proliferate.[60]

In the first half of the 20th century, the treatment in general focused on an improvement in the quality of life by controlling the symptoms attributed to CML. In the early 1900s radiotherapy to the spleen was introduced and became popular for control of splenic enlargement.[61,62] Radioactive phosphorus was also used intermittently.[63] Other treatment modalities used, with very limited success, included antileukocyte sera in 1932, benzene in 1935, urethane in 1950, and leukapheresis.[64–67] Despite the significant mortality associated and controversial benefits achieved, the use of splenectomy continued well into the 20th century.[68,69] There were a number of other notable treatment attempts, but most, if not all, were unsuccessful.[70]

The first cytotoxic drug used was an alkylating agent, busulfan, which was introduced largely by David Galton in London, in 1953.[71] Galton then carried out a prospective comparison of busulfan and splenic radiation, and showed a significant survival advantage for the cohort subjected to busulfan. Thereafter busulfan became the preferred treatment for all patients with CML. In 1961, Institorisz and colleagues introduced 1,6-dibromomannitol, as a possible alternative for patients who did not respond or became refractory to busulfan.[72]

Hydroxycarbamide (previously hydroxyurea), a ribonucleotide reductase inhibitor, was introduced into clinics in the early 1960s, largely as a result of efforts by Kennedy and colleagues, and it gradually became the treatment of choice for newly diagnosed patients in chronic phase.[73] A randomized study confirmed the superiority of hydroxycarbamide over busulfan, but neither drug reduced the proportion of Ph-positive cells in the bone marrow or prolonged the overall survival significantly.[74] The next major development in the treatment of CML was the introduction of the first biological therapy, interferon alfa, by Moshe Talpaz and colleagues in 1983.[75,76] This agent was able to reduce the proportion of Ph-positive cells in the bone marrow in some patients and a minority achieved complete cytogenetic remission. Subsequent prospective randomized studies comparing interferon alfa with hydroxycarbamide and busulfan confirmed the drug's superiority, and it prolonged life by 1–2 years. Remarkably, some of the patients who achieved Ph negativity continued to remain Ph negative even years after the drug was discontinued. By the early 1990s, interferon alfa became the non-transplant treatment of choice for the majority of patients with CML in chronic phase.

Though the original concept of bone marrow transplant was probably first advocated by Thomas Fraser in 1894, when he famously recommended that patients eat bone marrow 'sandwiches' flavored with port wine (to improve taste), sporadic attempts at marrow transplantation were undertaken much earlier.[77] The modern era of bone marrow (now stem cell) transplant did not begin until research had gained a basic understanding of the histocompatibility system. Much of the pioneering work in stem cell transplantation was carried out by Don Thomas (who was subsequently awarded a Nobel prize for his contributions) and colleagues in Seattle in the early 1970s.[78,79] The early results were, for the most part, disappointing, largely because patients were in the advanced phases of the disease and succumbed to either the disease or the complications of the transplant. However, in 1979 the Seattle group reported successful treatment of four patients with CML in chronic phase who were transplanted with marrow cells collected from their respective normal genetically identical twins.[80] These efforts stimulated a number of investigators to initiate programs for transplanting CML patients in chronic phase using marrow cells from their respective HLA-identical sibling donors. The results were very encouraging and by early 1990s, the potential for allogeneic transplant to induce a cure for the majority of patients was recognized. The precise mechanisms by which this cure is achieved, however, remains unclear, though it must, in large part, be attributable to an immunological assault on residual leukemia cells in the patient, which has been designated the 'graft-versus-leukemia' effect.[81] Most, but not all, patients in whom BCR-ABL transcripts are repeatedly undetectable at 5 years after their allogeneic stem cell transplant will remain negative for long periods thereafter and will probably never relapse.[82]

In 1978 Goldman and colleagues in London showed that marrow-repopulating stem cells were present in the peripheral blood of untreated CML patients.[83] There was some hope that for patients ineligible for allografting the use of cytoreduction followed by autografting with peripheral blood stem cells might prolong life. In some patients marrow Ph-negative hematopoiesis was restored by this approach but very few patients remained Ph negative for extended periods. There appears to be some renewed interest in the possible role of autografting in the current tyrosine kinase inhibitor era.

Following the establishment of the central role of *BCR-ABL1* in CML in 1990, efforts were made to develop a small molecule that could inhibit the deregulated tyrosine kinase activity of the BCR-ABL oncoprotein. The initial results of the ultimately successful program led by Brian Druker in Portland, Oregon and Alex Matter in Basel, Switzerland, were published in 1996 (Figure 1.9).[84] They developed a small molecule, imatinib mesylate, which selectively inhibited the ABL tyrosine kinase and thereby disrupted the oncogenic signals which lead to the development of CML. Imatinib mesylate entered phase I trials in 1998 and phase II trials in 1999.[85] The results were considered convincing enough for regulatory agencies on both sides of the Atlantic to approve the use of this oral drug for the treatment of CML considered to be resistant or refractory to interferon alfa, in 2001, even though the results of a phase III study were still unavailable.[86,87]

THE 21st CENTURY

Though the observation that a small molecule such as imatinib mesylate could reverse the clinical and hematological features of CML constituted the final proof of the importance of the BCR-ABL oncoprotein to CML, there persisted some uncertainty about whether BCR-ABL was the initiating lesion or only a secondary event. Indirect evidence, collated by Fialkow and colleagues in 1981, had suggested that there may be a preceding predisposition to genomic instability in a Ph-negative population.[88] Clonal changes have now been seen in the Ph-negative populations in patients successfully treated for Ph-positive CML, especially +8, monosomy 7, and –Y. Occasional cases of Ph-negative acute myeloid leukemia (AML) were reported by Kovitz and colleagues in 2006, in patients responding to imatinib.[89] In 2007, Zaccaria and colleagues, in Rome, reported five CML patients who had multiple cytogenetic abnormalities coexisting in the Ph-positive cells of newly diagnosed CML patients; when the patients were treated with imatinib therapy the Ph chromosome was eliminated but the other abnormalities persisted.[90] The authors speculated that the non-Ph abnormalities must have preceded the acquisition of the Ph chromosome. Furthermore, in 2007, Brazma and colleagues in London demonstrated that some patients with CML had acquired

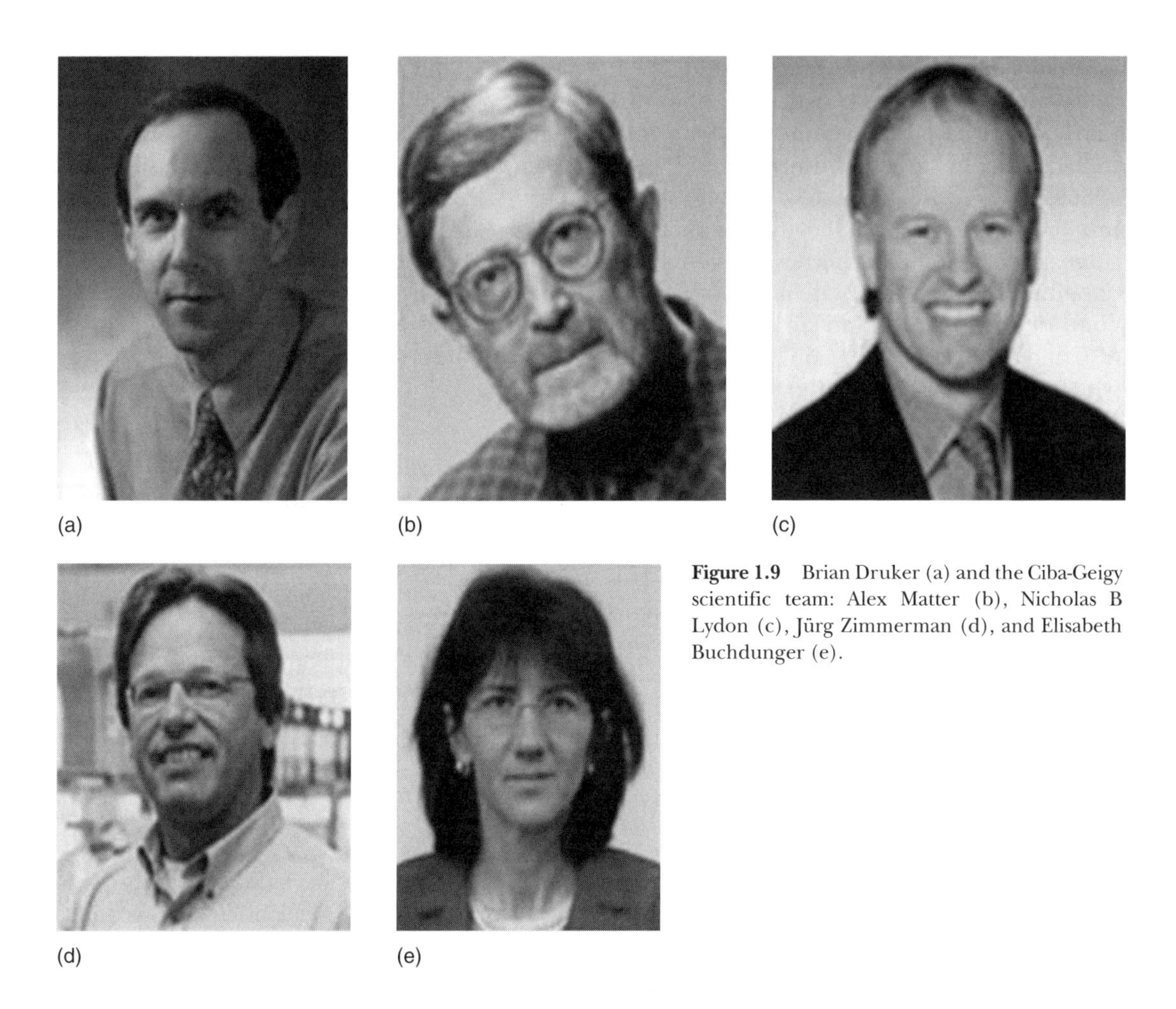

Figure 1.9 Brian Druker (a) and the Ciba-Geigy scientific team: Alex Matter (b), Nicholas B Lydon (c), Jürg Zimmerman (d), and Elisabeth Buchdunger (e).

molecular abnormalities identifiable by array comparative genomic hybridization.[91]

The recent 6-year follow-up results of the phase III data on previously untreated chronic phase patients were presented in December 2007, and published in abstract form. They clearly confirm not only the long-term efficacy of imatinib in inducing complete cytogenetic remission in about 64% of the original cohort, but also major molecular responses in a minority of these patients and an improved overall survival; the 5-year follow-up was published in December 2006.[92,93] Conversely resistance, both primary and secondary, is seen in a significant minority of patients in chronic phase.[94] Primary resistance is actually very rare and can be associated with low levels of the human organic cation transporter 1 (hOCT1), which are associated with poor intracellular uptake of imatinib. The mechanisms for secondary or 'acquired' resistance whereby patients respond well initially and then lose their response, appear to be quite different.[95] The best characterized mechanism underlying this secondary resistance appears to involve expansion of a Ph-clone bearing a BCR-ABL kinase domain mutation. Currently over 100 different mutations have been characterized in 50 amino acid residues and the precise significance of each appears to be different; not all are causally associated with resistance to imatinib. The first such mutation was described in 2001. This so-called 'gatekeeper' or T315I mutation remains a principal cause for resistance not only to the original ABL tyrosine kinase inhibitor, imatinib, but also to the second generation drugs such as dasatinib and nilotinib.[96] This mutation arises as a consequence of threonine being replaced by isoleucine at ABL residue position 315, where the isoleucine is much larger than the wild-type threonine and interferes with imatinib binding by steric hindrance.

Subsequent efforts to develop alternative inhibitors of ABL kinase activity have met with some success. Some of the newer agents, like dasatinib and bosutinib, are multikinases, in contrast to imatinib, and are active against SRC and ABL kinases.[97,98] Conversely nilotinib, which is essentially a modified version of imatinib, is also effective in imatinib-resistant patients with CML.[99,100] Preliminary findings of studies assessing the role of drugs which target the T315I mutant clone, such as MK-0457, an aurora kinase inhibitor, also appear interesting.[101] The notion that the graft-versus-leukemia effect is the principal reason for success in patients with CML subjected to an allograft has renewed interest in immunotherapy. Some evidence, collated since 2005, suggests that patients vaccinated with p210 multipeptides and the heat shock protein 70–peptide complexes generate immune responses that can be of clinical benefit.[102]

Finally, it is of note that more than 50 years after William Dameshek grouped a number of different diseases, including of course CML, under the heading of myeloproliferative disorders, four independent groups, Vainchenker in France, Gilliland in Boston, Skoda in Switzerland, and Green in England, reported in 2005 that a proportion of the patients with the so-called 'BCR-ABL-negative' myeloproliferative disorders carried a *JAK2* mutation (*JAK2*-V617F).[103–106] Many efforts are now being directed to establish the precise significance of such a mutation which actually unifies the diverse conditions. Furthermore, it would be of great interest if this mutation proved to be a useful target for therapeutic intervention.

CONCLUSIONS AND FUTURE DIRECTIONS

Clearly much has been learned over the past few centuries, but progress remains to be made. Imatinib has unequivocally established the principles that molecularly targeted treatment can work and the lessons learned are already being applied in the cancer field in general.[107] Compounds such as dasatinib, nilotinib, and bosutinib have been shown to have significant activity in selected patients resistant to imatinib and one or other of these newer agents could prove to be the preferred treatment for newly diagnosed patients in chronic phase.[108] Some of the current clinical outstanding issues include:

1. Is imatinib the best initial treatment for every chronic-phase patient?
2. At what dose should imatinib be started and how should response to treatment be monitored?
3. For how long should the drug be continued in patients who have achieved and maintain a complete molecular response?
4. What do we understand about the mechanisms of resistance to imatinib and how important is it?
5. What can we anticipate, if anything, from the next generation of tyrosine kinase inhibitors?
6. What is the role of an allograft and should conditioning be myeloablative or reduced intensity?
7. What is the precise significance of reducing the CML leukemia cell burden by more than 4 or 5 logs compared to the baseline?
8. What might immunotherapy and vaccines offer?

These and other issues, including biological questions, should keep CML aficionados busy for some time to come.

REFERENCES

1. Hooke R. Micrographia: Or, Some Physiological Descriptions of Minute Bodies Made by Magnifying Glasses, 1st edn. London: J Martyn and J Allestry, 1665.
2. van Leeuwenhoek A. Philosophical transactions of the Royal Society. London 1674; 9: 121–8.
3. Cobb M. Reading and Writing The Book of Nature: Jan Swammerdam (1637–1680). Endeavour 2000; 24: 122–8.

4. Lieutaud J. Elementa Physiologiae. Amsterdam, 1749: 82–4. [Translated and quoted in Dreyfus. Milestones in the History of Hematology. New York, 1957: 11–12].
5. Gulliver G. The works of William Hewson. FRS London, The Sydenham Society 1846; part III, lvi: 360pp, p 214.
6. Ehrlich P. Beitrag zur Kenntnis der Anilinfarbungen und ihrer Verwendung in der Microscopischen Technik. Archives Mikrochirurgie Anatomischer 1877; 13: 263–77.
7. Drew J. Paul Ehrlich: magister mundi. Nat Rev Drug Discov 2004; 3: 797–801.
8. Piller G. Leukaemia – a brief historical review from ancient times to 1950. Br J Haematol 2001; 112: 282–92.
9. Piller G. The history of leukemia: a personal perspective. Blood Cells 1993; 19: 521.
10. Bennett JH. Case of hypertrophy of the spleen and liver in which death took place from suppuration of the blood. Edinb Med Surg J 1845; 64: 413–23.
11. Velpeau A. Sur la resorption du puseat sur l'alteration du sang dans les maladies clinique de persection nenemant. Premier observation. Rev Med 1827; 2: 216.
12. Virchow R. Weisses Blut. Froriep's Notzien 1845; 36: 151–6.
13. Virchow R. Weisses Blut und Milztumoren. Med Z 1846; 15: 157.
14. Craigie D. Case of disease of the spleen in which death took place consequent on the presence of purulent matter in the blood. Edinb Med Surg J 1845; 64: 400–13.
15. Fuller H. Particulars of a case in which the enormous enlargement of the spleen and liver, together with dilatation of all vessels in the body were found coincident with a peculiarly altered condition of the blood. Lancet 1846; ii: 43.
16. Wood GB. Tran Coll Phys Philadelphia; 265: 1850–52.
17. Heuck G. Zwei Falle von Leukamie mit eigenthumlichem Blutresp. Knochenmarksbefund (two cases of leukemia with peculiar blood and bone marrow findings, respectively). Arch Pathol Anat Physiol Virchows 1879; 78: 475–96.
18. Assman H. Beitrage zur osteosklerotischen anamie. Beitr Pathol Anat Allgemeinen Pathologie (Jena) 1907; 41: 565–95.
19. Hirschfeld H. Die generalisierte aleukamische Myelose und ihre Stellung im System der leukamischen Erkrankungen. Z Klin Med 1914; 80: 126–73.
20. Epstein E, Goedel A. Hamorrhagische thrombozythamie bei vascularer schrumpfmilz (Hemorrhagic thrombocythemia with a vascular, sclerotic spleen). Virchows Archiv A Pathol Anat Histopathol 1934; 293: 233–48.
21. Jackson H Jr, Parker F Jr, Lemon HM. Agnogenic myeloid metaplasia of the spleen: a syndrome simulating other more definite hematological disorders. N Engl J Med 1940; 222: 985–94.
22. Jaffe ES, Harris NL, Stein H, Vardiman JW. World Health Organization Classification of Tumors of Hematopoietic and Lymphoid Tissues. Lyon, France: IARC Press, 2001: 1–351.
23. Mesa RA, Verstovsek S, Cervantes S et al. Primary myelofibrosis (PMF), post polycythemia vera myelofibrosis (post-PV MF), post essential thrombocythemia myelofibrosis (post-ET MF), blast phase PMF (PMF-BP): Consensus on terminology by the international working group for myelofibrosis research and treatment (IWG-MRT). Leuk Res 2007; 31: 737–40.
24. Donne A. De l'origine des globules du sang, de leur fin. CR Acad Sci 1842; 4: 366.
25. Brewer DB. Max Schultze (1865), G. Bizzozero (1882) and the discovery of the platelet. Br J Haematol 2006; 133: 251–8.
26. Neumann E. Ueber die Bedeutung des Knochenmarkes fur die Blutbildung. Ein Beitrag zur Entwicklungsgeschichte der Blutkorperchen. Archives Heilkunde 1869; 10: 68–102.
27. Drews J. Paul Ehrlich: magister mundi. Nat Rev Drug Discov 2004; 3: 797–801.
28. Neumann E. Uber myelogene Leukamie. Berliner Klin Wschr 15; 69: 1878.
29. Lissauer H. Zwei Fälle von Leukämie. Berliner Klinische Wochenshrift 1865; 2: 403–4.
30. Forkner CE. Leukemia and Allied Disorders, 1st edn. New York: Macmillan, 1938.
31. Vaquez H. Sur une forme speciale de cyanose s'accompnant d'hyperglobulie excessive et persistente. Compt rend Soc de biol and suppl note, Bull et mem Soc med d'hop de Paris, 3 ser 1892; 4: 384–8.
32. Cabot RC. A case of chronic cyanosis without discernible cause, ending in cerebral hemorrhage. Boston Med Surg J 1899; 141: 574–5.
33. Osler W. A clinical lecture on erythraemia (polycythaemia with cyanosis, maladie de Vaquez). Lancet 1908; 1: 143–6.
34. Turk W. Beitrage zur kenntnis des symptomenbildes polyzythamie mit milztumor and zyanose. Wiener medizinische Wochenschrift 1904; 17: 153–60, 189–93.
35. Weber FP, Watson JH. Chronic polycythemia with enlarged spleen, probably a disease of the bone marrow. Trans Clin Soc 1904; 37: 115.
36. Parkes-Weber F. Polycythemia, erythrocytosis and erythraemia. QJM 1908; 2: 85–134.
37. Di Guglielmo G. Richerche di ematologia. I. Un caso di eritroleucemia. megacariociti in circolo e loro funzione piastrinopoietico. Folio Med (Pavia) 1917; 13: 386.
38. Minot GR, Buckman TE, Isaacs R. Chronic myelogenous leukemia: age incidence, duration and benefit derived from irradiation. JAMA 1924; 82: 1489–94.
39. Vaughan JM, Harrison CV. Leuco-erythroblastic anaemia and myelosclerosis. J Pathol Bacteriol 1939; 48: 339–52.

40. Dameshek W. Some speculations on the myeloproliferative syndromes. Blood 1951; 6: 372–5.
41. Nowell PC, Hungerford DA. A minute chromosome in human granulocytic leukemia. Science 1960; 132: 1497.
42. Boveri T. Frage der Entstehung maligner Tumoren. Jena: Gustav Fischer; 1914.
43. Fialkow PJ, Garler SM, Yoshida A. Clonal origin of chronic myelocytic leukemia in man. Proc Natl Acad Sci USA 1967; 58: 1468–71.
44. Ohno S, Makino S. The single-X nature of sex chromatin in man. Lancet 1961; i: 78–9.
45. Fialkow PJ, Faguet GB, Jacobson RJ, Vaidya K, Murphy S. Evidence that essential thrombocythemia is a clonal disorder with origin in a multipotent stem cell. Blood 1981; 58: 916–19.
46. Rowley JD. A new consistent chromosome abnormality in chronic myelogenous leukaemia identified by quinacrine fluorescence and Giemsa banding. Nature 1973; 243: 290–3.
47. Heisterkamp N, Stephenson JR, Groffen J et al. Localization of the c-abl oncogene adjacent to a translocation break point in chronic myelocytic leukemia. Nature 1983; 306: 239–42.
48. De Klein A, van Kessel A, Grosveld G et al. A cellular oncogene is translocated to the Philadelphia chromosome in chronic myelocytic leukemia. Nature 1982; 300: 765–7.
49. Groffen J, Stephenson JR, Heisterkamp N et al. Philadelphia chromosome breakpoints are clustered within a limited region, bcr, on chromosome 22. Cell 1984; 36: 93–9.
50. Canaani E, Steiner-Saltz D, Aghai E et al. Altered transcription of an oncogene in chronic myeloid leukemia. Lancet 1984; i: 593–5.
51. Shtivelman E, Lifshitz B, Gale RP et al. Fused transcripts of bcr and abl genes in chronic myelogenous leukaemia. Nature 1985; 315: 550–4.
52. Ben-Neriah Y, Daley GQ, Mes-Masson A-M, Witte ON, Baltimore D. The chronic myelogenous leukemia specific p210 protein is the product of the bcr/abl hybrid gene. Science 1986; 223: 212–14.
53. Melo JV, Gordon DE, Cross NCP, Goldman JM. The ABL-BCR fusion gene is expressed in chronic myeloid leukemia. Blood 1993; 81: 158–65.
54. Kurzrock R, Gutterman JU, Talpaz M. The molecular genetics of Philadelphia chromosome positive leukemias. N Engl J Med 1988; 319: 990–8.
55. Daley GQ, Baltimore D. Transformation of an interleukin 3-dependent hematopoietic cell line by the chronic myelogenous leukemia-specific P210 bcr/abl protein. Proc Natl Acad Sci USA 1988; 85: 9312–16.
56. Daley GQ, van Etten RA, Baltimore D. Induction of chronic myelogenous leukemia in mice by the P210 BCR/ABL gene of the Philadelphia chromosome. Science 1990; 247: 824–30.
57. Elephanty AG, Hariharan IK, Cory S. Bcr-abl, the hallmark of chronic myeloid leukemia in man, induces multiple hemopoietic neoplasms in mice. EMBO J 1990; 9: 1069–78.
58. Pane F, Frigeri F, Sindona M et al. Neutrophilic – chronic myeloid leukemia: A distinct disease with a specific molecular marker (BCR/ABL with C3/A2 junction). Blood 1996; 88: 2410–14.
59. Mughal TI, Goldman JM. Chronic myeloid leukemia: why does it evolve from chronic phase to blast transformation? Front Biosci 2006; 1: 209–20.
60. Pellicano F, Holyoake T. Stem cells in chronic myeloid leukemia. Cancer Biomark 2007; 3: 181–91.
61. Pusey WA. Report of cases treated with Roentgen rays. JAMA 1902; 38: 911–19.
62. Senn N. Therapeutical value of Roentgen ray in treatment of pseudoleukemia. New York Med J 1903; 77: 665.
63. Osgood EE, Seaman AJ. Treatment of chronic leukemias: Results of therapy by titrated, regularly spaced total body radioactive phosphorus, or roentgen irradiation. JAMA 1952; 150: 1372–9.
64. Hueper WC, Russell M. Some immunological aspects of leukemia. Arch Intern Med 1932; 49: 113–22.
65. Kalapos I. Die Wirkung des Benzols bei der Leukamie. Klin Wochenschr 1935; 14: 864–7.
66. Cooper T, Watkins CH. Ethyl carbamate (urethane) in the treatment of chronic myelocytic leukemia: results of a three-year study. Med Clin North Am 1950; 34: 1205–15.
67. Buckner D, Graw RG Jr, Eisel RJ, Henderson ES, Perry S. Leukopheresis by continuous flow centrifugation (CFC) in patients with chronic myelocytic leukemia (CML). Blood 1969; 33: 353–69.
68. Cutting HO. The effect of splenectomy in chronic granulocytic leukemia. Report of a case. Arch Intern Med 1967; 120: 356–60.
69. Tura S, Baccarani M, Mandelli F et al. Splenectomy in chronic myeloid leukaemia: preliminary report on 37 cases. Haematologica 1974; 59: 428–39.
70. Tefferi A. The history of myeloproliferative disorders. Leukemia 2007: 1–11.
71. Galton DAG. Myleran in chronic myeloid leukaemia. Lancet 1953; 1: 208.
72. Institorisz L, Horvath IP, Csanyi E. Study of the distribution and metabolism of 82 Br-labelled dibromomannitol in normal and tumour bearing rats. Neoplasma 1964; 11: 245.
73. Kennedy BJ, Yarbro JW. Metabolic and therapeutic effects of hydroxyurea in chronic myelogenous leukemia. Trans Assoc Am Physicians 1965; 78: 391–9.
74. Hehlmann R, Heimpel H, Hasford J et al. Randomized comparison of busulfan and hydroxyurea in chronic myelogenous leukemia: prolongation of survival by hydroxyurea. The German CML Study Group. Blood 1993; 82: 398–407.

75. Talpaz M, McCredie KB, Malvigit GM, Gutterman JU. Leukocyte interferon-induced myeloid cytoreduction in chronic myelogenous leukaemia. Br Med J 1983; 1: 201.
76. Talpaz M, Kantarjian HM, McCredie K et al. Hematologic remission and cytogenetic improvement induced by recombinant human interferon alpha A in chronic myelogenous leukemia. N Engl J Med 1986; 314: 1065–9.
77. Fraser TR. Bone marrow in the treatment of pernicious anaemia. Br Med J 1894; 1: 1172.
78. Appelbaum FR. Hematopoietic-cell transplantation at 50. N Engl J Med 2007; 357: 1472–5.
79. Doney K, Buckner CD, Sale GE et al. Treatment of chronic granulocytic leukemia by chemotherapy, total body irradiation and allogeneic bone marrow transplantation. Exp Hematol 1978; 6: 738–47.
80. Fefer A, Cheever MA, Thomas ED et al. Disappearance of Ph[1]-positive cells in 4 patients with chronic granulocytic leukemia after chemotherapy, irradiation and marrow transplantation from an identical twin. N Engl J Med 1979; 300: 333–7.
81. Barrett J. Allogeneic stem cell transplantation for chronic myeloid leukemia. Semin Hematol 2003; 40: 59–71.
82. Mughal TI, Yong A, Szydlo R et al. The probability of long-term leukemia-free survival for patients in molecular remission 5 years after allogeneic stem cell transplantation for chronic myeloid leukaemia in chronic phase. Br J Haematol 2001; 115: 569–74.
83. Goldman JM, Thing KH, Park DS et al. Collection, cryopreservation and subsequent viability of hematopoietic stem cells intended for treatment of chronic granulocytic leukemia in blast-cell transformation. Br J Haematol 1978; 40: 185–95.
84. Druker BJ, Tamura S, Buchdunger E et al. Effects of a selective inhibitor of the Abl tyrosine kinase on the growth of Bcr-Abl positive cells. Nat Med 1996; 2: 561–6.
85. Druker BJ, Sawyers CL, Kantarjian HM et al. Activity of a specific inhibitor of the BCR-ABL tyrosine kinase in the blast crisis of chronic myeloid leukemia and acute lymphoblastic leukemia with the Philadelphia chromosome. N Engl J Med 2001; 344: 1038–42.
86. Mughal TI, Goldman JM. Chronic myeloid leukaemia: STI571 magnifies the therapeutic dilemma. Eur J Cancer 2001; 37: 561–8.
87. Goldman JM. Implications of imatinib mesylate for hematopoietic stem cell transplantation. Semin Hematol 2001; 38: 28–34.
88. Failkow P, Martin PJ, Najfield V et al. Evidence for a multistep pathogenesis of chronic myelogenous leukemia. Blood 1981; 58: 158–63.
89. Kovitz C, Kantarjian HM, Garcia-Manero G, Abbruzzo LV, Cortes J. Myelodysplastic syndromes and acute leukemia developing after imatinib mesylate therapy for chronic myeloid leukemia. Blood 2006; 108: 2811–13.
90. Zaccaria A, Valenti AM, Donti F et al. Persistence of chromosomal abnormalities additional to the Philadelphia chromosome after Philadelphia chromosome disappearance during imatinib treatment for chronic myeloid leukemia. Haematologica 2007; 4: 564–5.
91. Brazma D, Grace C, Howard J et al. Genomic profile of chronic myelogenous leukemia: imbalances associate with disease progression. Genes Chromosomes Cancer 2007; 46: 1039–50.
92. Hochhaus A, Druker BJ, Larson RA et al. IRIS 6-year-follow-up. Blood 2007; 110: 15a, abstract 25.
93. Druker BJ, Guilhot F, O'Brien SG et al. Five-year follow-up of patients receiving imatinib for chronic myeloid leukemia. N Engl J Med 2006; 355: 2408–17.
94. Druker BJ. Circumventing resistance to kinase-inhibitor therapy. N Engl J Med 2006; 354: 2594–6.
95. Shah NP, Tran C, Lee FY et al. Overriding imatinib resistance with a novel ABL kinase inhibitor. Science 2004; 305: 399–401.
96. Mughal TI, Goldman JM. Emerging strategies for the treatment of mutant Bcr-Abl T315I myeloid leukemias. Clin Lymphoma Myeloma 2007; (Suppl 2): S81–4.
97. Talpaz M, Shah NP, Kantarjian HM et al. Dasatinib in imatinib-resistant Philadelphia chromosome-positive leukemias. N Engl J Med 2006; 354: 2531–41.
98. Jabbour E, Cortes J, Ghanem H, O'Brien S, Kantarjian HM. Targeted therapy in chronic myeloid leukemia. Expert Rev Anticancer Ther 2008; 8: 99–110.
99. Kantarjian HM, Giles F, Wunderle L et al. Nilotinib in imatinib-resistant CML and Philadelphia chromosome-positive acute lymphoblastic leukemia. N Engl J Med 2006; 354: 2531–41.
100. Kantarjian HM, Giles F, Gatterman N et al. Nilotinib (formerly AMN107), a highly selective BCR-ABL tyrosine kinase inhibitor, is effective in patients with Philadelphia chromosome-positive CML in chronic phase following imatinib resistance or intolerance. Blood 2007; 10: 3540–6.
101. Giles F, Cortes J, Jones D et al. MK-0457, a novel kinase inhibitor, is active in patients with chronic myeloid leukemia or acute lymphoblastic leukemia with T315I BCR-ABL mutation. Blood 2007; 109: 500–2.
102. Bocchia M, Gentili S, Abruzzese E et al. Effect of a P210 multipeptide vaccine associated with imatinib or interferon in patients with chronic myelogenous leukaemia and persistent residual disease: a multicentre observational trial. Lancet 2005; 365: 657–9.
103. Levine RL, Wadleigh M, Cools J et al. Activating mutation in the tyrosine kinase JAK2 in polycythemia vera, essential thrombocythemia, and myeloid

metaplasia with myelofibrosis. Cancer Cell 2005; 7: 387–97.
104. James C, Ugo V, Couedic JP et al. A unique clonal JAK2 mutation leading to constitutive signaling causes polycythaemia vera. Nature 2005; 434: 1144–8.
105. Kralovics R, Passamonti F, Buser AS et al. A gain-of-function mutation of JAK2 in myeloproliferative disorders. N Engl J Med 2005; 352: 1779–90.
106. Baxter EJ, Scott LM, Campbell PJ et al. Acquired mutation of JAK2 in human myeloproliferative disorders. Lancet 2005; 365: 1779–90.
107. Mughal TI, Goldman JM. Targeting cancers with tyrosine kinase inhibitors: lessons learned from chronic myeloid leukaemia. Clin Med 2006; 6: 526–8.
108. Goldman JM. How I treat chronic myeloid leukemia in the imatinib era. Blood 2007; 110: 2828–37.

Cytogenetics and molecular biology of chronic myeloid leukemia

2

Paul La Rosée, Michael WN Deininger

INTRODUCTION

The efficacy of imatinib, a selective ABL-kinase inhibitor, for the treatment of chronic myeloid leukemia (CML) has set a paradigm for translational research in oncology.[1,2] This success would have been impossible without a detailed understanding of the molecular pathogenesis of CML, a story that took more than 150 years to unravel. CML was described in 1845 independently by Bennett and Virchow.[3,4] Progress was moderate for more than a century, until in 1960 Nowell and Hungerford reported the presence of a small (minute) chromosome 22 (22q−) in seven CML patients,[5] which was named the Philadelphia chromosome (Ph), according to the city of its discovery. The next four decades saw the identification of the (9;22)(q34;q11) reciprocal translocation by Janet Rowley and colleagues, and the identification of *BCR* and *ABL* genes as the translocation partners by Groffen and Bartram, respectively (Figure 2.1).[6–8] Even before the recognition of the *BCR-ABL* fusion it had been known that *ABL* is an oncogene. When studying the Moloney murine leukemia virus (M-MuLV) in neonatal mice, Abelson and Rabstein discovered a retrovirus with different oncogenic potential, which they termed Abelson-murine leukemia virus (A-MuLV).[9,10] Additional studies showed that the virus contained GAG sequences fused upstream of murine ABL.[11] Around the same time Collett and Erikson reported a correlation between the protein kinase activity of the Rous sarcoma virus (RSV) SRC protein and its transforming potency, which was subsequently characterized as specific tyrosine kinase activity by Hunter and Sefton.[12,13] The discovery that v-ABL is a tyrosine kinase and that the transforming potency of *BCR-ABL* is dependent on its tyrosine kinase activity led to the concept that transforming oncogenes can dysregulate target cells via aberrant tyrosine phosphorylation.[14,15] Recognizing the central role of *BCR-ABL* for disease pathogenesis, the World Health Organization has defined CML as a *BCR-ABL*-positive myeloproliferative disorder.

CML is probably the most extensively studied human malignancy and one might question the wisdom of yet another review. Surprisingly though, a number of questions remain unanswered. Moreover, recent developments such as the completion of the human genome project, advances in gene and protein analysis technology (genomics, proteomics), refinement of murine *in vivo* models of CML, progress in the analysis of CML stem cells, and reports on modification of CML disease biology by BCR-ABL-inhibitory drugs have added important new information.

ETIOLOGY OF THE BCR-ABL TRANSLOCATION

Epidemiological and *in vitro* data show a clear relationship between exposure to ionizing radiation and the risk of developing CML.[16–18] No hereditary, familial, geographic, ethnic, or economic associations have been linked to CML incidence. A hint as to why this translocation targets specifically hematopoietic cells was provided by nuclear gene topology studies.[19,20] The distance between the *BCR* and *ABL* genes in hematopoietic cell nuclei

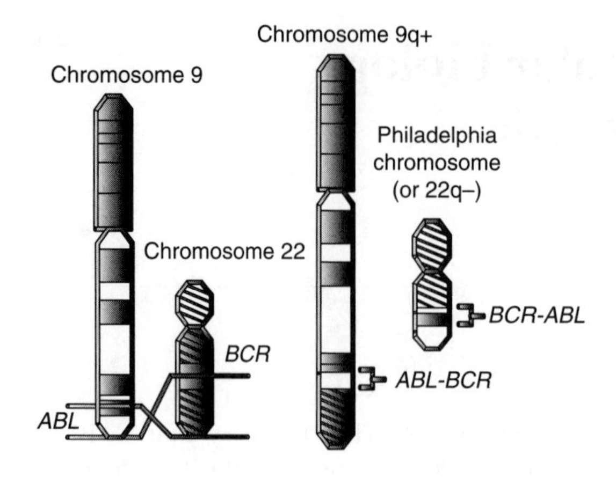

Figure 2.1 The Philadelphia translocation. Breakpoints in the long arms of chromosome 9 (q34) and chromosome 22 (q11) lead to the reciprocal translocation of the telomeric fragments. This results in an elongated chromosome 9q+ and a shortened chromosome 22q–, the so-called Philadelphia chromosome (Ph). The *ABL* and *BCR* genes reside on the long arms of chromosomes 9 and 22, respectively. As a result of the translocation, an *ABL-BCR* chimeric gene is formed on the derivative chromosome 9 and a *BCR-ABL* gene on the derivative chromosome 22.

varies considerably according to lineage and differentiation stage, but is significantly less than would be expected by chance. It is thought that this may favor translocation events between the two genes after double strand breaks occur. Another possibility is that repeat sequences in *BCR* may favor recombination events.[21] However, conflicting results on this issue have been published.[22]

THE TARGET CELL OF THE BCR-ABL TRANSLOCATION

Low levels of BCR-ABL mRNA have been detected in the blood of healthy individuals, raising the question of whether BCR-ABL itself is sufficient for leukemia initiation.[23–26] One could explain this finding by postulating that BCR-ABL is acquired by a hematopoietic progenitor cell that lacks the self-renewal capacity required to sustain the leukemic clone. Another possibility is that immunological surveillance mechanisms prevent the expansion of the leukemic cell clone. In support of this, it was found that certain HLA types are protective against CML.[27] A third possibility is that BCR-ABL alone is insufficient to induce CML and requires a cooperating genetic lesion to realize the chronic phase phenotype. In support of this, X-chromosome inactivation studies using expression of glucose-6-phosphate dehydrogenase isoenzymes as a clonality marker demonstrated the clonal origin of the Ph-positive cell clone.[28–30] Surprisingly however, skewing of the Ph-negative B-cell compartment towards the pattern observed in the CML clone was also observed, suggesting that a clonal state may predate the acquisition of Ph. This has been supported by mathematical modeling based on epidemiological data, which concluded that more than one event is required for the induction of the chronic phase of CML.[31]

The combination of fluorescence-activated cell sorting and fluorescence *in situ* hybridization revealed the presence of BCR-ABL in myeloid and lymphoid hematopoietic progenitor cells, consistent with a pluripotent hematopoietic stem cell (HSC) as the origin of CML.[32] The CML-like murine myeloproliferative disease that is generated by transplantation of bone marrow retrovirally infected with $p210^{BCR\text{-}ABL}$ into lethally irradiated recipients is characterized by multilineage involvement, consistent with a pluripotent HSC as the relevant BCR-ABL target.[33,34] Recently, the identification of the Ph rearrangement in *ex vivo* propagated endothelial cells of five out of six CML patients and the *in situ* detection of *BCR-ABL* in myocardium

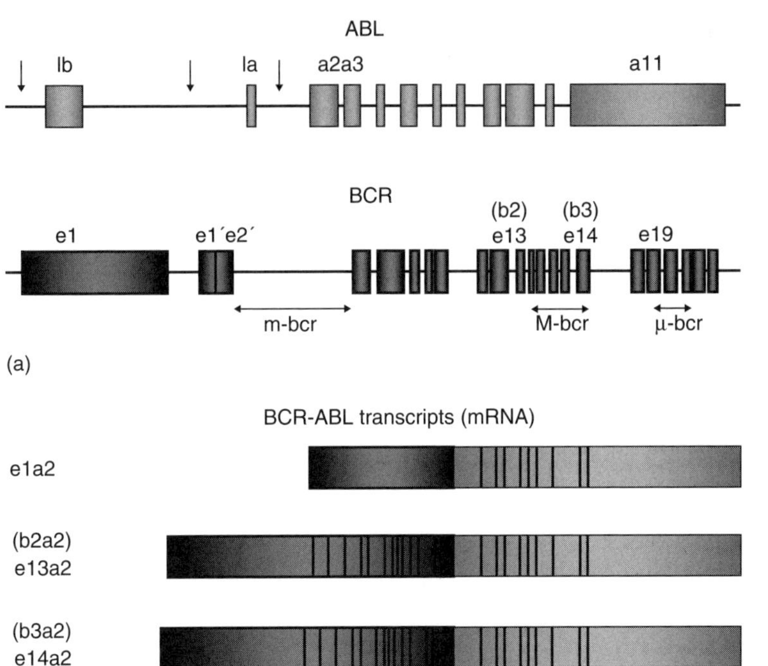

Figure 2.2 Molecular genetics of the BCR-ABL fusion. Locations of the breakpoints in the *ABL* and *BCR* genes (a) and the structure of the chimeric mRNAs derived from the various breakpoints (b). Arrows mark the three possible breakpoint locations that determine the length of the mRNA transcripts.

derived endothelial cells of one CML patient prompted the hypothesis that CML may originate in an even more primitive cell, the putative hemangioblast.[35] This is further supported by the detection of Ph in a very immature adherent fetal liver kinase-1 positive (Flk-1+), CD33–, CD34– cell with hematopoietic and endothelial differentiation capacity, and the ability to induce leukemia in mice.[36]

THE *BCR-ABL* GENE

The genomic anatomy of the fusion gene, its mRNA transcripts and the structure of the derivative fusion protein are depicted in Figure 2.2 (for a review see reference 37).

Breakpoints in the *ABL* gene on chromosome 9 (q34) are spread out over a 300-kb region at the 5′ end, most frequently between the two alternative exons Ib and Ia. Regardless of the genomic breakpoint, *ABL* exon I is spliced out during processing of the primary hybrid transcript. The *BCR* gene, in contrast, exhibits three so-called breakpoint cluster regions (BCR). The breakpoints most frequently detected in patients (almost all CML and one-third of Ph-positive acute lymphoblastic leukemia (ALL) patients) are located in a 5.8-kb area spanning *BCR* exons 12–16 (originally referred to as exons b1–b5). Fusion transcripts (Figure 2.2) derived from this so-called major breakpoint cluster region (M-bcr) show either e13a2 (b2a2) or e14a2 (b3a2) junctions, which code for the $p210^{BCR\text{-}ABL}$ chimeric protein. Breaks in the minor bcr (m-bcr), which is localized further 5′ between the alternative exons e2′and e2 and encompasses some 54.4 kb, give rise to an e1a2 transcript and $p190^{BCR\text{-}ABL}$ protein. e1a2 is the predominant transcript in most patients with Ph-positive ALL. The rare e1a2-positive CML patients tend to have high monocyte counts. With sensitive polymerase chain reaction (PCR) techniques e1a2 transcripts are detectable at a low level in a significant proportion of patients with $p210^{BCR\text{-}ABL}$, suggesting alternative splicing.[38] Finally, breaks in the micro bcr (μ-bcr) 3′ of e19 generate e19a2 transcripts and p230$^{BCR\text{-}ABL}$, which is associated with chronic neutrophilic leukemia.[39] Atypical transcripts such as e13a3, e14a3, e1a3, e6a2, e8a2 or e2a2 have been occasionally (<1%) reported in patients with ALL and CML.[40–42] The notion that ABL sequences are largely conserved in the different oncogenic fusions is in agreement with the role of ABL as the transforming principal. BCR, on the other hand, apparently modulates the disease phenotype. In simplistic terms, the less BCR sequence is conserved in the fusion protein, the more aggressive is the disease.[43]

THE BCR AND ABL PROTEINS

The BCR-ABL fusion protein was first detected in the CML cell line K562 by Konopka *et al.* and later identified as the product of the *BCR-ABL* fusion gene by Ben Neriah *et al.*[44,45] In analogy to v-ABL, aberrant tyrosine kinase activity was established as the transforming principle of BCR-ABL.[15] The 145-kDa ABL protein is a ubiquitously expressed non-receptor tyrosine kinase with a modular domain structure (Figure 2.3).[46–48] The N-terminus consists of three SRC-homology (SH) domains (SH1–SH3). The SH1 domain carries the tyrosine kinase function, whereas SH2 and

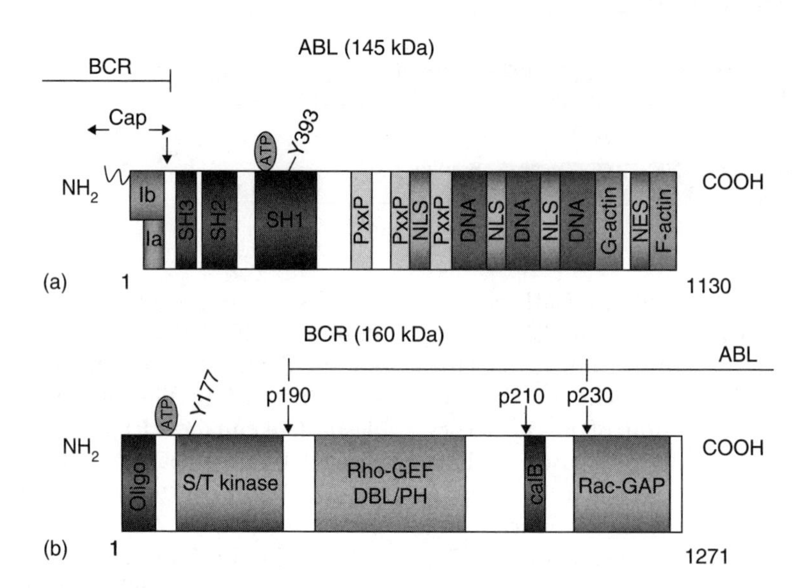

Figure 2.3 Structure of the ABL and the BCR proteins. (a) ABL type Ia is slightly shorter than type Ib. The Ib isoform contains a myristoyl residue that is believed to govern attachment to the plasma membrane, and plays a central role in autoinhibition of the protein. The N-terminus is also called 'cap', which recently was recognized to coordinate the myristoyl-phosphotyrosine switch for ABL autoregulation. The core part of the protein is composed of three SRC-homology (SH) domains situated towards the NH2 terminus. The SH1 domain comprises the catalytic domain for substrate phosphorylation (ATP), the SH2 and SH3 domains are regulatory subunits for docking proteins and autoregulatory intramolecular interactions of the enzyme. The SH2 domain binds to phosphorylated tyrosines in a sequence-specific context, the SH3 domain binds to proline-rich sequences. The center of ABL contains proline-rich (PxxP) regions capable of binding to SH3 domains, and it harbors one of three nuclear localization signals (NLS). The carboxy terminus contains two additional NLS, and DNA as well as G- and F-actin binding domains. The figure is not drawn to scale and multiple phosphorylation sites have been omitted for clarity reasons. (b) BCR is a 160-kDa serine/threonine kinase (S/T). The N-terminus consists of the coiled-coil oligomerization domain and the kinase domain. Tyrosine 177 (Y177) is an autophosphorylation site important for GRB2 binding. The center of the molecule contains a region homologous to Rho guanidine nucleotide exchange factors (Rho-GEF) as well as dbl-like and pleckstrin homology (PH) domains. Toward the C-terminus a putative site for calcium-dependent lipid binding (CalB) and a domain with activating function for Rac-GTPase (Rac-GAP) are found. Arrows indicate the position of the breakpoints in BCR-ABL fusion proteins.

SH3 bind other proteins through recognition of phosphotyrosine or proline-rich sequences, respectively. ABL kinase activity is tightly regulated in physiological conditions, but the precise mechanism of regulation had been elusive until recently. The N-terminus of ABL is very similar to the N-terminus of SRC. However, ABL lacks an equivalent of SRC tyrosine 527, which upon phosphorylation binds the SH2 domain in an intramolecular clamp that is crucial to SRC autoinhibition. Mutational studies have also implicated the SH3 domain and the N-terminal cap region in autoinhibition,[49–51] but the mechanism remained elusive until a combined biochemical and crystallographic approach solved the mystery.[52,53] The myristoylated ABL N-terminus binds to a hydrophobic pocket at the base of the SH1 domain, resulting in a clamp-like structure that resembles the autoinhibited conformation of SRC. In this conformation the kinase cannot 'breathe' and phosphorylation of the regulatory activation loop tyrosine 393 is impossible. Tyrosine phosphorylation of the linker between the SH2 and kinase domain abolishes the intramolecular clamping of the kinase domain, which allows for outward orientation and subsequent phosphorylation of the activation loop on tyrosine 393 (for review see references 48 and 54). The catalytic activity of ABL may additionally be fine tuned by co-inhibitory factors such as peroxiredoxin-I,[55] retinoblastoma protein (Rb)[56] or filamentous actin (f-actin).[57]

ABL shuttles between the nucleus and the cytoplasm, and participates in a diverse array of cellular signaling cascades. Cytoplasmic localization is associated with proliferation and survival.[58] In contrast, nuclear localization is observed after cell cycle arrest and apoptosis induced by DNA damage.[59] Overall, it appears that ABL serves a complex role as a cellular module that integrates signals from various extracellular (growth factors, cytokines, adhesions) and intracellular (oxidative stress, DNA damage) sources, and influences decisions in regard to cell cycle[60,61] and apoptosis.[62] The fact that ABL null mice show a severe phenotype, including high perinatal mortality, runting, skeletal abnormalities, and disturbed immune function indicates that ABL plays an important role in development.[63,64] Moreover, mice null for both ABL and ARG are embryonically lethal owing to lack of neurulation.[65]

BCR is a ubiquitously expressed 160-kD multidomain protein (Figure 2.3).[66] The N-terminus contains a coiled-coil domain capable of oligomerization, followed by a serine/threonine kinase domain.[66,67] The center of the protein contains a dbl homology (DH) and a pleckstrin homology (PH) domain that stimulate the exchange of guanidine triphosphate (GTP) for guanidine diphosphate (GDP) on small GTPases of the Rho family, while the C-terminus activates the GTPase activity of Rac.[68] The Rho-GEF and Rac-GAP functions suggest a role of BCR in cytoskeletal remodeling through regulation of small GTPases of the Rho family, such as Rac, cdc42, and Rho. Fibroblasts expressing p190$^{BCR\text{-}ABL}$, which lacks the DBL-like, cdc42, and PH domains, exhibit a more profound disruption of the actin cytoskeleton than cells expressing p210$^{BCR\text{-}ABL}$, and this has been linked to the more aggressive phenotype of p190$^{BCR\text{-}ABL}$ positive leukemia.[69] Recently, the demonstration of a BCR-dependent negative regulatory activity towards the RAS-ERK pathway ascribed potential tumor-suppressive properties to BCR.[70] Additionally, BCR was shown to negatively regulate the Wnt/β-catenin pathway.[71,72] The Wnt/β-catenin axis plays a role in proliferation and self-renewal of hematopoietic cells[73,74] and has also been implicated in regulation of CML progression.[75] Despite these findings it has been difficult to define BCR's true biological function, as BCR null mice are viable and a reduced neutrophil oxidative burst is the only identifiable defect.[76]

DEREGULATION OF BCR-ABL TYROSINE KINASE ACTIVITY

Central to BCR-ABL's oncogenicity is constitutive tyrosine kinase activity.[15] Several mechanisms have been implicated in the loss of regulation (Figure 2.4). An essential feature of

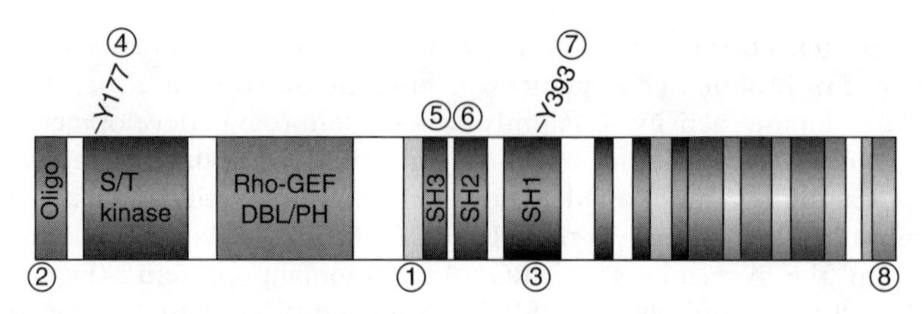

Figure 2.4 Molecular mechanisms underlying aberrant ABL kinase activity and sites of the BCR-ABL protein that govern the disease phenotype. (1) Fusion of the BCR moiety to the ABL N-terminus disrupts the autoinhibitory activity of the N-terminal myristoyl group that has been shown to be important for 'latching' the N-terminus to a hydrophobic pocket in the kinase domain, keeping ABL in a closed inactive conformation.[52,53] (2) The coiled-coil (CC) domain of the BCR N-terminus is central to the aberrant kinase activation of the ABL-kinase allowing oligomerization (dimerization, tetramerization) and subsequently *trans*-autophosphorylation.[51,67] Increased phosphotyrosine interferes with autoinhibitory constraints involved in the myristoyl-phosphotyrosine switch of ABL activation. Mutant CC-BCR-ABL fails to induce MPD in mice but induces T-cell leukemia/lymphoma with long latency. Combination of ΔCC-BCR-ABL with a kinase-activating mutation in the SH3 domain restores the MPD-inducing activity of BCR-ABL pointing to the significance of the aberrant kinase activity for leukemia induction.[77,78] (3) The tyrosine kinase activity located in the SH1 domain of BCR-ABL is central to the transformation potency in *in vitro* cell models.[15] Inactivation of the kinase by point mutations within the SH1 domain abrogates leukemogenicity in mice, further supporting the notion that the ABL kinase activity is absolutely essential for BCR-ABL leukemogenesis *in vivo*.[79] (4) Activation of the RAS and the PI3K-signaling pathways strongly depends on tyrosine-phosphorylation at Y177 of BCR.[80–82] *In vivo* induction of an MPD but not T-ALL or T-cell lymphoma depends on intact Y177.[77,78,83] (5) The SH3 domain is intramolecularly engaged in ABL autoinhibition.[49,51,52] c-ABL with a deleted SH3 domain shows increased tyrosine kinase activity and induces lymphoid lymphoma/leukemia in mice.[84] However, BCR-ABL lacking a functional SH3 domain still induces an MPD.[84] This points to the central role of the BCR moiety for the MPD phenotype. (6) The tight interaction between the SH2 domain and the kinase domain is involved in the so called 'clamping' of the autoinhibited c-ABL protein and can experimentally be disrupted by phosphopeptides.[52] Mutations in the SH2 domain of BCR-ABL reduce the ability of BCR-ABL to induce an MPD in mice,[85,86] but do not affect lymphoid leukemogenesis.[86] (7) The tyrosine residue Y393 decides on the intramolecular position of the activation loop, which in an unphosphorylated state folds into the substrate and ATP-binding pocket of the kinase domain.[87,88] Mutation of Y393 greatly impairs the leukemogenic activity of BCR-ABL in mice.[51] (8) Subcellular localization of BCR-ABL is governed by the F-actin binding domain (FABD).[89,90] The FABD is not essential for induction of MPD in mice,[91] but is believed to influence the adhesion properties of BCR-ABL-expressing cells.

oncogenic ABL derivatives such as GAG-ABL, BCR-ABL, and ETV6-ABL is the presence of an N-terminal oligomerization motif.[67,92,93] Deletion of the coiled-coil oligomerization motif suppresses kinase activity and leukemogenicity *in vivo*.[77,78,94] Crystal structure analysis revealed tetramer formation by the BCR N-terminus, which allows for transphosphorylation of the activation loop tyrosine.[95] This results in structural rearrangements that lead to full kinase activation. Tetramerization may also favor engagement of phosphotyrosine ligands important for ABL activation. While the dimerization domain has a central role in an otherwise unmutated BCR-ABL, kinase activity, transformation, and leukemogenesis of dimerization-defective BCR-ABL can be restored by mutations in ABL regulatory domains (SH3 ligand binding site, SH2-kinase domain linker), pointing to the complex regulation of the BCR-ABL molecule.[51] An additional consequence of replacing the ABL N-terminus with BCR sequences is the loss of the cap. In the B isoform of ABL the cap is myristoylated and serves as a key component of the intramolecular clamp that stabilizes the inactive conformation of ABL (Figure 2.4).[50,53] Therefore, critical structures regulating ABL autoinhibition are deleted in the fusion, favoring an uninhibited state of the kinase. Mechanisms acting in trans also contribute to kinase activation. The ABL SH3 domain negatively regulates ABL kinase activity through binding of trans-acting inhibitory proteins, including ABL interactor proteins 1 and 2 (ABI1, ABI2), and peroxiredoxin-I.[55,96–98] ABI1 and ABI2 are degraded in BCR-ABL-positive cells via the 26s proteasome in a kinase-dependent fashion, consistent with a positive feedback loop that enhances kinase activity.

BCR-ABL motifs other than SH1 with a critical role for leukemogenesis

The actin-binding domain

A large proportion of cytoplasmic ABL is associated with the f-actin cytoskeleton through the C-terminal actin-binding domain.[89] In noncycling cells f-actin exerts a negative effect on ABL tyrosine kinase activity.[57] BCR-ABL, which is primarily found in the cytoplasm, is closely associated with f-actin, but is not inhibited.[99,100] Several factors such as BCR-ABL autophosphorylation and binding of SH3-docking proteins were found to be able to abolish the actin-dependent inhibition of the ABL kinase activity.[101] Recently, the structural basis of molecular interaction between actin and BCR-ABL has been reported. This could open the possibility of pharmacologically interfering with this interaction to modulate the biological activity of BCR-ABL.[102]

TYROSINE 177 OF BCR

Autophosphorylation of Y177 generates a binding site for growth factor receptor binding protein 2 (GRB2). GRB2 binds SOS, a guanine-nucleotide exchanger of RAS, as well as the adapter GRB2-associated binding protein 2 (GAB2).[80,81,103,104] The resulting GRB2/GAB2 complex is required for full activation of the RAS/ERK pathway and recruitment of SHP2 and phosphatidylinositol 3-kinase (PI3K). Signal transduction downstream of PI3K leads to activation of AKT and mTOR.[81,105] A BCR-ABL mutant in which the Y177 phosphorylation site is disrupted by mutation of tyrosine to phenylalanine (Y177F) is defective for induction of CML-like disease, but retains the ability to induce T-ALL or T-cell lymphomas.[77,78,83] Similarly, loss of GAB2 abolishes myeloid transformation by BCR-ABL but only partially attenuates lymphoid transformation.[81] Besides being a target for autophosphorylation, Y177 is also transphosphorylated by the SRC family kinase HCK.[106] The role of SRC family kinases in the pathogenesis of BCR-ABL-positive leukemias is controversial. Mice lacking the SRC family kinases LYN, HCK, and FGR are selectively resistant to induction of lymphoid leukemia by BCR-ABL, while they readily develop CML.[107] Another study suggested a role for LYN in myeloid blast crisis.[108] These observations have received attention as a result of the availability of combined ABL/SRC inhibitors for the treatment of imatinib-resistant CML and ALL.[109,110]

CHRONIC MYELOID LEUKEMIA MODELS

When studying data on kinase activity, signaling, or functional oncogenicity of ABL or BCR-ABL mutants, it is important to reflect on the dependency of readouts on the cellular and intercellular context. Owing to the ease of manipulation and the abundant expression of relevant target proteins, cell lines provide a convenient platform for signaling and functional studies. On the minus side, they carry genetic lesions besides BCR-ABL, their differentiation is blocked and they are remote from the *in vivo* situation, where the leukemia cells are embedded in their microenvironment.

In vitro models of CML

Fibroblast lines were used extensively in the early stages of CML research for domain requirements and protein interaction studies as well as analysis of signaling pathways.[111–113] Fibroblast transformation – that is, anchorage-independent growth in soft agar – is the standard *in vitro* test for tumorigenicity.[114] BCR-ABL transforms Rat-1 fibroblasts,[115] while NIH3T3 cells are resistant.[116] Certain but not all fibroblast lines become serum-independent upon expression of BCR-ABL.[117] These partially conflicting findings indicate that the transforming capacity of BCR-ABL is dependent on the cellular context, which renders the interpretation of data difficult and has spurred the development of more physiological experimental systems. Expression of BCR-ABL induces factor-independent growth of cell lines that normally require cytokines such as interleukin-3 (IL-3), granulocyte-macrophage colony-stimulating factor (GM-CSF), IL-7, or erythropoietin (EPO) for their proliferation and survival.[118–120] Ba/F3 cells, a murine pre-B-cell line, and 32D cells, a murine myeloid progenitor cell line, have been used extensively to study BCR-ABL signal transduction and the requirement of BCR-ABL domains for transformation (for review see reference 121). Although the two lines show differences in BCR-ABL oncogenicity studies, these are not as pronounced as in fibroblasts, and may be related at least partially to their specific lineages. For example, a triple mutant lacking Y177 of BCR, Y393 in the ABL-kinase domain, and the ABL SH2-domain, rendered Ba/F3 but not 32D cells factor independent.[120] A cell line model that comes closer to primary cells is the multipotent murine hematopoietic FDCPmix cell line transduced with a BCR-ABL mutant, in which kinase activity is temperature dependent.[122] Even at the permissive temperature, the cells remain growth factor dependent and are responsive to differentiation stimuli, although they exhibit enhanced survival and proliferation. Yet another approach is the use of murine embryonic stem cells (ES) with potential to differentiate into multipotent hematopoietic progenitors.[123] In one such model, it was possible to reproduce one cardinal feature of the clinical disease, namely the expansion of the myeloid compartment at the expense of the erythroid compartment.[124] Similar to human proliferating CML progenitors, the increase in total cell numbers in the BCR-ABL-transduced ES was found to result from increased proliferation though there was little effect on apoptosis.[125]

Human CML cell lines

A number of human CML cell lines have been characterized. They are all derived from blast crisis patients and contain many genetic aberrations besides BCR-ABL, a reflection of the clonal evolution that characterizes disease progression.[126,127] Most are of myeloid (i.e. K562[128]), but some are of lymphoid lineage (i.e. BV173).[129] Their derivation from blast crisis makes them a reasonable model for CML-BC, but not for CML-CP. Attempts to immortalize chronic phase cells were not successful. EBV-transformed B-cell cultures from CML patients gradually become dominated by Ph-negative clones, consistent with a limited life span of the Ph-positive clones.[130]

Owing to the ease of maintaining CML cell lines in culture, these lines are very widely used and have undergone thousands of passages. Thus, frequently the lines housed in the various laboratories worldwide may not have much more in common than their name and BCR-ABL positivity. Contamination of newly generated cell lines, frequently with K562 cells, is not uncommon.[127] Surprisingly, despite their multiple aberrations, most of the CML lines still depend on BCR-ABL, as treatment with imatinib inhibits growth and induces apoptosis.[131] Nonetheless, caution is warranted when extrapolating from human CML cell line data to general CML biology.

Primary human hematopoietic cells

Only recently, the transduction of primary human CD34+ hematopoietic cells established an additional disease model with probably the closest relationship to the actual human disease.[132,133] Transduced cells recreate many of the phenotypic abnormalities seen in primary CML CD34+ cells, such as impaired control of proliferation by cell adhesion and delayed apoptosis after withdrawal of cytokines and serum.[133] These experiments also provided evidence that BCR-ABL-dependent autocrine production of IL-3 and GM-CSF is relevant to the the expansion of CML progenitor cells.[134]

Animal models of CML

In a pioneering study, Daley and colleagues showed that retroviral transduction of murine bone marrow followed by injection into lethally irradiated syngeneic recipient mice induced a myeloproliferative disorder (MPD) closely resembling CML.[34] The original model suffered from incomplete penetrance and produced a variety of hematological neoplasms besides MPD, but was subsquently optimized by modifications to the vector and infection conditions.[79] Current models are 100% effective in inducing a MPD that resembles the chronic phase of human CML.[33,79,135] The development of transgenic models was hampered by the fact that BCR-ABL expression from the BCR promoter during embryogenesis is lethal.[136] Transgenic mice in which BCR-ABL is expressed from a metallothionein-inducible promoter or the TEC promoter developed primarily T-cell ALL.[137–140] Studies targeting B-cell or megakaryocytic precursors with the *BCR-ABL* transgene demonstrated the importance of the precursor cell lineage for the leukemic phenotype (B-ALL versus megakaryocytic MPD).[141] Recently, a model has been described, where BCR-ABL is under the control of a tetracycline-repressible transactivator, which in turn is under the control of the SCL enhancer that targets expression to hematopoietic cells. Upon tetracycline withdrawal the mice develop a disease resembling chronic phase CML that is reversible upon re-challenge with tetracycline.[142] Together, these *in vivo* experiments provide the strongest evidence that BCR-ABL expression alone is sufficient to induce chronic phase CML.

BCR-ABL-DEPENDENT SIGNALING

Signal transduction downstream of BCR-ABL has been studied extensively (Figure 2.5). Many of the signaling cascades activated by BCR-ABL expression are common targets of oncogenic proteins.[143] They include pathways such as RAS/MAPK, PI3K/AKT or JAK/STAT, many of which are also activated by cytokine receptors involved in regulation of normal hematopoiesis and stem cell differentiation.[144–147] The list of BCR-ABL binding partners and tyrosine phosphorylated proteins is extensive and continues to expand,[54,148–151] but a comprehensive picture of how these proteins initiate leukemia and drive progression in patients is still lacking. This reflects the fact that signal transduction is not just a matter of yes or no (activation versus inactivation of target proteins), but rather a complex scenario of signal duration, signal attenuation, signal thresholds, and signal balances, which are in part governed by the cellular background.[143,152] This complexity accounts for the often confusing and sometimes contradictory data generated using different cell lines, mouse strains or primary patient cells harvested at various stages of the disease.

RAS/MAPK signaling

Circumstantial evidence that RAS activation is important for the pathogenesis of Ph-positive leukemias comes from the observation that activating mutations are uncommon, even in the blastic phase of the disease, unlike in most other tumors.[153,154] This implies that the RAS pathway is constitutively active, and no further activating mutations are necessary. Several lines of experimental evidence have put RAS/MAPK-dependent signaling in the frontline of CML pathogenesis. Expression of an oncogenic KRAS using a conditional knock-in line of mice was shown to induce MPD resembling human chronic myelomonocytic leukemia (CMML), indicating that RAS activation is sufficient for induction of myeloid leukemia.[155,156] Consistent with this, activating mutations of RAS or inactivating mutations of RAS inhibitory molecules are commonly found in CMML,[157] juvenile myelomonocytic leukemia (JMML),[158] and atypical (i.e. BCR-ABL negative) CML.[159] Inactivation of signal-induced proliferation-associated gene-1 (SIPA-1), a principal RAP1 GTPase-activating protein in hematopoietic progenitors, led to a spectrum of myeloid disorders in part resembling CML in mice.[160] There had been debate as to whether BCR-ABL kinase activity directly activates RAS/MAPK signaling or additional mutations are required.[161,162] At least three links between BCR-ABL and RAS have been described in various cellular contexts, including GRB2,[82] SHC,[163] and CRKL.[113] The most important connection is probably the aforementioned binding of GRB2 to phosphorylated tyrosine

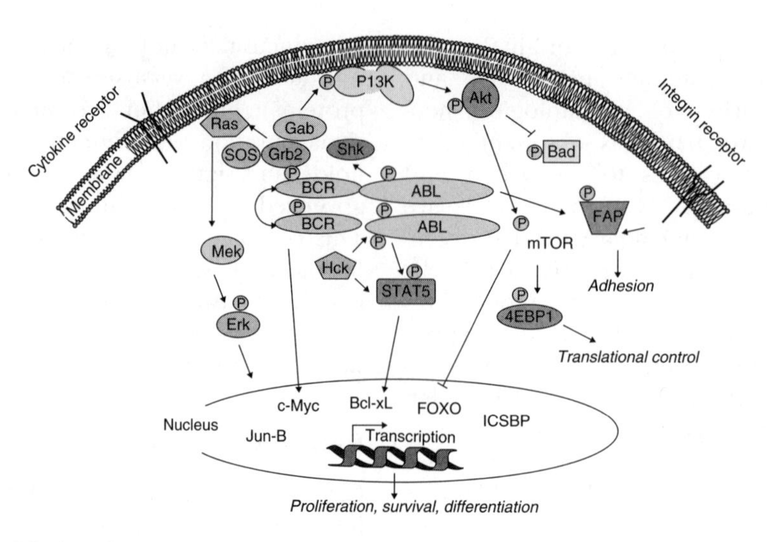

Figure 2.5 The BCR-ABL-dependent signaling complex. Depicted is a simplified cartoon of signaling and target molecules of BCR-ABL. Arrows indicate direct interaction or phosphorylation. The main pillars of BCR-ABL-dependent signaling cascades are the RAS/MEK/ERK, and the PI3K/Akt/mTOR pathways as well as signaling through STAT5. BCR-ABL disrupts normal cytokine signaling, which in many aspects shares the signaling events triggered by BCR-ABL. Modification of protein expression by either cytokines or BCR-ABL influences proliferation, survival or differentiation of hematopoietic cells. Interactions with the integrin receptor associated signaling complex (FAP: focal adhesion proteins and cytoskeletal proteins) are thought to be involved in the adhesion defects of BCR-ABL-expressing cells.

177 of BCR.[81] Recent data suggest that the regulatory network may be yet more complicated, extending to other RAS family members. For example, RAP1 is a small GTPase of the RAS family that is activated in response to IL-3 stimulation or BCR-ABL expression, thereby activating MEK/ERK signaling through activation of B-RAF.[164,165] JNK/SAPK activation by BCR-ABL has been demonstrated as well as suppression of pro-apoptotic MAPK p38 as yet another mechanism of how BCR-ABL enhances survival and proliferation.[166,167]

The net effect of BCR-ABL-dependent RAS-MAPK and RAS-independent MAPK activation includes a multitude of proliferative and anti-apoptotic responses that are regulated by phosphorylation of transcription factors such as c-Myc or c-Jun, frequently in a cell context-dependent fashion.[151,168] Thus, inhibition of BCR-ABL by imatinib rapidly inactivates ERK1/2 in BCR-ABL-transformed cell lines, leading to apoptotic cell death.[143] In contrast, imatinib treatment of CD34-enriched progenitor cells from CML patients in the presence of physiological growth factors leads to dose-dependent ERK1/2 activation, which protects the cells from apoptosis, an effect that can be abrogated by MAPK inhibitors and provides a rationale for combination therapies.[169–172]

PI3K and AKT

The phosphoinositol 3-kinase (PI3K) signaling pathway is commonly deregulated in cancer and is considered an attractive therapeutic target (Figure 2.6).[173] PI3K is a lipid kinase that converts phosphatidylinositol-4, 5-bisphosphate to phosphatidylinositol-3,4,5-trisphosphate (PIP3).[174] Membrane-bound PIP3 is a docking site for pleckstrin homology domain containing proteins such as phosphoinositide-dependent kinase-1 (PDK-1) and AKT (also known as protein kinase B).[175] PI3K activation occurs via phosphorylation of its p85 regulatory subunit by BCR-ABL and is crucial for the growth of Ph-positive cells.[176] Importantly, the observation that inactivation of phosphatase and tensin homolog deleted on chromosome 10 (PTEN), the lipid phosphatase that degrades PIP3, turns normal stem cells into leukemia initiating stem

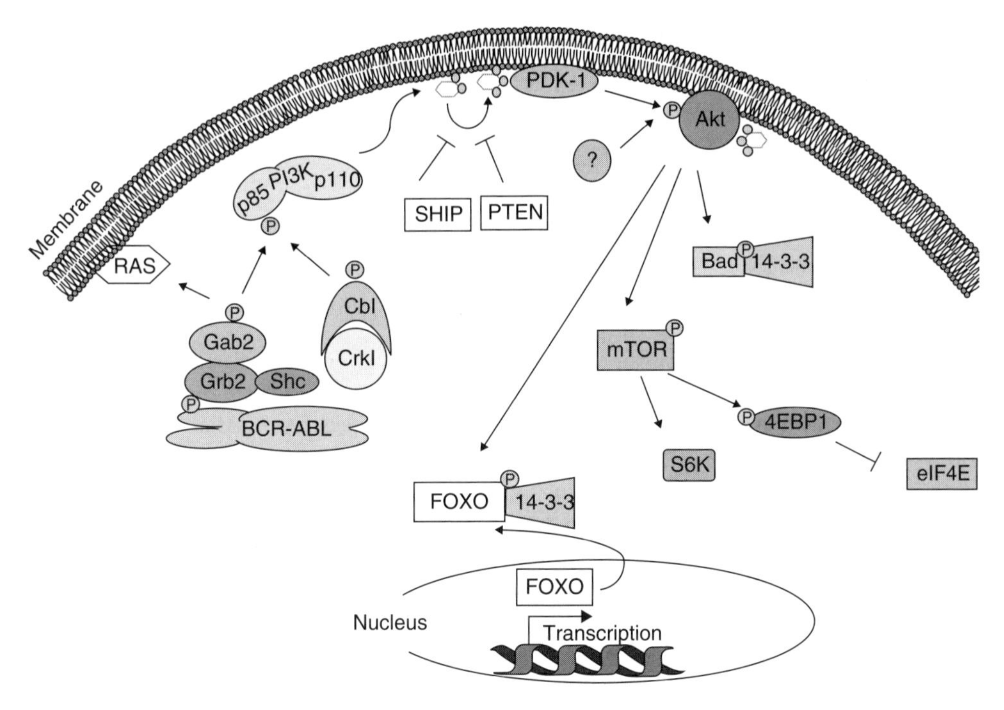

Figure 2.6 PI3K signaling. BCR-ABL activates PI3K by two well-characterized protein complexes, the GRB2/GAB2, or the CRKL/CBL adaptor complexes. Second messenger lipid products (depicted as membrane-bound hexamers) and phosphoinositide-dependent kinase-1 (PDK-1) activate AKT downstream of PI3K. AKT has a variety of downstream target proteins that promote cell growth, proliferation, and survival. For more details see paragraph PI3K and AKT.

cells suggests a profound role for PI3K signaling in leukemogenesis.[177] Another counterplayer of PI3K is the SH2-containing inositol-5-phosphatase (SHIP), which is suppressed by BCR-ABL expression in murine Ba/F3 cells.[178] Consistent with this, mice lacking SHIP develop a lethal CML-like myeloproliferative disease.[179] PI3K activation in BCR-ABL-expressing cells is mediated through phosphorylation of Y177 and recruitment of the adapter proteins GRB2 and GAB2.[81] Alternative mechanisms involve recruitment of the GRB2–GAB2 complex via SHC[180,181] or formation of a multimeric complex between BCR-ABL, CRKL, CBL, and the p85 regulatory subunit of PI3K.[182] Genetic approaches were explored to define more precisely the relevance of the various pathways for leukemogenesis. CRKL overexpressing transgenic mice show enhanced sensitivity to p190$^{BCR\text{-}ABL}$-induced lymphoid leukemia, but deletion of CRKL does not impair leukemic transformation.[183,184] Similarily, BCR-ABL is fully leukemogenic in CBL null mice.[185] In contrast, BCR-ABL fails to induce MPD in GAB2 null mice.[81]

PI3K activation leads to PIP3 accumulation, which recruits AKT to the membrane, where it is phosphorylated and activated by PDK1 and a yet unidentified serine/threonine kinase.[174] Expression of dominant-negative AKT greatly diminishes BCR-ABL-dependent myeloid leukemogenesis, and constitutively active AKT can complement a transformation-deficient variant of BCR-ABL.[186] AKT phosphorylates diverse substrates in transformed cells promoting cell growth, proliferation, and survival. A major target is the forkhead box subgroup O (FOXO) family of transcription factors. PI3K-AKT-dependent phosphorylation directs cytoplasmic sequestration and/or degradation of FOXO leading to suppression of FOXO target proteins.[187] It has been shown that BCR-ABL mediates suppression of tumor necrosis factor-related apoptosis-inducing ligand (TRAIL)-induced apoptosis through inhibition of the

FOXO member FOXO3a.[188] Other relevant targets of AKT include pro-apoptitic Bcl-2 family member BAD,[145,189] which is inactivated by phosphorylation and possibly the transcription factor nuclear factor-κB (NF-κB).[190] The mechanism for NF-κB activation is not fully understood, and seems to depend on cooperative effects between the RAS- and AKT-dependent signaling pathways.[191] From a therapeutic standpoint the most important AKT target is the serine/threonine kinase mammalian target of rapamycin (mTOR) owing to the availability of approved clinical inhibitors such as rapamycin, an immunosuppressant that is currently in clinical trials of CML.[105,192–195] mTOR in turn phosphorylates ribosomal S6 kinases (S6K1/2) and the translation inhibitor protein 4EBP-1, which are part of an ancient system to regulate protein translation.[105,196] Figure 2.6 gives a simplified overview of this central signaling cascade in CML pathogenesis.

JAK/STAT (or SRC/STAT, or BCR-ABL/STAT)

The JAK/STAT-pathway (janus kinase, signal transducer and activator of transcription) connects cytokine receptors such as the IL-3 or GM-CSF receptors and gene transcription.[197] JAKs are stimulated by activation of cytokine receptors and phosphorylate STATs, which translocate to the nucleus, where they regulate transcription. Although activation of STAT5 in BCR-ABL-expressing cell lines and primary leukemia cells was recognized almost a decade ago, the precise mechanism involved remains somewhat controversial.[198,199] BCR-ABL may either directly bind and phosphorylate STAT5,[200] or the phosphorylation may be mediated by JAK2[201] or HCK.[202] Genetic inactivation of STAT5*a* attenuates the induction of murine CML-like MPD, and fetal liver hematopoietic progenitors from STAT5*ab*-/- mice fail to induce leukemia in recipient mice after retroviral transduction with BCR-ABL.[203,204] In primary human CD34+ cells, Ph-positive myeloid colony formation is impaired by treatment with siRNA against STAT5.[205] The effect of STAT5 may be primarily anti-apoptotic, and involve Bcl-X as a critical mediator.[206] Together, these data suggest that STAT5 signaling contributes to BCR-ABL leukemogenesis.

GENETIC ENGINEERING OF THE CHRONIC MYELOID LEUKEMIA-LIKE PHENOTYPE IN MICE

Research over recent years has added valuable insights into candidate genes the deregulation of which has the potential of inducing a CML-like disease in mice. In many instances, these genes are negative regulators of hematopoiesis and their disruption induces a hyperproliferative state of the hematopoietic system that paves the way to MPD. For example, mice null for the interferon consensus sequence binding protein (ICSBP, also known as IRF-8) develop CML-like disease with 100% penetrance, the expression of ICSBP is downregulated in BCR-ABL-induced murine CML-like disease, and forced co-expression of ICSBP inhibits BCR-ABL-induced MPD.[207,208] Downregulation of ICSBP transcripts was also found in patients with CML, and this reduction could be reversed by treatment with interferon alfa.[209] *In vitro*, co-expression of ICSBP and BCR-ABL antagonizes the leukemogenic effects of BCR-ABL, possibly by downregulation of the anti-apoptotic factor Bcl-2.[210] Along the same lines, mice null for the *Alox15* gene, the coding locus for 12/15-lipoxygenase, develop MPD, and this is associated with reduced levels of nuclear ICSBP, Akt activation, and elevated expression of Bcl-2. Further research is needed to clarify the role of *Alox15* in MPD, in particular in Ph-positive MPD.[211,212]

Another transcriptional factor important for myelopoiesis that has been shown to induce a MPD closely resembling CML after genetic knock-out in mice is the AP-1 transcription factor JunB.[213,214] In CML patient samples, JunB expression is downregulated, and downregulation is correlated with progression of disease to blast crisis.[215,216] The mechanism of downregulation seems to be promoter hypermethylation, and treatment with the demethylating agent decitabine in part re-induces JunB expression *in vitro*.[215]

Another example of a negative regulator the deletion of which is leukemogenic is the lipid phosphatase SHIP.[179] Consistent with this, BCR-ABL inhibits expression of SHIP in hematopoietic cells.[178]

BCR-ABL AND THE HALLMARKS OF CANCER

A widely accepted notion first put forward by Hanahan and Weinberg is that during their development most if not all cancers have acquired a similar set of functional capabilities.[217] These include self-sufficiency in growth signals, the ability to evade programmed cell death (apoptosis), insensitivity to growth-inhibitory signals, sustained angiogenesis, limitless replicative potential, and the ability to invade tissue and metastasize.

CML provides an opportunity to observe the process of carcinogenesis from the adenoma-like chronic phase through the accelerated phase CML to the completely transformed state of blastic crisis, which satisfies all of the Weinberg criteria.

Self-sufficiency in growth signals

Mammalian cells are susceptible to regulation by extracellular signals during the early/mid G1 phase of the proliferative cell cycle. Once the so-called restriction point (R) in mid/late G1 has been passed, the cells complete the cycle independent of extrinsic signals.[218] Expression of BCR-ABL induces factor-independent growth of cell lines that normally require cytokines such as IL-3, GM-CSF or EPO.[216,217] Primary CML progenitor cells are not growth factor independent, but do have reduced growth factor requirements compared with normal cells.[219] The critical cytokine may be IL-3, which is produced by CML cells in a BCR-ABL kinase-dependent fashion and stimulates their growth in an autocrine loop.[79,220–222] Additionally, ligand-independent activation of the IL-3 receptor can be induced by BCR-ABL.[223] However, there is controversy regarding the role of IL-3, as BCR-ABL is fully leukemogeneic in IL-3 null mice.[224] It is conceivable that this reflects the aggressive nature of the transduction/transplantation model of CML, where the animals succumb to MPD derived from BCR-ABL expressing progenitor cells, whereas the effect of IL-3 may be critical at an earlier stage of differentiation.[225] What has been said for BCR-ABL and the IL-3 receptor pathway, in many aspects is also valid for other cytokine pathways such as GM-CSF or EPO.[121,148] Major effector molecules of growth factor signals include D-cyclins that activate cyclin-dependent kinases (CDK). Cyclin D1 and ABL oncogenes are synergistic in the transformation of fibroblasts and hematopoietic cells in culture. More recent papers have shown BCR-ABL- and IL-3-dependent upregulation of cyclin D2.[226,227] Conversely, BCR-ABL downregulates the CDK inhibitor $p27^{Kip1}$.[227–231] $p27^{Kip1}$ is highly expressed and stable in quiescent, non-cycling cells, but undergoes degradation as cells progress into S-phase.[232,233] BCR-ABL decreases $p27^{Kip1}$-protein levels by increasing its degradation by the proteasome, probably by upregulating SKP2, which provides the p27 recognition moiety (F-box) of the E3 ubiquitin ligase SCF^{SKP2}.[230] Recently, direct tyrosine phosphorylation of $p27^{Kip1}$ by BCR-ABL was shown to allow for subsequent phosphorylation by CDK2, which in turn promotes SCF-SKP2-dependent proteasomal degradation of $p27^{Kip1}$.[231] In primary progenitor cells BCR-ABL was shown to induce sequestration of $p27^{Kip1}$ into the cytoplasm, where it is unavailable for inhibition of nuclear CDK2.[234]

Insensitivity to growth-inhibitory signals

In addition to positive signals, quiescence, cycling, and differentiation of hematopoietic cells are subject to negative regulation by cytokines and the microenvironment, and there is evidence that BCR-ABL blocks growth inhibitory signals. For example, $p27^{Kip1}$ induction by transforming growth factor (TGF)β is completely blocked in BCR-ABL-transformed human MO7e cells.[229] As yet this has not been confirmed in primary cells,[235] the TGFβ sensitivity of which appears to be increased rather than reduced, which may maintain the cells in a quiescent, imatinib-resistant state.[236]

In contrast to normal progenitors, CML progenitors proliferate continuously even when in contact with bone marrow stroma, which is a potent inhibitor of progenitor proliferation.[237–239] The unresponsiveness of CML progenitors to negative regulatory signals from the bone marrow is thought to be caused by their inability to signal via β1 integrins.[240]

Evading programmed cell death (apoptosis)

The ability of leukemia cells to expand in number is determined not only by the rate of cell proliferation but also by the rate of cell death. Partially conflicting results have been reported on evasion of programmed cell death in CML cells. For example, responses to cytokine deprivation or ionizing irradiation have been reported to be similar in normal and in chronic phase CML progenitors in one study, while another study came to the opposite conclusion.[241,242] All in all, however, it appears to be an accepted notion that inhibition of apotosis is one of the key effects of BCR-ABL. Pathways involved in transducing the anti-apoptotic signals include PI3K/AKT/mTOR, RAS/MAPK, and JAK/STAT.[145,174,206,243,244] Important effector molecules are BCL-X, BAD, survivin, and MCL-1.[145,245–247] Apoptosis-related molecules are currently the target of intense research aiming at overcoming the apoptosis-inhibiting function of BCR-ABL.[248,249]

Another important mechanism by which BCR-ABL kinase negatively regulates apoptotic responses is downregulation of p53 by enhancing the translation of Mdm2, the ubiquitin ligase that promotes p53 degradation.[250,251] Since the p53/Mdm2 pathway plays an important role in the induction of cell cycle arrest or apoptosis in response to genotoxic stress, the corruption of the p53 response may contribute to the genomic instability that characterizes CML cells and underlies progression to blast crisis.

Sustained angiogenesis

Angiogenesis, a requirement for solid tumors to maintain viability and growth is regulated by angiogenic factors such as vascular endothelial growth factor (VEGF).[252,253] The potential role of angiogenesis in CML has attracted attention owing to the high microvessel density in the bone marrow of CML patients.[254,255] High VEGF levels in the plasma of CML patients have also been reported.[256] Treatment of CML patients with imatinib leads to normalization of bone marrow microvessel density and reduction of plasma VEGF levels.[257,258] Consistent with clinical observations, expression of BCR-ABL in hematopoietic cells induces VEGF secretion, which can be blocked by rapamycin, consistent with an mTOR-dependent mechanism.[194] Other angiogenic factors such as interleukin-8 (IL-8), hepatocyte growth factor (HGF), fibroblast growth factor-2 (FGF-2) or metalloproteinases (MMPs) have been reported to be released by BCR-ABL-expressing cells and are assumed to stimulate leukemia cell growth.[259] Whether anti-angiogenic therapy will be effective in CML therapy remains to be determined.

Limitless replicative potential

Stem cells are defined by their ability to self-renew, a feature that is required to sustain hematopoiesis over a lifespan. Human cancer stem cells have been detected in a variety of malignant disorders and share functional properties with normal stem cells.[260] Primitive CML cells harvested from chronic phase patients exhibit increased turnover, in part induced by autocrine cytokine stimulation, and defective adhesion control.[222,238,261] The increased cycling rate is reflected by increased telomere shortening, which is assumed to contribute to chromosomal instability as the disease progresses.[262] In analogy to normal hematopoietic cells the self-renewal capacity of chronic phase CML cells is apparently confined to the most primitive compartment, while committed progenitors have limited replicative potential.[263] Moreover, it seems that BCR-ABL itself is unable to confer self-renewal capacity, unlike MOZ-TIF2, a chimeric protein associated with AML, which implies that the BCR-ABL translocation must occur in a cell with innate self-renewal capacity.[264,265] In contrast, there is evidence that blast crisis granulocyte-macrophage progenitors (GMP) acquire the ability to self-renew. This is associated with activation of the Wnt-signaling pathway and characterized by accumulation of nuclear β-catenin, which seems to be critical for hematopoietic stem cell (HSC) self-renewal.[73,75]

The ability to invade tissues and metastasize

Ph-positive stem cells are presumed to have partially escaped the normal requirement for close association with specialized marrow regulatory stromal cells, because of defective adhesion control and altered cytoskeletal function.[238,266] The result is a massively expanded pool of myeloid progenitor cells in the blood and hematopoiesis in the spleen and other extramedullary sites outside the physiological stem cell niche in the bone marrow.[267] Several constituents of the bone marrow microenvironment have been analyzed for their interaction with CML progenitors and significant differences between normal and CML-derived progenitors have been observed.[239] There is evidence that β1 integrin function is defective in CML CD34+ cells, which may impair binding to cell adhesion molecules (CAM) such as vascular cell adhesion molecule (VCAM) or matrix proteins such as fibronectin (FN).[268] The molecular mechanisms underlying abnormal integrin function involve the well-established effects of BCR-ABL on the cytoskeleton, such as binding to f-actin, and phosphorylation of cytoskeletal proteins such as paxillin, talin, vinculin, focal adhesion kinase (FAK), and CRKL or tensin.[83,90,91,269–273] Besides defective β1 integrin signaling, homing of CML progenitors is impaired owing to a perturbation of chemotaxis mediated through stroma derived factor 1 (SDF-1), and the corresponding surface receptor CXCR4.[274] Whether this is as a result of downregulation of CXCR4 or a signaling defect downstream of CXCR4 has yet to be determined.[275,276] A recent publication suggests that interfering with homing and adhesion may be exploited therapeutically. Thus, homing and engraftment of transplanted BCR-ABL-expressing cells was inhibited in mice null for the hyaluronan receptor CD44, suggesting that interference with CD44 binding may prevent CML stem cells from engrafting after autologous stem cell transplantation.[277]

MECHANISMS OF DISEASE PROGRESSION

The distinct feature of blast crisis CML (CML-BC) is the differentiation arrest of hematopoietic precursor cells with inherently high proliferation rate and resistance to apoptosis. Recent years have added many pieces to the still unresolved puzzle of disease progression from chronic phase to accelerated phase and eventually blast crisis.[278,279] Clonal cytogenetic evolution occurs in 60–80% of patients. The most frequent abnormalities are trisomy 8 (34%), duplication of Ph, trisomy 19, and isochromosome 17.[280] The specific role of chromosomal abnormalities in CML disease progression is not clear. One may expect that the *MYC* gene located at 8q24 is involved in disease progression in cases with trisomy 8, yet no correlation between trisomy 8 and MYC amplification/overexpression has been observed.[281] Similarly, an association between p53 mutations and the appearance of an isochromosome 17 was hypothesized, owing to the loss of the corresponding 17p coding for p53. However, no mutations in the remaining p53 allele were found in i(17q) positive patients.[282] Mutational events below the detection level of cytogenetics are thought to play an important role in transformation to blast crisis.[126] Consistent with the importance of genetic abnormalities below the detection level of cytogenetics, patients with a normal karyogram do not do significantly better in treatment studies compared with patients with an aberrant karyotype.[283]

The underlying mutator phenotype of CML cells is probably the result of diverse mechanisms that cooperate to destabilize the genome of the leukemia cells. Evidently, the high cell turnover itself combined with the anti-apoptotic activity of BCR-ABL must increase the mutation risk per unit of time. At the biochemical level, BCR-ABL negatively affects DNA repair. For example, downregulation of the DNA repair protein DNA-PKCS, upregulation of DNA polymerase β, the mammalian DNA polymerase with the least fidelity, or modulation of nucleotide excision repair (NER) was shown.[284–286] Deutsch and colleagues reported an association of BCR-ABL expression in primary CML cells and cell lines with downregulation of BRCA1, a protein involved in surveillance of genomic integrity.[287] Other mechanisms that may enhance the mutation rate are the reported accelerated telomere shortening,[262] or the generation of reactive oxygen species, which are potent mutagens.[288] Important tumor suppressors disrupted in blast crisis are the cell cycle regulators p53 and INK4/ARF. Whereas p53 mutations are found in approximately 30% of myeloid blast crisis patients, the INK4/ARF locus is mutated exclusively in lymphoid blast crisis.[289,290] However, these lesions do not readily explain the most prominent feature of blastic transformation, namely the loss of differentiation capacity. Surprisingly, mutations in key regulators of hematopoietic differentiation are rarely found in blast crisis.[289,291,292] Thus, other mechanisms must be responsible for the differentiation block. For example, it has been demonstrated that BCR-ABL perturbs the translational control of C/EBPα, an important myeloid transcription factor.[279] However, as BCR-ABL is expressed in all phases of CML, one would have to postulate an additional event to explain why the differentiation block occurs at the time of transformation. Alternatively, there could be a dose effect of BCR-ABL; since levels increase with disease progression, this could eventually overcome a critical threshold.[293]

The efficacy of ABL inhibitors in patients with blast crisis indicates that in many cases the disease remains dependent on BCR-ABL, despite its genetic diversity.[294] Unfortunately, almost all patients eventually relapse owing to BCR-ABL kinase domain mutations or other mutations that reactivate BCR-ABL activity or confer BCR-ABL independence.[295]

Prior to the availability of imatinib, CML often progressed within 5 years from diagnosis, which is now rare.[296,297] This observation fits the concept that accumulation of additional mutations depends on BCR-ABL kinase activity. This suggests that more complete suppression of BCR-ABL kinase activity with more potent second-line ABL inhibitors such as dasatinib or nilotinib in conjunction with a rapid reduction of the leukemia burden may further reduce the risk of blast crisis. For this to be fully effective, it will be crucial to inhibit BCR-ABL in the most primitive leukemia (stem) cells.

SUMMARY AND FUTURE DIRECTIONS

CML research continues to break new ground, opening new views and perspectives on cancer biology. The importance of understanding the disease biology has been demonstrated impressively by the success of imatinib for the treatment of CML. The lessons that continue to be learned from the imatinib experience will serve as a model for target cancer treatments with other molecules.[297] Despite the durability of most imatinib responses in patients treated in early chronic phase, persistence of residual disease is the rule,[298] suggesting that current therapy may be unable to efficiently target leukemic stem cells. If we define cure as the eradication of all leukemia cells then few patients may be curable with imatinib therapy. The key to overcome this will be a better understanding of CML stem cell biology and the mechanisms that allow the most critical cells to survive in the presence of imatinib.[261,299] Most importantly, defining whether persistence is a BCR-ABL-dependent or -independent phenomenon will be necessary to guide the development of rational therapeutic approaches. Are there additional, non-redundant molecules that can be targeted with reasonable selectivity against leukemic stem cells? Or is it the case that only the combination of molecular therapy with an immunological approach that is targeted against the leukemia stem cell rather than the BCR-ABL kinase will ultimately allow for disease eradication? If so, what is the appropriate antigen to be targeted by such an immunological approach? Eventually, only clinical trials will be able to answer these questions. Besides questions related to CML therapy, much remains to be learned about its biology. Is there really a Ph-negative clonal state that pre-dates the acquisition of Ph? What is the relation of lymphoid blast crisis and Ph-positive ALL? What is the molecular basis of the differentiation block? Answering these questions will require close collaboration between clinical and basic research scientists.

REFERENCES

1. Savage DG, Antman KH. Imatinib mesylate – a new oral targeted therapy. N Engl J Med 2002; 346: 683–93.
2. Druker BJ, Lydon NB. Lessons learned from the development of an Abl tyrosine kinase inhibitor for chronic myelogenous leukemia. J Clin Invest 2000; 105: 3–7.
3. Virchow R. Weisses Blut. Frorieps Notizen 1845; 36: 151–6.
4. Bennett JH. Case of hypertrophy of the spleen and liver, in which death took place from suppuration of the blood. Edinburgh Med Surg J 1845; 64: 413–23.
5. Nowell PC, Hungerford DA. A minute chromosome in human chronic granulocytic leukemia. Science 1960; 132: 1497–501.
6. Rowley JD. A new consistent chromosome abnormality in chronic myelogenous leukaemia detected by quinacrine fluorescence and Giemsa staining. Nature 1973; 243: 290–3.
7. Bartram CR, de Klein A, Hagemeijer A et al. Translocation of c-abl oncogene correlates with the presence of a Philadelphia chromosome in chronic myelocytic leukaemia. Nature 1983; 306: 277–80.
8. Groffen J, Stephenson JR, Heisterkamp N et al. Philadelphia chromosomal breakpoints are clustered within a limited region, bcr, on chromosome 22. Cell 1984; 36: 93–9.
9. Abelson HT, Rabstein LS. Lymphosarcoma: virus induced thymic-independent disease in mice. Cancer Res 1970; 30: 2213–22.
10. Scher CD, Siegler R. Direct transformation of 3T3 cells by Abelson murine leukaemia virus. Nature 1975; 253: 729–31.
11. Witte ON, Rosenberg NE, Baltimore D. A normal cell protein cross-reactive to the major Abelson murine leukaemia virus gene product. Nature 1979; 281: 396–8.
12. Collett MS, Erikson RL. Protein kinase activity associated with the avian sarcoma virus src gene product. Proc Natl Acad Sci U S A 1978; 75: 2021–4.
13. Hunter T, Sefton BM. Transforming gene product of Rous sarcoma virus phosphorylates tyrosine. Proc Natl Acad Sci U S A 1980; 77: 1311–15.
14. Witte ON, Dasgupta A, Baltimore D. Abelson murine leukaemia virus protein is phosphorylated in vitro to form phosphotyrosine. Nature 1980; 283: 826–31.
15. Lugo TG, Pendergast AM, Muller AJ, Witte ON. Tyrosine kinase activity and transformation potency of bcr-abl oncogene products. Science 1990; 247: 1079–82.
16. Tanaka K, Takechi M, Hong J et al. 9;22 translocation and bcr rearrangements in chronic myelocytic leukemia patients among atomic bomb survivors. J Radiat Res Tokyo 1989; 30: 352–8.
17. Corso A, Lazzarino M, Morra E et al. Chronic myelogenous leukemia and exposure to ionizing radiation – a retrospective study of 443 patients. Ann Hematol 1995; 70: 79–82.
18. Deininger MWN, Bose S, Gora-Tybor J et al. Selective induction of leukemia-associated fusion genes by high-dose ionizing radiation. Cancer Res 1998; 58: 421–5.
19. Neves H, Ramos C, da Silva MG et al. The nuclear topography of ABL, BCR, PML, and RARa genes. Evidence for gene proximity in specific phases of the cell cycle and stages of hematopoietic differentiation. Blood 1999; 93: 1197–207.
20. Kozubek S, Lukasova E, Ryznar L et al. Distribution of ABL and BCR genes in cell nuclei of normal and irradiated lymphocytes. Blood 1997; 89: 4537–45.
21. Chen SJ, Chen Z, d'Auriol L et al. Ph1+bcr- acute leukemias: implication of Alu sequences in a chromosomal translocation occurring in the new cluster region within the BCR gene. Oncogene 1989; 4: 195–202.
22. Jeffs AR, Wells E, Morris CM. Nonrandom distribution of interspersed repeat elements in the BCR and ABL1 genes and its relation to breakpoint cluster regions. Genes Chromosomes Cancer 2001; 32: 144–54.
23. Bose S, Deininger M, Gora-Tybor J et al. The presence of typical and atypical BCR-ABL fusion genes in leukocytes of normal individuals: biological

significance and implications for the assessment of minimal residual disease. Blood 1998; 92: 3362–7.
24. Biernaux C, Loos M, Sels A et al. Detection of major bcr-abl gene expression at a very low level in blood cells of some healthy individuals. Blood 1995; 88: 3118–22.
25. Matioli GT. BCR-ABL insufficiency for the transformation of human stem cells into CML. Med Hypotheses 2002; 59: 588–9.
26. Michor F, Iwasa Y, Nowak MA. The age incidence of chronic myeloid leukemia can be explained by a one-mutation model. Proc Natl Acad Sci U S A 2006; 103: 14931–4.
27. Posthuma EFM, Falkenburg JHF, Apperley JF et al. HLA-B8 and HLA-A3 coexpressed with HLA-B8 are associated with areduced risk of the development of chronic myeloid leukemia. Blood 1999; 93: 3863–5.
28. Raskind WH, Steinmann L, Najfeld V. Clonal development of myeloproliferative disorders: clues to hematopoietic differentiation and multistep pathogenesis of cancer. Leukemia 1998; 12: 108–16.
29. Fialkow PJ, Jacobson RJ, Papayannopoulou T. Chronic myelocytic leukemia: clonal origin in a stem cell common to the granulocyte, erythrocyte, platelet and monocyte/macrophage. Am J Med 1977; 63: 125–30.
30. Fialkow PJ, Gartler SM, Yoshida A. Clonal origin of chronic myelocytic leukemia in man. Proc Natl Acad Sci U S A 1967; 58: 1468–71.
31. Vickers M. Estimation of the number of mutations necessary to cause chronic myeloid leukaemia from epidemiological data. Br J Haematol 1996; 94: 1–4.
32. Takahashi N, Miura I, Saitoh K, Miura AB. Lineage involvement of stem cells bearing the philadelphia chromosome in chronic myeloid leukemia in the chronic phase as shown by a combination of fluorescence-activated cell sorting and fluorescence in situ hybridization. Blood 1998; 92: 4758–63.
33. Li S, Ilaria RL Jr, Million RP et al. The P190, P210, and P230 forms of the BCR/ABL oncogene induce a similar chronic myeloid leukemia-line syndrome in mice but have different lymphoid leukemogenic activity. J Exp Med 1999; 189: 1399–412.
34. Daley GQ, van Etten RA, Baltimore D. Induction of chronic myelogenous leukemia in mice by the P210bcr/abl gene of the Philadelphia chromosome. Science 1990; 247: 824–30.
35. Gunsilius E, Duba HC, Petzer AL et al. Evidence from a leukaemia model for maintenance of vascular endothelium by bone-marrow-derived endothelial cells. Lancet 2000; 355: 1688–91.
36. Fang B, Zheng C, Liao L et al. Identification of human chronic myelogenous leukemia progenitor cells with hemangioblastic characteristics. Blood 2005; 105: 2733–40.
37. Melo JV. The diversity of BCR-ABL fusion proteins and their relationship to leukemia phenotype. Blood 1996; 88: 2375–84.
38. van Rhee F, Hochhaus A, Lin F et al. p190 BCR-ABL mRNA is expressed at low levels in p210-positive chronic myeloid and acute lymphoblastic leukemias. Blood 1996; 87: 5213–17.
39. Pane F, Frigeri F, Sindona M et al. Neutrophilic-chronic myelogenous leukemia (CML-N): a distinct disease with a specific marker (BCR-ABL with c3a2 junction). Blood 1996; 88: 2410–14.
40. Hochhaus A, Reiter A, Skladny H et al. A novel BCR-ABL fusion gene (e6a2) in a patient with Philadelphia chromosome negative chronic myelogenous leukemia. Blood 1996; 88: 2236–40.
41. Advani AS, Pendergast AM. Bcr-Abl variants: biological and clinical aspects. Leuk Res 2002; 26: 713–20.
42. Demehri S, Paschka P, Schultheis B et al. e8a2 BCR-ABL: more frequent than other atypical BCR-ABL variants? Leukemia 2005; 19: 681–4.
43. Barnes DJ, Melo JV. Cytogenetic and molecular genetic aspects of chronic myeloid leukaemia. Acta Haematol 2002; 108: 180–202.
44. Konopka JB, Watanabe SM, Witte ON. An alteration of the human c-abl protein in K562 leukemia cells unmasks associated tyrosine kinase activity. Cell 1984; 37: 1035–42.
45. Ben Neriah Y, Daley GQ, Mes-Masson AM et al. The chronic myelogenous leukemia-specific P210 protein is the product of the bcr/abl hybrid gene. Science 1986; 233: 212–14.
46. van Etten RA. Cycling, stressed-out and nervous: cellular functions of c-Abl. Trends Cell Biol 1999; 9: 179–86.
47. Pendergast AM. The Abl family kinases: mechanisms of regulation and signaling. Adv Cancer Res 2002; 85: 51–100.
48. Hantschel O, Superti-Furga G. Regulation of the c-Abl and Bcr-Abl tyrosine kinases. Nat Rev Mol Cell Biol 2004; 5: 33–44.
49. Barila D, Superti-Furga G. An intramolecular SH3-domain interaction regulates c-Abl activity. Nat Genet 1998; 18: 280–2.
50. Pluk H, Dorey K, Superti-Furga G. Autoinhibition of c-Abl. Cell 2002; 108: 247–59.
51. Smith KM, Yacobi R, van Etten RA. Autoinhibition of Bcr-Abl through its SH3 domain. Mol Cell 2003; 12: 27–37.
52. Nagar B, Hantschel O, Young MA et al. Structural basis for the autoinhibition of c-Abl tyrosine kinase. Cell 2003; 112: 859–71.
53. Hantschel O, Nagar B, Guettler S et al. A myristoyl/phosphotyrosine switch regulates c-Abl. Cell 2003; 112: 845–57.
54. Wong S, Witte ON. The BCR-ABL story: bench to bedside and back. Annu Rev Immunol 2004; 22: 247–306.

55. Wen ST, van Etten RA. The PAG gene product, a stress-induced protein with antioxidant properties, is an Abl SH3-binding protein and a physiological inhibitor of c-Abl tyrosine kinase activity. Genes Dev 1997; 11: 2456–67.
56. Welch PJ, Wang JYJ. A C-terminal protein-binding domain in the retinoblastoma protein regulates nuclear c-Abl tyrosine kinase in the cell cycle. Cell 1993; 75: 779–90.
57. Woodring PJ, Hunter T, Wang JY. Inhibition of c-Abl tyrosine kinase activity by filamentous actin. J Biol Chem 2001; 276: 27104–10.
58. Zhu J, Wang JY. Death by Abl: a matter of location. Curr Top Dev Biol 2004; 59: 165–92.
59. Yoshida K, Yamaguchi T, Natsume T et al. JNK phosphorylation of 14-3-3 proteins regulates nuclear targeting of c-Abl in the apoptotic response to DNA damage. Nat Cell Biol 2005; 7: 278–85.
60. Kipreos ET, Wang JY. Differential phosphorylation of c-Abl in cell cycle determined by cdc2 kinase and phosphatase activity. Science 1990; 248: 217–20.
61. Sawyers CL, McLaughlin J, Goga A et al. The nuclear tyrosine kinase c-Abl negatively regulates cell growth. Cell 1994; 77: 121–31.
62. Yuan ZM, Shioya H, Ishiko T et al. p73 is regulated by tyrosine kinase c-Abl in the apoptotic response to DNA damage. Nature 1999; 399: 814–17.
63. Schwartzberg PL, Stall AM, Hardin JD et al. Mice homozygous for the ablm1 mutation show poor viability and depletion of selected B and T cell populations. Cell 1991; 65: 1165–75.
64. Tybulewicz VL, Crawford CE, Jackson PK et al. Neonatal lethality and lymphopenia in mice with a homozygous disruption of the c-abl proto-oncogene. Cell 1991; 65: 1153–63.
65. Koleske AJ, Gifford AM, Scott ML et al. Essential roles for the Abl and Arg tyrosine kinases in neurulation. Neuron 1998; 21: 1259–72.
66. Maru Y, Witte ON. The BCR gene encodes a novel serine/threonine kinase activity within a single exon. Cell 1991; 67: 459–68.
67. McWhirter JR, Galasso DL, Wang JY. A coiled-coil oligomerization domain of Bcr is essential for the transforming function of Bcr-Abl oncoproteins. Mol Cell Biol 1993; 13: 7587–95.
68. Boguski MS, McCormick F. Proteins regulating Ras and its relatives. Nature 1993; 366: 643–54.
69. Chuang TH, Xu X, Kaartinen V et al. Abr and Bcr are multifunctional regulators of the Rho GTP-binding protein family. Proc Natl Acad Sci U S A 1995; 92: 10282–6.
70. Radziwill G, Erdmann RA, Margelisch U, Moelling K. The Bcr kinase downregulates Ras signaling by phosphorylating AF-6 and binding to its PDZ domain. Mol Cell Biol 2003; 23: 4663–72.
71. Ress A, Moelling K. Bcr interferes with beta-catenin-Tcf1 interaction. FEBS Lett 2006; 580: 1227–30.
72. Ress A, Moelling K. Bcr is a negative regulator of the Wnt signalling pathway. EMBO Rep 2005; 6: 1095–100.
73. Reya T, Duncan AW, Ailles L et al. A role for Wnt signalling in self-renewal of haematopoietic stem cells. Nature 2003; 423: 409–14.
74. Willert K, Brown JD, Danenberg E et al. Wnt proteins are lipid-modified and can act as stem cell growth factors. Nature 2003; 423: 448–52.
75. Jamieson CH, Ailles LE, Dylla SJ et al. Granulocyte-macrophage progenitors as candidate leukemic stem cells in blast-crisis CML. N Engl J Med 2004; 351: 657–67.
76. Voncken JW, van Schaick H, Kaartinen V et al. Increased neutrophil respiratory burst in bcr-null mutants. Cell 1995; 80: 719–28.
77. Zhang X, Subrahmanyam R, Wong R et al. The NH(2)-terminal coiled-coil domain and tyrosine 177 play important roles in induction of a myeloproliferative disease in mice by Bcr-Abl. Mol Cell Biol 2001; 21: 840–53.
78. He Y, Wertheim JA, Xu L et al. The coiled-coil domain and Tyr177 of bcr are required to induce a murine chronic myelogenous leukemia-like disease by bcr/abl. Blood 2002; 99: 2957–68.
79. Zhang X, Ren R. Bcr-Abl efficiently induces a myeloproliferative disease and production of excess interleukin-3 and granulocyte-macrophage colony-stimulating factor in mice: a novel model for chronic myelogenous leukemia. Blood 1998; 92: 3829–40.
80. Puil L, Liu J, Gish G et al. Bcr-Abl oncoproteins bind directly to activators of the Ras signalling pathway. EMBO J 1994; 13: 764–73.
81. Sattler M, Mohi MG, Pride YB et al. Critical role for Gab2 in transformation by BCR/ABL. Cancer Cell 2002; 1: 479–92.
82. Pendergast AM, Quilliam LA, Cripe LD et al. BCR-ABL-induced oncogenesis is mediated by direct interaction with the SH2 domain of the GRB-2 adaptor protein. Cell 1993; 75: 175–85.
83. Million RP, van Etten RA. The Grb2 binding site is required for the induction of chronic myeloid leukemia-like disease in mice by the Bcr/Abl tyrosine kinase. Blood 2000; 96: 664–70.
84. Gross AW, Zhang X, Ren R. Bcr-Abl with an SH3 deletion retains the ability to induce a myeloproliferative disease in mice, yet c-Abl activated by an SH3 deletion induces only lymphoid malignancy. Mol Cell Biol 1999; 19: 6918–28.
85. Zhang X, Wong R, Hao SX et al. The SH2 domain of bcr-Abl is not required to induce a murine myeloproliferative disease; however, SH2 signaling influences disease latency and phenotype. Blood 2001; 97: 277–87.
86. Roumiantsev S, de Aos IE, Varticovski L et al. The src homology 2 domain of Bcr/Abl is required for efficient induction of chronic myeloid leukemia-like disease in mice but not for lymphoid

leukemogenesis or activation of phosphatidylinositol 3-kinase. Blood 2001; 97: 4–13.
87. Schindler T, Bornmann W, Pellicena P et al. Structural mechanism for STI-571 inhibition of abelson tyrosine kinase. Science 2000; 289: 1938–42.
88. Dorey K, Engen JR, Kretzschmar J et al. Phosphorylation and structure-based functional studies reveal a positive and a negative role for the activation loop of the c-Abl tyrosine kinase. Oncogene 2001; 20: 8075–84.
89. van Etten RA, Jackson PK, Baltimore D et al. The COOH terminus of the c-Abl tyrosine kinase contains distinct F- and G-actin binding domains with bundling activity. J Cell Biol 1994; 124: 325–40.
90. McWhirter JR, Wang JY. An actin-binding function contributes to transformation by the Bcr-Abl oncoprotein of Philadelphia chromosome-positive human leukemias. EMBO J 1993; 12: 1533–46.
91. Wertheim JA, Perera SA, Hammer DA et al. Localization of BCR-ABL to F-actin regulates cell adhesion but does not attenuate CML development. Blood 2003; 102: 2220–8.
92. Golub TR, Goga A, Barker GF et al. Oligomerization of the ABL tyrosine kinase by the Ets protein TEL in human leukemia. Mol Cell Biol 1996; 16: 4107–16.
93. Muller AJ, Young JC, Pendergast AM et al. BCR first exon sequences specifically activate the BCR/ABL tyrosine kinase oncogene of Philadelphia chromosome-positive human leukemias. Mol Cell Biol 1991; 11: 1785–92.
94. Heisterkamp N, Voncken JW, Senadheera D et al. The Bcr N-terminal oligomerization domain contributes to the full oncogenicity of P190 Bcr/Abl in transgenic mice. Int J Mol Med 2001; 7: 351–7.
95. Zhao X, Ghaffari S, Lodish H et al. Structure of the Bcr-Abl oncoprotein oligomerization domain. Nat Struct Biol 2002; 9: 117–20.
96. Franz WM, Berger P, Wang JY. Deletion of an N-terminal regulatory domain of the c-abl tyrosine kinase activates its oncogenic potential. EMBO J 1989; 8: 137–47.
97. Dai Z, Quackenbush RC, Courtney KD et al. Oncogenic Abl and Src tyrosine kinases elicit the ubiquitin-dependent degradation of target proteins through a Ras-independent pathway. Genes Dev 1998; 12: 1415–24.
98. Shi Y, Alin K, Goff SP. Abl-interactor-1, a novel SH3 protein binding to the carboxy-terminal portion of the Abl protein, suppresses v-abl transforming activity. Genes Dev 1995; 9: 2583–97.
99. Wetzler M, Talpaz M, van Etten RA et al. Subcellular localization of Bcr, Abl, and Bcr-Abl proteins in normal and leukemic cells and correlation of expression with myeloid differentiation. J Clin Invest 1993; 92: 1925–39.
100. McWhirter JR, Wang JY. Activation of tyrosinase kinase and microfilament-binding functions of c-abl by bcr sequences in bcr/abl fusion proteins. Mol Cell Biol 1991; 11: 1553–65.
101. Woodring PJ, Hunter T, Wang JY. Mitotic phosphorylation rescues Abl from F-actin-mediated inhibition. J Biol Chem 2005; 280: 10318–25.
102. Hantschel O, Wiesner S, Guttler T et al. Structural basis for the cytoskeletal association of Bcr-Abl/c-Abl. Mol Cell 2005; 19: 461–73.
103. Gishizky ML, Cortez D, Pendergast AM. Mutant forms of growth factor-binding protein-2 reverse BCR-ABL- induced transformation. Proc Natl Acad Sci U S A 1995; 92: 10889–93.
104. Tauchi T, Boswell HS, Leibowitz D, Broxmeyer HE. Coupling between p210bcr-abl and Shc and Grb2 adaptor proteins in hematopoietic cells permits growth factor receptor-independent link to ras activation pathway. J Exp Med 1994; 179: 167–75.
105. Ly C, Arechiga AF, Melo JV et al. Bcr-Abl kinase modulates the translation regulators ribosomal protein S6 and 4E-BP1 in chronic myelogenous leukemia cells via the mammalian target of rapamycin. Cancer Res 2003; 63: 5716–22.
106. Stanglmaier M, Warmuth M, Kleinlein I et al. The interaction of the Bcr-Abl tyrosine kinase with the Src kinase Hck is mediated by multiple binding domains. Leukemia 2003; 17: 283–9.
107. Hu Y, Liu Y, Pelletier S et al. Requirement of Src kinases Lyn, Hck and Fgr for BCR-ABL1-induced B-lymphoblastic leukemia but not chronic myeloid leukemia. Nat Genet 2004; 36: 453–61.
108. Ptasznik A, Nakata Y, Kalota A et al. Short interfering RNA (siRNA) targeting the Lyn kinase induces apoptosis in primary, and drug-resistant, BCR-ABL1(+) leukemia cells. Nat Med 2004; 10: 1187–9.
109. Hochhaus A, Kantarjian HM, Baccarani M et al. Dasatinib induces notable hematologic and cytogenetic responses in chronic-phase chronic myeloid leukemia after failure of imatinib therapy. Blood 2007; 109: 2303–9.
110. Talpaz M, Shah NP, Kantarjian H et al. Dasatinib in imatinib-resistant Philadelphia chromosome-positive leukemias. N Engl J Med 2006; 354: 2531–41.
111. Afar DE, Goga A, McLaughlin J et al. Differential complementation of Bcr-Abl point mutants with c-Myc. Science 1994; 264: 424–6.
112. Ilaria RL Jr, van Etten RA. The SH2 domain of P210BCR/ABL is not required for the transformation of hematopoietic factor-dependent cells. Blood 1995; 86: 3897–904.
113. Senechal K, Halpern J, Sawyers CL. The CRKL adaptor protein transforms fibroblasts and functions in transformation by the BCR-ABL oncogene. J Biol Chem 1996; 271: 23255–61.

114. Tordaro GJ, Green H. An assay for cellular transformation by SV40. Virology 1964; 23: 117–19.
115. Lugo TG, Witte ON. The BCR-ABL oncogene transforms Rat-1 cells and cooperates with v-myc. Mol Cell Biol 1989; 9: 1263–70.
116. Daley GQ, McLaughlin J, Witte ON, Baltimore D. The CML-specific P210 bcr/abl protein, unlike v-abl, does not transform NIH/3T3 fibroblasts. Science 1987; 237: 532–5.
117. Renshaw MW, Kipreos ET, Albrecht MR, Wang JYJ. Oncogenic v-Abl tyrosine kinase can inhibit or stimulate growth, depending on the cell context. EMBO J 1992; 11: 3941–51.
118. Daley GQ, Baltimore D. Transformation of an interleukin 3-dependent hematopoietic cell line by the chronic myelogenous leukemia-specific P210bcr/abl protein. Proc Natl Acad Sci U S A 1988; 85: 9312–16.
119. Ghaffari S, Wu H, Gerlach M et al. BCR-ABL and v-SRC tyrosine kinase oncoproteins support normal erythroid development in erythropoietin receptor-deficient progenitor cells. Proc Natl Acad Sci U S A 1999; 96: 13186–90.
120. Cortez D, Kadlec L, Pendergast AM. Structural and signaling requirements for BCR-ABL-mediated transformation and inhibition of apoptosis. Mol Cell Biol 1995; 15: 5531–41.
121. Ghaffari S, Daley GQ, Lodish HF. Growth factor independence and BCR/ABL transformation: promise and pitfalls of murine model systems and assays. Leukemia 1999; 13: 1200–6.
122. Pierce A, Owen-Lynch PJ, Spooncer E et al. p210 Bcr-Abl expression in a primitive multipotent haematopoietic cell line models the development of chronic myeloid leukaemia. Oncogene 1998; 17: 667–72.
123. Nakano T, Kodama H, Honjo T. Generation of lymphohematopoietic cells from embryonic stem cells in culture. Science 1994; 265: 1098–101.
124. Era T, Witte ON. Regulated expression of P210 Bcr-Abl during embryonic stem cell differentiation stimulates multipotential progenitor expansion and myeloid cell fate. Proc Nat Acad Sci U S A 2000; 97: 1737–42.
125. Albrecht T, Schwab R, Henkes M et al. Primary proliferating immature cells from CML patients are not resistant to induction of apoptosis by DNA damage and growth factor withdrawal. Br J Haematol 1996; 95: 501–7.
126. Johansson B, Fioretos T, Mitelman F. Cytogenetic and molecular genetic evolution of chronic myeloid leukemia. Acta Haematol 2002; 107: 76–94.
127. Drexler HG. The Leukemia-Lymphoma Cell Line FactsBook. San Diego, London: Academic Press, 2001.
128. Lozzio CB, Lozzio BB. Human chronic myelogenous leukemia cell-line with positive Philadelphia chromosome. Blood 1975; 45: 321–34.
129. Pegoraro L, Matera L, Ritz J et al. Establishment of a Ph1-positive human cell line (BV173). J Natl Cancer Inst 1983; 70: 447–51.
130. Spencer A, Yan XH, Chase A et al. BCR-ABL-positive lymphoblastoid cells display limited proliferative capacity under in vitro culture conditions. Br J Haematol 1996; 94: 654–8.
131. Deininger MWN, Goldman JM, Lydon N, Melo JV. The tyrosine kinase inhibitor CGP57148B selectively inhibits the growth of BCR-ABL-positive cells. Blood 1997; 90: 3691–8.
132. Conneally E, Eaves CJ, Humphries RK. Efficient retroviral-mediated gene transfer to human cord blood stem cells with in vivo repopulating potential. Blood 1998; 91: 3487–93.
133. Zhao RC, Jiang Y, Verfaillie CM. A model of human p210(bcr/ABL)-mediated chronic myelogenous leukemia by transduction of primary normal human CD34(+) cells with a BCR/ABL-containing retroviral vector. Blood 2001; 97: 2406–12.
134. Chalandon Y, Jiang X, Loutet S et al. Growth autonomy and lineage switching in BCR-ABL-transduced human cord blood cells depend on different functional domains of BCR-ABL. Leukemia 2004; 18: 1006–12.
135. Pear WS, Miller JP, Xu L et al. Efficient and rapid induction of a chronic myelogenous leukemia-like myeloproliferative disease in mice receiving P210 bcr/abl-transduced bone marrow. Blood 1998; 92: 3780–92.
136. Heisterkamp N, Jenster G, Kioussis D et al. Human bcr-abl gene has a lethal effect on embryogenesis. Transgenic Res 1991; 1: 45–53.
137. Heisterkamp N, Jenster G, ten Hoeve J et al. Acute leukaemia in bcr/abl transgenic mice. Nature 1990; 344: 251–3.
138. Voncken JW, Griffiths S, Greaves MF et al. Restricted oncogenicity of BCR/ABL p190 in transgenic mice. Cancer Res 1992; 52: 4534–9.
139. Voncken JW, Kaartinen V, Pattengale PK et al. BCR/ABL P210 and P190 cause distinct leukemia in transgenetic mice. Blood 1995; 86: 4603–11.
140. Honda H, Fujii T, Takatoku M et al. Expression of p210bcr/abl by metallothionein promoter induced T- cell leukemia in transgenic mice. Blood 1995; 85: 2853–61.
141. Huettner CS, Zhang P, van Etten RA, Tenen DG. Reversibility of acute B-cell leukaemia induced by BCR-ABL1. Nat Genet 2000; 24: 57–60.
142. Koschmieder S, Gottgens B, Zhang P et al. Inducible chronic phase of myeloid leukemia with expansion of hematopoietic stem cells in a transgenic model of BCR-ABL leukemogenesis. Blood 2005; 105: 324–34.
143. Sharma SV, Gajowniczek P, Way IP et al. A common signaling cascade may underlie "addiction" to the Src, BCR-ABL, and EGF receptor oncogenes. Cancer Cell 2006; 10: 425–35.

144. Nieborowska-Skorska M, Wasik MA, Slupianek A et al. Signal transducer and activator of transcription (STAT)5 activation by BCR/ABL is dependent on intact Src homology (SH)3 and SH2 domains of BCR/ABL and is required for leukemogenesis. J Exp Med 1999; 189: 1229–42.
145. Neshat MS, Raitano AB, Wang HG et al. The survival function of the Bcr-Abl oncogene is mediated by Bad-dependent and -independent pathways: roles for phosphatidylinositol 3-kinase and Raf. Mol Cell Biol 2000; 20: 1179–86.
146. Pendergast AM, Gishizky ML, Havlik MH, Witte ON. SH1 domain autophosphorylation of P210 BCR/ABL is required for transformation but not growth factor independence. Mol Cell Biol 1993; 13: 1728–36.
147. Pendergast AM, Muller AJ, Havlik MH et al. BCR sequences essential for transformation by the BCR-ABL oncogene bind to the ABL SH2 regulatory domain in a non-phosphotyrosine-dependent manner. Cell 1991; 66: 161–71.
148. Sattler M, Salgia R. Activation of hematopoietic growth factor signal transduction pathways by the human oncogene BCR/ABL. Cytokine Growth Factor Rev 1997; 8: 63–79.
149. Sawyers CL. Signal transduction pathways involved in BCR-ABL transformation. Baillieres Clin Haematol 1997; 10: 223–31.
150. Deininger MW, Goldman JM, Melo JV. The molecular biology of chronic myeloid leukemia. Blood 2000; 96: 3343–56.
151. Steelman LS, Pohnert SC, Shelton JG et al. JAK/STAT, Raf/MEK/ERK, PI3K/Akt and BCR-ABL in cell cycle progression and leukemogenesis. Leukemia 2004; 18: 189–218.
152. Stork PJ. ERK signaling: duration, duration, duration. Cell Cycle 2002; 1: 315–17.
153. Watzinger F, Gaiger A, Karlic H et al. Absence of N-ras mutations in myeloid and lymphoid blast crisis of chronic myeloid leukemia. Cancer Res 1994; 54: 3934–8.
154. Bos JL. ras oncogenes in human cancer: a review. Cancer Res 1989; 49: 4682–9.
155. Chan IT, Kutok JL, Williams IR et al. Conditional expression of oncogenic K-ras from its endogenous promoter induces a myeloproliferative disease. J Clin Invest 2004; 113: 528–38.
156. Braun BS, Tuveson DA, Kong N et al. Somatic activation of oncogenic Kras in hematopoietic cells initiates a rapidly fatal myeloproliferative disorder. Proc Natl Acad Sci U S A 2004; 101: 597–602.
157. Hirsch Ginsberg C, LeMaistre AC, Kantarjian H et al. RAS mutations are rare events in Philadelphia chromosome-negative/bcr gene rearrangement-negative chronic myelogenous leukemia, but are prevalent in chronic myelomonocytic leukemia. Blood 1990; 76: 1214–19.
158. Flotho C, Valcamonica S, Mach-Pascual S et al. RAS mutations and clonality analysis in children with juvenile myelomonocytic leukemia (JMML). Leukemia 1999; 13: 32–7.
159. Cogswell PC, Morgan R, Dunn M et al. Mutations of the ras protooncogenes in chronic myelogenous leukemia: a high frequency of ras mutations in bcr/abl rearrangement-negative chronic myelogenous leukemia. Blood 1989; 74: 2629–33.
160. Ishida D, Kometani K, Yang H et al. Myeloproliferative stem cell disorders by deregulated Rap1 activation in SPA-1-deficient mice. Cancer Cell 2003; 4: 55–65.
161. Cortez D, Reuther G, Pendergast AM. The Bcr-Abl tyrosine kinase activates mitogenic signaling pathways and stimulates G1-to-S phase transition in hematopoietic cells. Oncogene 1997; 15: 2333–42.
162. Kabarowski JH, Allen PB, Wiedemann LM. A temperature sensitive p210 BCR-ABL mutant defines the primary consequences of BCR-ABL tyrosine kinase expression in growth factor dependent cells. EMBO J 1994; 13: 5887–95.
163. Goga A, McLaughlin J, Afar DEH et al. Alternative signals to RAS for hematopoietic transformation by the BCR-ABL oncogene. Cell 1995; 82: 981–8.
164. Stork PJ, Dillon TJ. Multiple roles of Rap1 in hematopoietic cells: complementary versus antagonistic functions. Blood 2005; 106: 2952–61.
165. Jin A, Kurosu T, Tsuji K et al. BCR/ABL and IL-3 activate Rap1 to stimulate the B-Raf/MEK/Erk and Akt signaling pathways and to regulate proliferation, apoptosis, and adhesion. Oncogene 2006; 25: 4332–40.
166. Raitano AB, Halpern JR, Hambuch TM, Sawyers CL. The Bcr-Abl leukemia oncogene activates Jun kinase and requires Jun for transformation. Proc Natl Acad Sci U S A 1995; 92: 11746–50.
167. Wong S, McLaughlin J, Cheng D, Witte ON. Cell context-specific effects of the BCR-ABL oncogene monitored in hematopoietic progenitors. Blood 2003; 101: 4088–97.
168. Notari M, Neviani P, Santhanam R et al. A MAPK/HNRPK pathway controls BCR/ABL oncogenic potential by regulating MYC mRNA translation. Blood 2006; 107: 2507–16.
169. Chu S, Holtz M, Gupta M, Bhatia R. BCR/ABL kinase inhibition by imatinib mesylate enhances MAP kinase activity in chronic myelogenous leukemia CD34+ cells. Blood 2004; 103: 3167–74.
170. Bhatia R, Holtz M, Niu N et al. Persistence of malignant hematopoietic progenitors in chronic myelogenous leukemia patients in complete cytogenetic remission following imatinib mesylate treatment. Blood 2003; 101: 4701–7.
171. Yu C, Krystal G, Varticovksi L et al. Pharmacologic mitogen-activated protein/extracellular signal-regulated kinase kinase/mitogen-activated protein kinase inhibitors interact synergistically with STI571

to induce apoptosis in Bcr/Abl-expressing human leukemia cells. Cancer Res 2002; 62: 188–99.

172. La Rosee P, Jia T, Demehri S et al. Antileukemic activity of lysophosphatidic acid acyltransferase-beta inhibitor CT32228 in chronic myelogenous leukemia sensitive and resistant to imatinib. Clin Cancer Res 2006; 12: 6540–6.
173. Vivanco I, Sawyers CL. The phosphatidylinositol 3-kinase AKT pathway in human cancer. Nat Rev Cancer 2002; 2: 489–501.
174. Kharas MG, Fruman DA. ABL oncogenes and phosphoinositide 3-kinase: mechanism of activation and downstream effectors. Cancer Res 2005; 65: 2047–53.
175. Storz P, Toker A. 3′-phosphoinositide-dependent kinase-1 (PDK-1) in PI 3-kinase signaling. Front Biosci 2002; 7: d886–902.
176. Skorski T, Kanakaraj P, Nieborowska Skorska M et al. Phosphatidylinositol-3 kinase activity is regulated by BCR/ABL and is required for the growth of Philadelphia chromosome-positive cells. Blood 1995; 86: 726–36.
177. Yilmaz OH, Valdez R, Theisen BK et al. Pten dependence distinguishes haematopoietic stem cells from leukaemia-initiating cells. Nature 2006; 441: 475–82.
178. Sattler M, Verma S, Byrne CH et al. BCR/ABL directly inhibits expression of SHIP, an SH2-containing polyinositol-5-phosphatase involved in the regulation of hematopoiesis. Mol Cell Biol 1999; 19: 7473–80.
179. Helgason CD, Damen JE, Rosten P et al. Targeted disruption of SHIP leads to hemopoietic perturbations, lung pathology, and a shortened life span. Genes Dev 1998; 12: 1610–20.
180. Raffel GD, Parmar K, Rosenberg N. In vivo association of v-Abl with Shc mediated by a non-phosphotyrosine-dependent SH2 interaction. J Biol Chem 1996; 271: 4640–5.
181. Harrison-Findik D, Susa M, Varticovski L. Association of phosphatidylinositol 3-kinase with SHC in chronic myelogeneous leukemia cells. Oncogene 1995; 10: 1385–91.
182. Sattler M, Salgia R, Okuda K et al. The proto-oncogene product p120CBL and the adaptor proteins CRKL and c-CRK link c-ABL, p190BCR/ABL and p210BCR/ABL to the phosphatidylinositol-3′ kinase pathway. Oncogene 1996; 12: 839–46.
183. Hemmeryckx B, Reichert A, Watanabe M et al. BCR/ABL P190 transgenic mice develop leukemia in the absence of Crkl. Oncogene 2002; 21: 3225–31.
184. Hemmeryckx B, van Wijk A, Reichert A et al. Crkl enhances leukemogenesis in BCR/ABL P190 transgenic mice. Cancer Res 2001; 61: 1398–405.
185. Dinulescu DM, Wood LJ, Shen L et al. c-CBL is not required for leukemia induction by Bcr-Abl in mice. Oncogene 2003; 22: 8852–60.
186. Skorski T, Bellacosa A, Nieborowska-Skorska M et al. Transformation of hematopoietic cells by BCR/ABL requires activation of a PI-3k/Akt-dependent pathway. EMBO J 1997; 16: 6151–61.
187. Kops GJ, Burgering BM. Forkhead transcription factors: new insights into protein kinase B (c-akt) signaling. J Mol Med 1999; 77: 656–65.
188. Ghaffari S, Jagani Z, Kitidis C et al. Cytokines and BCR-ABL mediate suppression of TRAIL-induced apoptosis through inhibition of forkhead FOXO3a transcription factor. Proc Natl Acad Sci U S A 2003; 100: 6523–8.
189. Salomoni P, Condorelli F, Sweeney SM, Calabretta B. Versatility of BCR/ABL-expressing leukemic cells in circumventing proapoptotic BAD effects. Blood 2000; 96: 676–84.
190. Reuther JY, Reuther GW, Cortez D et al. A requirement for NF-kappaB activation in Bcr-Abl-mediated transformation. Genes Dev 1998; 12: 968–81.
191. Gelfanov VM, Burgess GS, Litz-Jackson S et al. Transformation of interleukin-3-dependent cells without participation of Stat5/bcl-xL: cooperation of akt with raf/erk leads to p65 nuclear factor kappaB-mediated antiapoptosis involving c-IAP2. Blood 2001; 98: 2508–17.
192. Mohi MG, Boulton C, Gu TL et al. Combination of rapamycin and protein tyrosine kinase (PTK) inhibitors for the treatment of leukemias caused by oncogenic PTKs. Proc Natl Acad Sci U S A 2004; 101: 3130–5.
193. Mayerhofer M, Aichberger KJ, Florian S et al. Identification of mTOR as a novel bifunctional target in chronic myeloid leukemia: dissection of growth-inhibitory and VEGF-suppressive effects of rapamycin in leukemic cells. FASEB J 2005; 19: 960–2.
194. Mayerhofer M, Valent P, Sperr WR et al. BCR/ABL induces expression of vascular endothelial growth factor and its transcriptional activator, hypoxia inducible factor-1alpha, through a pathway involving phosphoinositide 3-kinase and the mammalian target of rapamycin. Blood 2002; 100: 3767–75.
195. Burchert A, Wang Y, Cai D et al. Compensatory PI3-kinase/Akt/mTor activation regulates imatinib resistance development. Leukemia 2005; 19: 1774–82.
196. Hay N, Sonenberg N. Upstream and downstream of mTOR. Genes Dev 2004; 18: 1926–45.
197. Reddy EP, Korapati A, Chaturvedi P, Rane S. IL-3 signaling and the role of Src kinases, JAKs and STATs: a covert liaison unveiled. Oncogene 2000; 19: 2532–47.
198. Ilaria RL Jr, van Etten RA. P210 and P190(BCR/ABL) induce the tyrosine phosphorylation and DNA binding activity of multiple specific STAT family members. J Biol Chem 1996; 271: 31704–10.
199. Shuai K, Halpern J, ten Hoeve J et al. Constitutive activation of STAT5 by the BCR-ABL oncogene in

chronic myelogenous leukemia. Oncogene 1996; 13: 247–54.
200. Nieborowska-Skorska M, Wasik MA, Slupianek A et al. Signal transducer and activator of transcription (STAT)5 activation by BCR/ABL is dependent on intact Src homology (SH)3 and SH2 domains of BCR/ABL and is required for leukemogenesis. J Exp Med 1999; 189: 1229–42.
201. Samanta AK, Lin H, Sun T et al. Janus kinase 2: a critical target in chronic myelogenous leukemia. Cancer Res 2006; 66: 6468–72.
202. Klejman A, Schreiner SJ, Nieborowska-Skorska M et al. The Src family kinase Hck couples BCR/ABL to STAT5 activation in myeloid leukemia cells. EMBO J 2002; 21: 5766–74.
203. Ye D, Wolff N, Li L et al. STAT5 signaling is required for the efficient induction and maintenance of CML in mice. Blood 2006; 107: 4917–25.
204. Hoelbl A, Kovacic B, Kerenyi MA et al. Clarifying the role of Stat5 in lymphoid development and Abelson-induced transformation. Blood 2006; 107: 4898–906.
205. Scherr M, Chaturvedi A, Battmer K et al. Enhanced sensitivity to inhibition of SHP2, STAT5, and Gab2 expression in chronic myeloid leukemia (CML). Blood 2006; 107: 3279–87.
206. Gesbert F, Griffin JD. Bcr/Abl activates transcription of the Bcl-X gene through STAT5. Blood 2000; 96: 2269–76.
207. Holtschke T, Löhler J, Kanno Y et al. Immunodefiency and chronic myelogenous leukemia-like syndrome in mice with atargeted mutation of the ICSBP gene. Cell 1996; 87: 307–17.
208. Hao SX, Ren RB. Expression of interferon consensus sequence binding protein (ICSBP) is downregulated in Bcr-Abl-induced murine chronic myelogenous leukemia-like disease, and forced coexpression of ICSBP inhibits Bcr-Abl-induced myeloproliferative disorder. Mol Cell Biol 2000; 20: 1149–61.
209. Schmidt M, Nagel S, Proba J et al. Lack of interferon consensus sequence binding protein (ICSBP) transcripts in human myeloid leukemias. Blood 1998; 91: 22–9.
210. Burchert A, Cai D, Hofbauer LC et al. Interferon consensus sequence binding protein (ICSBP; IRF-8) antagonizes BCR/ABL and down-regulates bcl-2. Blood 2004; 103: 3480–9.
211. Middleton MK, Zukas AM, Rubinstein T et al. Identification of 12/15-lipoxygenase as a suppressor of myeloproliferative disease. J Exp Med 2006; 203: 2529–40.
212. van Etten RA. Oncogenic signaling: new insights and controversies from chronic myeloid leukemia. J Exp Med 2007; 204: 461–5.
213. Passegue E, Jochum W, Schorpp-Kistner M et al. Chronic myeloid leukemia with increased granulocyte progenitors in mice lacking junB expression in the myeloid lineage. Cell 2001; 104: 21–32.
214. Passegue E, Wagner EF, Weissman IL. JunB deficiency leads to a myeloproliferative disorder arising from hematopoietic stem cells. Cell 2004; 119: 431–43.
215. Yang MY, Liu TC, Chang JG et al. JunB gene expression is inactivated by methylation in chronic myeloid leukemia. Blood 2003; 101: 3205–11.
216. Radich JP, Dai H, Mao M et al. Gene expression changes associated with progression and response in chronic myeloid leukemia. Proc Natl Acad Sci U S A 2006; 103: 2794–9.
217. Hanahan D, Weinberg RA. The hallmarks of cancer. Cell 2000; 100: 57–70.
218. Pardee AB. G1 events and regulation of cell proliferation. Science 1989; 246: 603–8.
219. Jonuleit T, Peschel C, Schwab R et al. Bcr-Abl kinase promotes cell cycle entry of primary myeloid CML cells in the absence of growth factors. Br J Haematol 1998; 100: 295–303.
220. Hariharan IK, Adams JM, Cory S. bcr-abl oncogene renders myeloid cell line factor independent: potential autocrine mechanism in chronic myeloid leukemia. Oncogene Res 1988; 3: 387–99.
221. Peters DG, Klucher KM, Perlingeiro RC et al. Autocrine and paracrine effects of an ES-cell derived, BCR/ABL-transformed hematopoietic cell line that induces leukemia in mice. Oncogene 2001; 20: 2636–46.
222. Jiang X, Lopez A, Holyoake T et al. Autocrine production and action of IL-3 and granulocyte colony-stimulating factor in chronic myeloid leukemia. Proc Natl Acad Sci U S A 1999; 96: 12804–9.
223. Wong S, McLaughlin J, Cheng D et al. Sole BCR-ABL inhibition is insufficient to eliminate all myeloproliferative disorder cell populations. Proc Natl Acad Sci U S A 2004; 101: 17456–61.
224. Wong S, McLaughlin J, Cheng D et al. IL-3 receptor signaling is dispensable for BCR-ABL-induced myeloproliferative disease. Proc Natl Acad Sci U S A 2003; 100: 11630–5.
225. Li S, Gillessen S, Tomasson MH et al. Interleukin 3 and granulocyte-macrophage colony-stimulating factor are not required for induction of chronic myeloid leukemia-like myeloproliferative disease in mice by BCR/ABL. Blood 2001; 97: 1442–50.
226. Deininger MW, Vieira SA, Parada Y et al. Direct relation between BCR-ABL tyrosine kinase activity and cyclin D2 expression in lymphoblasts. Cancer Res 2001; 61: 8005–13.
227. Parada Y, Banerji L, Glassford J et al. BCR-ABL and interleukin 3 promote haematopoietic cell proliferation and survival through modulation of cyclin D2 and p27Kip1 expression. J Biol Chem 2001; 276: 23572–80.
228. Gesbert F, Sellers WR, Signoretti S et al. BCR/ABL regulates expression of the cyclin-dependent kinase inhibitor p27Kip1 through the phosphatidylinositol

3-Kinase/AKT pathway. J Biol Chem 2000; 275: 39223–30.
229. Jonuleit T, van der KH, Miething C et al. Bcr-Abl kinase down-regulates cyclin-dependent kinase inhibitor p27 in human and murine cell lines. Blood 2000; 96: 1933–9.
230. Andreu EJ, Lledo E, Poch E et al. BCR-ABL induces the expression of Skp2 through the PI3K pathway to promote p27Kip1 degradation and proliferation of chronic myelogenous leukemia cells. Cancer Res 2005; 65: 3264–72.
231. Grimmler M, Wang Y, Mund T et al. Cdk-inhibitory activity and stability of p27Kip1 are directly regulated by oncogenic tyrosine kinases. Cell 2007; 128: 269–80.
232. Hengst L, Reed SI. Translational control of p27Kip1 accumulation during the cell cycle. Science 1996; 271: 1861–4.
233. Pagano M, Tam SW, Theodoras AM et al. Role of the ubiquitin-proteasome pathway in regulating abundance of the cyclin-dependent kinase inhibitor p27. Science 1995; 269: 682–5.
234. Jiang Y, Zhao RC, Verfaillie CM. Abnormal integrin-mediated regulation of chronic myelogenous leukemia CD34+ cell proliferation: BCR/ABL up-regulates the cyclin-dependent kinase inhibitor, p27Kip, which is relocated to the cell cytoplasm and incapable of regulating cdk2 activity. Proc Natl Acad Sci U S A 2000; 97: 10538–43.
235. Dong M, Blobe GC. Role of transforming growth factor-beta in hematologic malignancies. Blood 2006; 107: 4589–96.
236. Moller GM, Frost V, Melo JV, Chantry A. Upregulation of the TGFbeta signalling pathway by Bcr-Abl: implications for haemopoietic cell growth and chronic myeloid leukaemia. FEBS Lett 2007; 581: 1329–34.
237. Hurley RW, McCarthy JB, Verfaillie CM. Direct adhesion to bone marrow stroma via fibronectin receptors inhibits hematopoietic progenitor proliferation. J Clin Invest 1995; 96: 511–19.
238. Gordon MY, Dowding CR, Riley GP et al. Altered adhesive interactions with marrow stroma of haematopoietic progenitor cells in chronic myeloid leukaemia. Nature 1987; 328: 342–4.
239. Verfaillie CM, McCarthy JB, McGlave PB. Mechanisms underlying abnormal trafficking of malignant progenitors in chronic myelogenous leukemia. Decreased adhesion to stroma and fibronectin but increased adhesion to the basement membrane components laminin and collagen type IV. J Clin Invest 1992; 90: 1232–41.
240. Lundell BI, McCarthy JB, Kovach NL, Verfaillie CM. Activation-dependent alpha5beta1 integrin-mediated adhesion to fibronectin decreases proliferation of chronic myelogenous leukemia progenitors and K562 cells. Blood 1996; 87: 2450–8.
241. Amos TA, Lewis JL, Grand FH et al. Apoptosis in chronic myeloid leukaemia: normal responses by progenitor cells to growth factor deprivation, X-irradiation and glucocorticoids. Br J Haematol 1995; 91: 387–93.
242. Bedi A, Barber JP, Bedi GC et al. BCR-ABL-mediated inhibition of apoptosis with delay of G2/M transition after DNA damage: a mechanism of resistance to multiple anticancer agents. Blood 1995; 86: 1148–58.
243. Thompson JE, Thompson CB. Putting the rap on Akt. J Clin Oncol 2004; 22: 4217–26.
244. McCubrey JA, Steelman LS, Chappell WH et al. Roles of the Raf/MEK/ERK pathway in cell growth, malignant transformation and drug resistance. Biochim Biophys Acta 2007; 1773: 1263–84.
245. Horita M, Andreu J, Benito A et al. Blockade of the Bcr-Abl Kinase activity induces apoptosis of chronic myelogenous leukemia cells by suppressing signal transducer and activator of transcription 5-dependent expression of Bcl-xL. J Exp Med 2000; 191: 977–84.
246. Wang Z, Sampath J, Fukuda S, Pelus LM. Disruption of the inhibitor of apoptosis protein survivin sensitizes Bcr-abl-positive cells to STI571-induced apoptosis. Cancer Res 2005; 65: 8224–32.
247. Aichberger KJ, Mayerhofer M, Krauth MT et al. Identification of mcl-1 as a BCR/ABL-dependent target in chronic myeloid leukemia (CML): evidence for cooperative antileukemic effects of imatinib and mcl-1 antisense oligonucleotides. Blood 2005; 105: 3303–11.
248. Kuroda J, Puthalakath H, Cragg MS et al. Bim and Bad mediate imatinib-induced killing of Bcr/Abl+ leukemic cells, and resistance due to their loss is overcome by a BH3 mimetic. Proc Natl Acad Sci U S A 2006; 103: 14907–12.
249. Aichberger KJ, Mayerhofer M, Krauth MT et al. Low-level expression of proapoptotic Bcl-2-interacting mediator in leukemic cells in patients with chronic myeloid leukemia: role of BCR/ABL, characterization of underlying signaling pathways, and reexpression by novel pharmacologic compounds. Cancer Res 2005; 65: 9436–44.
250. Goetz AW, van der KH, Maya R et al. Requirement for Mdm2 in the survival effects of Bcr-Abl and interleukin 3 in hematopoietic cells. Cancer Res 2001; 61: 7635–41.
251. Trotta R, Vignudelli T, Candini O et al. BCR/ABL activates mdm2 mRNA translation via the La antigen. Cancer Cell 2003; 3: 145–60.
252. Folkman J. Clinical applications of research on angiogenesis. N Engl J Med 1995; 333: 1757–63.
253. Ferrara N. Vascular endothelial growth factor. Eur J Cancer 1996; 32A: 2413–22.
254. Lundberg LG, Lerner R, Sundelin P et al. Bone marrow in polycythemia vera, chronic myelocytic

leukemia, and myelofibrosis has an increased vascularity. Am J Pathol 2000; 157: 15–19.
255. Aguayo A, Kantarjian H, Manshouri T et al. Angiogenesis in acute and chronic leukemias and myelodysplastic syndromes. Blood 2000; 96: 2240–5.
256. Liu P, Li J, Han ZC et al. Elevated plasma levels of vascular endothelial growth factor is associated with marked splenomegaly in chronic myeloid leukemia. Leuk Lymphoma 2005; 46: 1761–4.
257. Kvasnicka HM, Thiele J, Staib P et al. Reversal of bone marrow angiogenesis in chronic myeloid leukemia following imatinib mesylate (STI571) therapy. Blood 2004; 103: 3549–51.
258. Legros L, Bourcier C, Jacquel A et al. Imatinib mesylate (STI571) decreases the vascular endothelial growth factor plasma concentration in patients with chronic myeloid leukemia. Blood 2004; 104: 495–501.
259. Janowska-Wieczorek A, Majka M, Marquez-Curtis L et al. Bcr-abl-positive cells secrete angiogenic factors including matrix metalloproteinases and stimulate angiogenesis in vivo in Matrigel implants. Leukemia 2002; 16: 1160–6.
260. Passegue E, Jamieson CH, Ailles LE, Weissman IL. Normal and leukemic hematopoiesis: are leukemias a stem cell disorder or a reacquisition of stem cell characteristics? Proc Natl Acad Sci U S A 2003; 100: 11842–9.
261. Holyoake TL, Jiang X, Drummond MW et al. Elucidating critical mechanisms of deregulated stem cell turnover in the chronic phase of chronic myeloid leukemia. Leukemia 2002; 16: 549–58.
262. Brümmendorf TH, Holyoake TL, Rufer N et al. Prognostic implications of differences in telomere length between normal and malignant cells from patients with chronic myeloid leukemia measured by flow cytometry. Blood 2000; 95: 1883–90.
263. Clarkson B, Strife A, Wisniewski D et al. Chronic myelogenous leukemia as a paradigm of early cancer and possible curative strategies. Leukemia 2003; 17: 1211–62.
264. Huntly BJ, Shigematsu H, Deguchi K et al. MOZ-TIF2, but not BCR-ABL, confers properties of leukemic stem cells to committed murine hematopoietic progenitors. Cancer Cell 2004; 6: 587–96.
265. Huntly BJ, Gilliland DG. Cancer biology: summing up cancer stem cells. Nature 2005; 435: 1169–70.
266. Salgia R, Li JL, Ewaniuk DS et al. BCR/ABL induces multiple abnormalities of cytoskeletal function. J Clin Invest 1997; 100: 46–57.
267. Salesse S, Verfaillie CM. Mechanisms underlying abnormal trafficking and expansion of malignant progenitors in CML: BCR/ABL-induced defects in integrin function in CML. Oncogene 2002; 21: 8605–11.
268. Schwartz MA, Schaller MD, Ginsberg MH. Integrins: emerging paradigms of signal transduction. Annu Rev Cell Dev Biol 1995; 11: 549–99.
269. Sattler M, Salgia R, Shrikhande G et al. Differential signaling after beta1 integrin ligation is mediated through binding of CRKL to p120(CBL) and p110(HEF1). J Biol Chem 1997; 272: 14320–6.
270. Salgia R, Brunkhorst B, Pisick E et al. Increased tyrosine phosphorylation of focal adhesion proteins in myeloid cell lines expressing p210BCR/ABL. Oncogene 1995; 11: 1149–55.
271. Gotoh A, Miyazawa K, Ohyashiki K et al. Tyrosine phosphorylation and activation of focal adhesion kinase (p125FAK) by BCR-ABL oncoprotein. Exp Hematol 1995; 23: 1153–9.
272. Salgia R, Uemura N, Okuda K et al. CRKL links p210BCR/ABL with paxillin in chronic myelogenous leukemia cells. J Biol Chem 1995; 270: 29145–50.
273. Oda T, Heaney C, Hagopian JR et al. Crkl is the major tyrosine-phosphorylated protein in neutrophils from patients with chronic myelogenous leukemia. J Biol Chem 1994; 269: 22925–8.
274. Salgia R, Quackenbush E, Lin J et al. The BCR/ABL oncogene alters the chemotactic response to stromal-derived factor-1alpha. Blood 1999; 94: 4233–46.
275. Kronenwett R, Butterweck U, Steidl U et al. Distinct molecular phenotype of malignant CD34(+) hematopoietic stem and progenitor cells in chronic myelogenous leukemia. Oncogene 2005; 24: 5313–24.
276. Durig J, Rosenthal C, Elmaagacli A et al. Biological effects of stroma-derived factor-1 alpha on normal and CML CD34+ haemopoietic cells. Leukemia 2000; 14: 1652–60.
277. Krause DS, Lazarides K, von Andrian UH, van Etten RA. Requirement for CD44 in homing and engraftment of BCR-ABL-expressing leukemic stem cells. Nat Med 2006; 12: 1175–80.
278. Ilaria RL Jr. Pathobiology of lymphoid and myeloid blast crisis and management issues. Hematology Am Soc Hematol Educ Program 2005: 188–94.
279. Calabretta B, Perrotti D. The biology of CML blast crisis. Blood 2004; 103: 4010–22.
280. Johansson B, Mertens F, Fioretos T et al. Remarkably long survival of a patient with Ph1-positive chronic myeloid leukemia and 5′ bcr rearrangement. Leukemia 1990; 4: 448–9.
281. Jennings BA, Mills KI. c-myc locus amplification and the acquisition of trisomy 8 in the evolution of chronic myeloid leukaemia. Leuk Res 1998; 22: 899–903.
282. Fioretos T, Strombeck B, Sandberg T et al. Isochromosome 17q in blast crisis of chronic myeloid leukemia and in other hematologic malignancies is the result of clustered breakpoints in 17p11 and is not associated with coding TP53 mutations. Blood 1999; 94: 225–32.

283. Kantarjian HM, Keating MJ, Talpaz M et al. Chronic myelogenous leukemia in blast crisis: an analysis of 242 patients. Am J Med 1987; 83: 445–54.
284. Deutsch E, Dugray A, AbdulKarim B et al. BCR-ABL down-regulates the DNA repair protein DNA-PKcs. Blood 2001; 97: 2084–90.
285. Canitrot Y, Lautier D, Laurent G et al. Mutator phenotype of BCR–ABL transfected Ba/F3 cell lines and its association with enhanced expression of DNA polymerase beta. Oncogene 1999; 18: 2676–80.
286. Canitrot Y, Falinski R, Louat T et al. p210 BCR/ABL kinase regulates nucleotide excision repair (NER) and resistance to UV radiation. Blood 2003; 102: 2632–7.
287. Deutsch E, Jarrousse S, Buet D et al. Down-regulation of BRCA1 in BCR-ABL-expressing hematopoietic cells. Blood 2003; 101: 4583–8.
288. Sattler M, Verma S, Shrikhande G et al. The BCR/ABL tyrosine kinase induces production of reactive oxygen species in hematopoietic cells. J Biol Chem 2000; 275: 24273–8.
289. Feinstein E, Cimino G, Gale RP et al. p53 in chronic myelogenous leukemia in acute phase. Proc Natl Acad Sci U S A 1991; 88: 6293–7.
290. Sill H, Goldman JM, Cross NCP. Homozygous deletions of the p16 tumor-suppressor gene are associated with lymphoid transformation of chronic myeloid leukemia. Blood 1995; 85: 2013–16.
291. Pabst T, Stillner E, Neuberg D et al. Mutations of the myeloid transcription factor CEBPA are not associated with the blast crisis of chronic myeloid leukaemia. Br J Haematol 2006; 133: 400–2.
292. Deguchi K, Gilliland DG. Cooperativity between mutations in tyrosine kinases and in hematopoietic transcription factors in AML. Leukemia 2002; 16: 740–4.
293. Chang JS, Santhanam R, Trotta R et al. High levels of the BCR/ABL oncoprotein are required for the MAPK-hnRNP E2-dependent suppression of C/EBPalpha-driven myeloid differentiation. Blood 2007; 110: 994–1003.
294. Sawyers CL, Hochhaus A, Feldman E et al. Imatinib induces hematologic and cytogenetic responses in patients with chronic myelogenous leukemia in myeloid blast crisis: results of a phase II study. Blood 2002; 99: 3530–9.
295. Hochhaus A, La Rosee P. Imatinib therapy in chronic myelogenous leukemia: strategies to avoid and overcome resistance. Leukemia 2004; 18: 1321–31.
296. Sawyers CL. Chronic myeloid leukemia. N Engl J Med 1999; 340: 1330–40.
297. Druker BJ, Guilhot F, O'Brien SG et al. Five-year follow-up of patients receiving imatinib for chronic myeloid leukemia. N Engl J Med 2006; 355: 2408–17.
298. Hughes TP, Kaeda J, Branford S et al. Frequency of major molecular responses to imatinib or interferon alfa plus cytarabine in newly diagnosed chronic myeloid leukemia. N Engl J Med 2003; 349: 1423–32.
299. Jamieson CH, Weissman IL, Passegue E. Chronic versus acute myelogenous leukemia: a question of self-renewal. Cancer Cell 2004; 6: 531–3.

Risk stratification models and prognostic variables for chronic myeloid leukemia

3

Michele Baccarani, Fausto Castagnetti, Ilaria Iacobucci, Francesca Palandri, Anna Pusiol

PHILADELPHIA-POSITIVE CHRONIC MYELOID LEUKEMIA

The genetic lesion that causes Philadelphia (Ph)-positive chronic myeloid leukemia (CML) is the same in all patients and is unique, in spite of many well-founded hypotheses that more than one genetic abnormality is required for leukemic transformation of the hemopoietic stem cells.[1–4] Consistent with the uniformity of the defect, the clinical and laboratory features of CML, and the patterns of evolution towards accelerated and blast phases are rather homogeneous. In the absence of effective treatment, the annual death rate was about 10% during the first year and about 20% from the second year onwards, with a median survival of 3–4 years and with about 5%of patients alive at 10 years.[5] Nonetheless, it was recognized more than 30 years ago that some clinical and laboratory features could be associated with a significant difference in overall survival.[5] The factors that were prognostically significant in univariate analysis included age, sex, spleen size, hemoglobin level, platelet count, white blood cell (WBC) count, and differential blood count.[5] More than 20 years ago, Joseph Sokal, working at Duke University, North Carolina, collected data on 813 patients who had been treated by chemotherapy (conventional and non-conventional) in the US and Europe, and elaborated a prognostic classification that was first named 'international', but was renamed 'Sokal' after the death of its inventor.[6] This prognostic classification can separate patients into three groups, low risk, intermediate risk, and high risk, where the term 'risk' was not related to the probability of dying, which was close to 100% in all groups, but to the time to death. After the introduction of interferon alfa (IFNα), Sokal's prognostic classification was reviewed and refined by an European group of investigators, based on the course of the disease in patients treated with IFNα-based regimens.[7] Contemporarily, the European Group for Blood and Marrow Transplantation (EBMT) worked out and proposed a risk score for patients submitted to allogeneic stem cell transplantation (alloSCT).[8] Soon after, the protein tyrosine kinase inhibitor (TKI) imatinib mesylate was established as the front-line treatment of Ph-positive CML,[9–17] calling into question all prior prognostic formulations and highlighting the need to identify new and TKI-related prognostic features.[18–20] All the above prognostic classifications and scores, with the exception of the EBMT score, apply only to patients in early chronic phase (ECP). The prognosis of the patients in accelerated phase (AP) or in blast crisis (BC) is much poorer, and a shared and updated definition of AP and BC is required.[20]

DEFINITION OF ACCELERATED PHASE AND BLAST CRISIS

According to the World Health Organization (WHO)[21] AP is defined by any one of the following criteria: increasing spleen size, increasing WBC count or a platelet count $>1000 \times 10^9/l$ unresponsive to therapy, a platelet count $<100 \times 10^9/l$ unrelated to therapy,

Table 3.1 Definition of accelerated phase and blast crisis according to WHO,[21] and according to the criteria reported by the European LeukemiaNet (ELN) expert panel[20]

	Accelerated phase		*Blast crisis*	
	WHO	*ELN*	*WHO*	*ELN*
Extramedullary involvement	NA	NA	Yes	Yes
Spleen size	Increasing*	NA	NA	NA
Platelet count (× 10^9/l)	<100† or >1000*	<100†	NA	NA
WBC count	Increasing*	NA	NA	NA
Blast cells in blood or marrow (%)	10–19	15–29	≥20‡	≥30
Basophils in blood (%)	≥20	≥20	NA	NA
Cytogenetics	Clonal evolution	NA	NA	NA

*Unresponsive to therapy; †unrelated to therapy; ‡or large focus or clusters of blast cells in the bone marrow biopsy.
NA, not applicable.

blast cells in blood or marrow 10–19%, basophils in blood >20%, or clonal evolution (additional chromosome abnormalities in the Ph-positive clone). Currently, these recommendations are not universally used, and several recent reports on the treatment of CML have used different criteria,[20] that have been reviewed and adopted provisionally by an expert panel appointed by European LeukemiaNet,[18] namely a platelet count <100 × 10^9/l unrelated to therapy, a blood or marrow blast cell percentage between 15 and 29, or a blood basophil percentage ≥20 (Table 3.1). Table 3.1 also lists the criteria for the definition of BC, focusing on extramedullary leukemic involvement (such as lymph nodes, skin, bone, central nervous system (CNS), etc.) and on the blast cell percentage in marrow or blood, with an upper limit of 20% for WHO and of 30% for several recent reports.[18,20] Clearly, a shared definition of AP and BC is required. This was not critical until a few years ago, when treatment was ineffective and the prognosis was universally very poor; however, it may be critical today and may become even more critical tomorrow, following the introduction of imatinib mesylate, of second generation TKI, and other targeted agents, which may influence significantly response and survival. The next round of definitions will probably include more use of cytogenetics, as well as new molecular data, with focus on point mutations in the BCR-ABL kinase domain and on gene profile.

INTERNATIONAL (SOKAL) AND EUROPEAN (HASFORD) SCORES

The International, or Sokal score was developed in 1983, based on 813 patients who were treated with conventional chemotherapy at six American and European centers.[6] By multivariable analysis, four prognostic variables were identified at diagnosis, namely age, spleen size, platelet count, and the percentage of blast cells in blood. These four variables were incorporated as continuous variables in a formula that allowed calculation of the relative risk (RR) of each patient (Table 3.2). It was proposed to divide the patients according to the value of the RR into a low-risk group (39% of patients, median survival 5 years), an intermediate-risk group (38% of patients, median survival 3.7 years), and a high-risk group (23% of patients, median survival 2.5 years). Such was the survival of Ph-positive CML patients treated with chemotherapy. The International or Sokal score was confirmed in several subsequent studies of patients treated with chemotherapy or with IFNα-based regimens.[22–25] Later, it was shown to predict

Table 3.2 Calculation of the relative risk according to Sokal[6] and Hasford.[7] All data must be collected prior to any treatment

	International/Sokal score	*European/Hasford score*
Age (years)	0.116 (age – 43.4)	0.666 when age >50 years
Spleen size (cm)*	0.0345 × (spleen – 7.51)	0.042 × spleen
Platelet count (× 10^9/l)	0.188 × [(platelet/700)^2 – 0.563]	1.0956 when platelet count ≥1500
Blood blast cells (%)	0.0887 × (blast cells – 2.10)	0.0584 × blast cells
Blood basophils (%)	NA	0.20399 when basophils >3%
Blood eosinophils (%)	NA	0.0413 × eosinophils
Relative risk	(Exponential of the total)	(Total × 1000)
Low	<0.8	≤780
Intermediate	0.8–1.2	781–1480
High	>1.2	>1480

*Maximum distance from costal margin.

response and survival also in imatinib mesylate-treated patients.[14,17,25,26]

The European, or Hasford, score was developed in 1997 based on 1573 patients who were treated with IFNα-based regimens at 12 European institutions.[7] By multivariable analysis, six prognostic variables were identified, including the four prognostic variables of Sokal score (age, spleen size, platelet count, and the percentage of blast cells in blood), and the percentage of basophils and eosinophils in blood. All six variables were included in a formula that allowed calculation of the RR of each patient (Table 3.2). It was proposed to divide the patients according to the value of RR into a low-risk group (41% of patients, median survival 8.2 years), an intermediate-risk group (44% of patients, median survival 5.4 years), and a high-risk group (14% of patients, median survival 3.5 years). These figures clearly reflect advances in treatment, owing to the introduction of IFNα. The European or Hasford score was confirmed in several subsequent studies of patients treated with IFNα-based regimens,[27–30] and was reported to predict cytogenetic response in imatinib mesylate-treated patients.[26]

It must be pointed out that all the variables necessary to calculate these scores must be collected at diagnosis and before any treatment. A short course of hydroxyurea would modify spleen size, platelet count, and blood differential, and would make it impossible to calculate the risk. Neither of the two formulae can be applied to patients in late chronic phase (LCP), and neither was ever shown to predict survival in patients who received alloSCT.

EUROPEAN GROUP FOR BLOOD AND MARROW TRANSPLANTATION RISK SCORE

The EBMT risk score (also known as Gratwohl score) was developed in 1997 by the EBMT group, based on 3142 patients submitted to alloSCT in any phase of CML and from any donor.[8] Five independent prognostic variables were identified, including age, the interval from diagnosis to SCT, the phase of the disease, the donor–recipient sex match, and the donor type (Table 3.3). It was proposed to divide the patients into five risk groups, according to the overall risk score (Table 3.3). The EBMT risk score was validated by the Center for International Blood and Marrow Transplant Research (CIBMTR) in an independent series of patients[31] (Table 3.3). Overall, 5-year survival of low-risk and high-risk patients ranged between 69 and 72%, and between

Table 3.3 European Group for Blood and Marrow Transplantation (EBMT) risk score (Gratwohl score).[8] The risk is assigned based on five independent prognostic variables, and the patients are divided into five different risk groups. The table shows 5-year overall survival of the original 3142 patients analyzed by the EBMT group[8] and of the 3211 patients subsequently analyzed by the Center for International Blood and Marrow Transplant Research (CIBMTR)[31]

		5-Year overall survival		
Risk factors	*Risk score*	*Total risk score*	*EBMT series*	*CIBMTR series*
Age				
<20 years	0			
20–40 years	1	0–1	72%	69%
>40 years	2			
Interval from diagnosis to SCT				
≤1 year	0	2	62%	63%
>1 year	1			
Disease phase				
Chronic	0	3	48%	44%
Accelerated	1			
Blastic	2			
Donor–recipient sex match		4	40%	26%
Female donor, male recipient	1			
Any other match	0			
Donor type		5–7	22%	11%
HLA-identical sibling	0			
Any other	1			

SCT, stem cell transplantation.

11 and 21%, respectively (Table 3.3). The EBMT risk score was also applied to a series of 187 patients who were submitted to reduced intensity conditioning alloSCT.[32] In that series, 3-year overall survival was 70% for the patients with an EBMT score of 0–2, 50% for the patients with a score of 3–4, and about 30% for those with a score of 5 or higher.

PROGNOSIS OF IMATINIB MESYLATE-TREATED PATIENTS

Baseline prognostic factors

Since the molecular basis of the therapeutic effects of imatinib mesylate differs from that of conventional cytotoxic agents, IFNα and alloSCT, it is expected that in patients treated with imatinib mesylate the response to treatment and the effect of treatment on survival may be related to other factors, different from the prognostic variables which have been identified so far. However, with imatinib mesylate as with any other treatment, the major prognostic variables are the phase of the disease and the time lapsed from diagnosis to treatment. ECP patients respond much better to imatinib mesylate than LCP patients, who respond much better than AP patients, who in turn respond much better than BC patients (Table 3.4). The reasons for such a strong prognostic value of phase and time have not been fully elucidated but can be easily understood, based on the knowledge that the natural progression of CML, from CP to BC, is a function of time. While it may be difficult to

Table 3.4 Summary of the results of imatinib mesylate treatment in early and late chronic phase (400 mg daily), and in accelerated phase and in blast crisis (600–800 mg daily)[10–17]

	Complete hematological response	*Complete cytogenetic reponse*	*Major molecular response*
Early chronic phase, first-line	>95%	75–90%	50–60%
Late chronic phase, second-line (IFNα resistant or intolerant)	>90%	45–60%	30–40%
Accelerated phase	30–40%	10–20%	<10%
Blast crisis	10–15%	5–10%	NA

NA, not available.

Table 3.5 Complete cytogenetic response rate according to Sokal's risk score[6] in three independent studies of previously untreated early chronic phase patients[14,17,33,34]

	Sokal risk group		
	Low	*Intermediate*	*High*
IRIS study, 400 mg daily			
12 months[14]	76%	67%	49%
60 months[17]	89%	82%	69%
ICSG on CML, 400 mg daily[34]*			
3 months	35%	33%	11%
6 months	73%	75%	17%
12 months	79%	87%	28%
60 months	88%	96%	72%
MD Anderson Hospital, 400–800 mg daily[33]			
12–24 months	96%	94%	86%

All the differences are significant ($p < 0.01$). *The data from reference 34 have been updated.

detect the biological and molecular marker of progression during CP, they become more and more detectable in AP, and overt in BC.

In ECP patients treated with imatinib mesylate first-line, only one variable has been consistently found to affect the response, with a potential of influencing the long-term outcomes, such as progression-free survival (PFS) and overall survival (OS). Rather surprisingly, in the era of molecular hematology and targeted treatment, the variable is the relative risk according to Sokal.[17,26,33,34] The complete cytogenetic response rate according to Sokal is reported in Table 3.5, showing that in high-risk patients the response rate is lower and slower. Since PFS is strongly related with cytogenetic response, high-risk patients differ also in PFS.[35] Increasing the imatinib mesylate dose to 800 mg daily can increase the response rate in all risk groups, but the difference remains significant.[36]

Two other baseline variables were proposed to have a prognostic value, namely BCR-ABL amplification and the deletions of the long arm of chromosome 9 (del 9q+).[18] If a leukemic cell has more than one copy of the *BCR-ABL* gene, it is expected that the cell will have more BCR-ABL transcripts, hence more BCR-ABL protein molecules, and will be more resistant to TKI. This expectation is well founded, but to date there have been no reports proving or disproving this expectation. Del 9q+ was found to have a negative prognostic value before the introduction of imatinib mesylate,[37–39] while the data in imatinib mesylate-treated patients were controversial.[40,41] A prospective study of the Italian CML Working Party in more than 400 Ph-positive ECP CML patients treated first-line with imatinib mesylate 400 mg daily showed that the complete cytogenetic response rate and the major molecular response rate after 6 and 12 months of therapy are the same in the patients with and without del 9q+.[42] Therefore, del 9q+ should no longer be considered as a warning feature in the treatment of CML with imatinib mesylate, although is it possible that a more subtle relationship with prognosis could depend on the size of the deletion, and that small subgroups of patients may respond less well.[37–39] The expression and functional activity of a transmembrane protein belonging to the organic cation transporter family (OCT1), have been reported to influence the outcome of imatinib mesylate treatment, because OCT1, by transporting imatinib mesylate into the cells, affects the intracellular concentration of the drug. Experimental data and clinical observations show that low expression of OCT1 is associated with a lower sensitivity to imatinib mesylate of Ph-positive cells and with a lower response rate.[43–45] The biological and clinical role of the transporters of the family of the ATP binding cassette, such as P-glycoprotein, MDR1 and 2, MRP, BCP, and other molecules with the capacity of exporting imatinib mesylate outside the cells and reducing the imatinib mesylate intracellular concentration, has also been investigated, with contrasting results, but it is expected that the expression and activity of these transporters could contribute to a decreased sensitivity of Ph-positive cells, and particularly of Ph-positive stem cells, to TKI.[43–54]

The sensitivity of Ph-positive cells to imatinib mesylate and other TKI can be assessed by measuring the effects downstream of BCR-ABL, namely the phosphotyrosine content of the cells and the phosphorylation status of Crkl, which is one of the first messengers downstream of BCR-ABL.[55,56] Moreover, BCR-ABL inhibition is accompanied by inhibition of other gene transcripts, including the WT1 (Wilms tumor) gene, so that measuring *in vitro* and also *in vivo* the WT1 transcript level can help to assess the sensitivity to imatinib mesylate and to predict treatment outcome.[57]

The molecular basis of the sensitivity to TKI has not yet been fully elucidated, apart from BCR-ABL kinase domain point mutations,[58–64] but some studies have begun to focus on gene expression profiling as an important area of investigation; it has already been reported that the profile of gene expression is different in different phases, and is different in cases of sensitivity or resistance to TKI.[65–70] This area is still investigational, but is very promising, not only to refine prognosis, but also, more important, to understand the causes of resistance and to provide biological guidelines to overcome resistance with other targeted agents.

RESPONSE-RELATED PROGNOSTIC FACTORS

Response to treatment is a potent prognostic factor. The response can be defined at three levels, hematological, cytogenetic, and molecular (Table 3.6). All the studies have shown that achieving a hematological response predicts for cytogenetic response, and that achieving a cytogenetic response predicts for molecular response. All the studies have shown that a complete hematological response, a complete cytogenetic response, and a major molecular response predict for a better event-free, progression-free, and overall survival. Many studies have shown that the earlier the response the better the subsequent responses, as well as progression-free, or event-free survival.[73–78] However, while the time to achieve a complete hematological response is short in almost all cases, the time to achieve a complete cytogenetic response and a major molecular response is much more variable, and may range between 3 and 24 months. Moreover, the progression-free survival of late responders is likely to be as good as that of early responders.[79] Therefore, it is critical to

Table 3.6 Working definitions of the three response levels, hematological, cytogenetic, and molecular. Cytogenetic response is assessed by conventional morphological techniques on at least 20 marrow cell metaphases. Molecular response is assessed on blood cells (buffy coat cells) and is expressed according to the international scale, where a ratio of 0.10% equals a 3-log reduction from an international standard.[71,72] The housekeeping gene is usually ABL, but others can be used such as G6PD, GUS, β-2M or BCR. A complete hematological response, a complete cytogenetic response, and a major or a complete molecular response, must be confirmed in two subsequent tests

Hematological response	
Complete	
WBC count $<10 \times 10^9/l$	
no immature granulocytes	
basophils <5%	
platelet count $<450 \times 10^9/l$	
spleen non-palpable	
Cytogenetic response	
Complete	Ph-positive 0
Partial	Ph-positive 1–35%
Minor	Ph-positive 36–65%
Minimal	Ph-positive 66–95%
None	Ph-positive >95%
Molecular response	
Major	BCR-ABL : ABL <0.10%
Complete	BCR-ABL undetectable by RTQ-PCR and nested RT-PCR

RTQ-PCR, real-time quantitative polymerase chain reaction; RT-PCR, reverse transcriptase polymerase chain reaction.

assign a prognostic value to the response as a function of time. This issue was analyzed and discussed by a panel of experts appointed by European LeukemiaNet;[18] they proposed identifying three levels of response, namely optimal, suboptimal, and failure (Table 3.7). The basis for this proposal was that the goal of imatinib mesylate treatment should be the achievement of a complete hematological response in 6 months, a complete cytogenetic response in 12 months, and a major molecular response in 18 months, in all patients. Any inferior results would be defined as suboptimal or failure, depending on time. A patient who 'fails' to respond may still have a long-term benefit from continuing imatinib mesylate at a standard dose, but it is believed that the outcome would not be as good as expected, and it is recommended that such a patient should be moved to other available treatments, whenever they are available. A patient who has a 'suboptimal' response is likely to have a yet undefined long-term benefit from continuing imatinib mesylate, but is eligible for investigational treatments and studies. While the evolution of the response as a function of time may require some degree of flexibility, the loss of any response, from complete or major to less than complete or major, should always raise the suspicion that treatment may be failing, and that alternative treatment is required. These considerations highlight the importance of diligent and regular monitoring, hematological, cytogenetic and molecular.[18,19,80] Cytogenetic monitoring requires marrow cells, but once a complete cytogenetic response has been achieved and confirmed, fluorescence *in situ* hybridization (FISH) on blood cells may be sufficient, and marrow cells can be required only in selected cases.[18,81] Molecular monitoring of BCR-ABL transcript levels by reverse transcriptase, real-time, quantitative polymerase chain reaction (RTQ-PCR) is also mandatory; it is performed on blood cells (buffy coat cells). It is not expensive but requires careful harmonization of current methodologies and reagents, and a unique international scale for the expression of the results.[71,72] Overall, the cost of monitoring is not negligible, but is always much lower than the cost of treatment, and treatment with TKI must be optimized, both in the interest of the patients, and to be cost effective.[82] Monitoring should also include pharmacokinetic data, namely the determination of trough imatinib mesylate plasma levels, because they correlate with cytogenetic and molecular response,[83,84] and confirm that the patient is complying with treatment recommendations.

The confirmation of the prognostic value of the responses as well as the identification of new response-related variables, is important

Table 3.7 Definition of the response to imatinib mesylate (modified from reference 18). The detection of BCR-ABL kinase domain point mutations defines suboptimal response or failure, but mutations are almost always associated with response loss or with primary resistance. The detection of additional chromosome abnormalities in the Ph-positive clone or of other chromosome abnormalities in Ph-negative cells suggests that the response is at least suboptimal

Time on imatinib mesylate treatment	*Optimal response*	*Suboptimal response*	*Failure*
3 months	CHR	Less than CHR	No HR (stable disease or disease progression)
6 months	PCgR	Less than PCgR	No CgR
12 months	CCgR	PCgR	Less than PCgR
18 months	MMolR	Less than MMolR	Less than CCgR
Any time	Stable CCgR and MMolR	Loss of MMolR	Loss of CHR, loss of CCgR

CHR, complete hematological response; PCgR, partial cytogenetic response (Ph-positive 1–35%); CCgR, complete cytogenetic response; MMolR, major molecular response (BCR-ABL : ABL ratio <0.1% by the International Scale).

not only for improving treatment outcome, but also to provide early surrogate markers of response and survival, which may help to speed clinical studies of new agents or new treatment modalities. However, it should not be overlooked that the prognostic value of the baseline variables and of the responses that have been discussed and identified for imatinib mesylate may not apply in cases of other TKI, other targeted agents, and other treatment modalities.

ACKNOWLEDGMENTS

This work was supported by the Italian Association against Leukemia, Lymphoma and Myeloma, Bologna Section (BolognAIL), and by European LeukemiaNet.

REFERENCES

1. Deininger MWN, Goldman JM, Melo JV. The molecular biology of chronic myeloid leukemia. Blood 2000; 96: 3343–56.
2. Holyoake TL. Recent advances in the molecular and cellular biology of chronic myeloid leukaemia: lessons to be learned from the laboratory. Br J Haematol 2001; 113: 11–23.
3. Goldman J, Mahon F, Reiffers J. Imatinib for chronic myeloid leukemia. Semin Hematol 2003; 40(Suppl 2): 1–113.
4. Hehlmann R, Berger U, Hochhaus A. Chronic myeloid leukemia: a model for oncology. Ann Hematol 2005; 84: 487–97.
5. Sokal JE, Baccarani M, Russo D et al. Staging and prognosis in chronic myelogenous leukemia. Semin Hematol 1988; 25: 49–61.
6. Sokal JE, Cox EB, Baccarani M et al. Prognostic discrimination in "good-risk" chronic granulocytic leukemia. Blood 1984; 63: 789–99.
7. Hasford J, Pfirrmann M, Hehlmann R et al. A new prognostic score for survival of patients with chronic myeloid leukemia treated with interferon alfa. J Natl Cancer Inst 1998; 90: 850–8.
8. Gratwohl A, Hermans J, Goldman JM et al. Risk assessment for patients with chronic myeloid leukaemia before allogeneic blood or marrow transplantation. Chronic Leukemia Working Party of the European Group for Blood and Marrow Transplantation. Lancet 1998; 352: 1087–92.
9. Druker BJ, Talpaz M, Resta DJ et al. Efficacy and safety of a specific inhibitor of the BCR-ABL tyrosine kinase in chronic myeloid leukemia. N Engl J Med 2001; 344: 1031–7.
10. Kantarjian H, Sawyers C, Hochhaus A et al. Hematologic and cytogenetic responses to imatinib mesylate in chronic myelogenous leukemia. N Engl J Med 2002; 346: 645–52.
11. Talpaz M, Silver RT, Druker BJ et al. Imatinib induces durable hematologic and cytogenetic responses in patients with accelerated phase chronic myeloid leukemia: results of a phase 2 study. Blood 2002; 99: 1928–37.
12. Sawyers CL, Hochhaus A, Feldman E et al. Imatinib induces hematologic and cytogenetic responses in patients with chronic myelogenous leukemia in myeloid blast crisis: results of a phase II study. Blood 2002; 99: 3530–9.

13. O'Brien SG, Guilhot F, Larson RA et al. Imatinib compared with interferon and low-dose cytarabine for newly diagnosed chronic-phase chronic myeloid leukemia. N Engl J Med 2003; 348: 994–1004.
14. Hughes TP, Kaeda J, Branford S et al. Frequency of major molecular responses to imatinib or interferon alfa plus cytarabine in newly diagnosed chronic myeloid leukemia. N Engl J Med 2003; 349: 1421–32.
15. Silver RT, Talpaz M, Sawyers CL et al. Four years of follow-up of 1027 patients with late chronic phase, accelerated phase, or blast crisis chronic myeloid leukemia treated with Imatinib in three large phase II trials. Blood 2004; 104: 11a, abstract 23.
16. Deininger M, Buchdunger E, Druker BJ. The development of imatinib as a therapeutic agent for chronic myeloid leukemia. Blood 2005; 105: 2640–53.
17. Druker BJ, Guilhot F, O'Brien SG et al. Five-years follow-up of patients receiving imatinib for chronic myeloid leukemia. N Engl J Med 2006; 355: 2408–17.
18. Baccarani M, Saglio G, Goldman J et al. Evolving concepts in the management of chronic myeloid leukemia: recommendations from an expert panel of behalf of the European LeukemiaNet. Blood 2006; 108: 1809–20.
19. Hehlmann R, Hochhaus A, Baccarani M. Chronic myeloid leukemia. Lancet Oncol 2007; 369: 1–9.
20. Cortes JE, Talpaz M, O'Brien S et al. Staging of chronic myeloid leukemia in the imatinib era. Cancer 2006; 106: 1306–15.
21. Jaffe ES, Harris NL, Stein H et al. World Health Organization Classification of Tumours. Pathology and Genetics of Tumours of Hematopoietic and Lymphoid Tissues. Lyon, France: IARC Press, 2001.
22. Guilhot F, Chastang C, Michallet M et al. Interferon alfa-2b combined with cytarabine versus interferon alone in chronic myelogenous leukemia. French Chronic Myeloid Leukemia Study Group. N Engl J Med 1997; 337: 223–9.
23. Bonifazi F, de Vivo A, Rosti G et al. Chronic myeloid leukemia and interferon-alpha: a study of complete cytogenetic responders. Blood 2001; 98: 3074–81.
24. Baccarani M, Rosti G, de Vivo A et al. A randomized study of interferon-alpha versus interferon-alpha and low-dose arabinosyl cytosine in chronic myeloid leukemia. Blood 2002; 99: 1527–35.
25. Baccarani M, Russo D, Rosti G et al. Interferon-alfa for chronic myeloid leukemia. Semin Hematol 2003; 40: 22–33.
26. Rosti G, Trabacchi E, Bassi S et al. Risk and early cytogenetic response to imatinib and interferon in chronic myeloid leukemia. Haematologica 2003; 88: 256–9.
27. Guilhot F, on behalf of the IRIS study group. Sustained durability of responses plus high rates of cytogenetic responses result in long term benefit for newly diagnosed chronic phase chronic myeloid leukemia treated with Imatinib therapy: update from the IRIS study. Blood 2004; 104: 10a, abstract 21.
28. Hehlmann R, Ansari H, Hasford J et al. Comparative analysis of the impact of risk profile and of drug therapy on survival in CML using Sokal's index and a new score. Br J Haematol 1997; 97: 76–85.
29. Bonifazi F, de Vivo A, Rosti G et al. Testing Sokal's and the new prognostic score for chronic myeloid leukaemia treated with α-interferon. Br J Haematol 2000; 111: 587–95.
30. Hasford J, Pfirrmann M, Hehlmann R et al. Prognosis and prognostic factors for patients with chronic myeloid leukemia: nontransplant therapy. Semin Hematol 2003; 40: 4–12.
31. Passweg JR, Walker I, Sobocinski KA et al. Validation and extension of the EBMT Risk Score for patients with chronic myeloid leukaemia receiving allogeneic haematopoietic stem cell transplants. Br J Haematol 2004; 125: 613–20.
32. Crawley C, Szydlo R, Lalancette M et al. Outcomes of reduced-intensity transplantation for chronic myeloid leukemia: an analysis of prognostic factors from the Chronic Leukemia Working Party of the EBMT. Blood 2005; 106: 2969–76.
33. Kantarjian HM, O'Brien S, Cortes J et al. Imatinib mesylate therapy improves survival in patients with newly diagnosed Philadelphia chromosome-positive chronic myelogenous leukemia in the chronic phase. Cancer 2003; 98: 2636–42.
34. Baccarani M, Martinelli G, Rosti G et al. Imatinib and pegylated human recombinant interferon-alpha2b in early chronic-phase chronic myeloid leukemia. Blood 2004; 104: 4245–51.
35. Simonsson B, on behalf of the IRIS study group. Beneficial effects of cytogenetic and molecular response on long term outcome in patients with newly diagnosed chronic myeloid leukemia in chronic phase (CML-CP) treated with Imatinib (IM): update from the IRIS study. Blood 2005; 106: 52a, abstract 166.
36. Kantarjian H, Talpaz M, O'Brien S et al. High-dose imatinib mesylate therapy in newly diagnosed Philadelphia chromosome-positive chronic phase chronic myeloid leukemia. Blood 2004; 103: 2873–8.
37. Guilbert ND, Morel F, Quemener S et al. Deletion size characterization of der(9) deletions in Philadelphia-positive chronic myeloid leukemia. Cancer Genet Cytogenet 2006; 170: 89–92.
38. Lee YK, Kim YR, Min HC et al. Deletion of any part of the BCR or ABL gene on the derivative chromosome 9 in a poor prognostic marker in chronic myelogenous leukemia. Cancer Genet Cytogenet 2006; 166: 65–73.

39. Kreil S, Pfirrmann M, Haferlach C et al. Heterogeneous prognostic impact of derivative chromosome 9 deletions in chronic myelogenous leukemia. Blood 2007; 110: 1283–90.
40. Huntly BJ, Guilhot F, Reid AG et al. Imatinib improves but may not fully reverse the poor prognosis of patients with CML with derivative chromosome 9 deletions. Blood 2003; 102: 2205–12.
41. Quintas-Cardama A, Kantarjian H, Talpaz M et al. Imatinib mesylate therapy may overcome the poor prognostic significance of deletions of derivative chromosome 9 in patients with chronic myelogenous leukemia. Blood 2005; 105: 2281–6.
42. Castagnetti F, Marzocchi G, Luatti S et al. Deletions of the derivative chromosome 9 do not influence response to imatinib of early chronic phase chronic myeloid leukemia patients. Blood 2006; 108: 599a, abstract 2112.
43. Thomas J, Wang L, Clark RE et al. Active transport of imatinib into and out of cells: implications for drug resistance. Blood 2004; 104: 3739–45.
44. Crossman LC, Druker BJ, Deininger MW. hOCT 1 and resistance to imatinib. Blood 2005; 106: 1133–4.
45. White DL, Saunders VA, Dang P et al. OCT-1-mediated influx is a key determinant of the intracellular uptake of imatinib but not nilotinib (AMN107): reduced OCT-1 activity is the cause of low in vitro sensitivity to imatinib. Blood 2006; 108: 697–704.
46. Mahon FX, Deininger MW, Schultheis B et al. Selection and characterization of BCR-ABL positive cell lines with differential sensitivity to the tyrosine kinase inhibitor STI571: diverse mechanisms of resistance. Blood 2000; 96: 1070–9.
47. Mahon FX, Belloc F, Lagarde V et al. MDR1 gene overexpression confers resistance to imatinib mesylate in leukemia cell line models. Blood 2003; 101: 2368–73.
48. Ferrao PT, Frost MJ, Siah SP et al. Overexpression of P-glycoprotein in K562 cells does not confer resistance to the growth inhibitory effects of imatinib (STI571) in vitro. Blood 2003; 102: 4499–4503.
49. Burger H, van Tol H, Boersma AWM et al. Imatinib mesylate (STI571) is a substrate for the breast cancer resistance protein (BCRP)/ABCG2 drug pump. Blood 2004; 104: 2940–2.
50. Illmer T, Schaich M, Platzbecker U et al. P-glycoprotein-mediated drug efflux is a resistance mechanism of chronic myelogenous leukemia cells to treatment with imatinib mesylate. Leukemia 2004; 18: 401–8.
51. Zong Y, Zhou S, Sorrentino BP. Loss of P-glycoprotein expression in hematopoietic stem cells does not improve responses to imatinib in a murine model of chronic myelogenous leukemia. Leukemia 2005; 19: 1590–6.
52. Rumpold H, Wolf AM, Gruenewald K et al. RNAi-mediated knockdown of P-glycoprotein using a transposon-based vector system durably restores imatinib sensitivity in imatinib-resistant CML cell lines. Exp Hematol 2005; 33: 767–75.
53. Nakanishi T, Shiozawa K, Hassel BA et al. Complex interaction of BCRP/ABCG2 and imatinib in BCR-ABL-expression cells: BCRP-mediated resistance to imatinib is attenuated by imatinib-induced reduction of BCRP expression. Blood 2006; 108: 678–84.
54. Jordanides NE, Jorgensen HG, Holyoake TL et al. Functional ABCG2 is overexpression on primary CML CD34+ cells and is inhibited by imatinib mesylate. Blood 2006; 108: 1370–3.
55. Schultheis B, Szydlo R, Mahon FX et al. Analysis of total phosphotyrosine levels in CD34+ cells from CML patients to predict the response to imatinib mesylate treatment. Blood 2005; 105: 4893–4.
56. White D, Saunders V, Lyons AB et al. In vitro sensitivity to imatinib-induced inhibition of ABL kinase activity is predictive of molecular response in patients with de novo CML. Blood 2005; 106: 2520–6.
57. Cilloni D, Messa F, Gottardi E et al. Sensitivity to imatinib therapy may be predicted by testing Wilms tumor gene expression and colony growth after a short in vitro incubation. Cancer 2004; 101: 979–88.
58. Branford S, Rudzki Z, Walsh S et al. High frequency of point mutations clustered within the adenosine triphosphate-binding region of BCR/ABL in patients with chronic myeloid leukemia or Ph-positive acute lymphoblastic leukemia who develop imatinib (STI571) resistance. Blood 2002; 99: 3472–5.
59. Branford S, Rudzki Z, Walsh S et al. Detection of BCR-ABL mutations in patients with CML treated with imatinib is virtually always accompanied by clinical resistance, and mutations in the ATP phosphate-binding loop (P-loop) are associated with a poor prognosis. Blood 2003; 102: 276–83.
60. Branford S, Rudzki Z, Parkinson I et al. Real-time quantitative PCR analysis can be used as a primary screen to identify patients with CML treated with imatinib who have BCR-ABL kinase domain mutations. Blood 2004; 104: 2926–32.
61. Soverini S, Martinelli G, Rosti G et al. ABL mutations in late chronic phase chronic myeloid leukemia patients with up-front cytogenetic resistance to imatinib are associated with a greater likelihood of progression to blast crisis and shorter survival: a study by the GIMEMA Working Party on Chronic Myeloid Leukemia. J Clin Oncol 2005; 23: 4100–9.
62. Kantarjian HM, Talpaz M, Giles F et al. New insights into the pathophysiology of chronic myeloid leukemia and imatinib resistance. Ann Intern Med 2006; 145: 913–23.

63. Khorashad JS, Anand M, Marin D et al. The presence of a BCR-ABL mutant allele in CML does not always explain clinical resistance to imatinib. Leukemia 2006; 20: 658–63.
64. Jabbour E, Kantarjian H, Jones D et al. Frequency and clinical significance of BCR-ABL mutations in patients with chronic myeloid leukemia treated with imatinib mesylate. Leukemia 2006; 20: 1767–73.
65. Tipping AJ, Deininger MW, Goldman JM et al. Comparative gene expression profile of chronic myeloid leukemia cells innately resistant to imatinib mesylate. Exp Hematol 2003; 31: 1073–80.
66. McLean LA, Gathmann I, Capdeville R et al. Pharmacogenomic analysis of cytogenetic response in chronic myeloid leukemia patients treated with imatinib. Clin Cancer Res 2004; 10: 155–65.
67. Oehler V, Branford S, Pogosova-Agadjanyan E et al. Gene expression signatures associated with treatment and resistance to Imatinib mesylate in chronic myeloid leukemia patients. Blood 2005; 106: 131a, abstract 433.
68. Yong AS, Szydlo RM, Goldman JM et al. Molecular profiling of CD34+ cells identifies low expression of CD7, along with high expression of proteinase 3 or elastase, as predictors of longer survival in patients with CML. Blood 2006; 107: 205–12.
69. Villuendas R, Steegmann JL, Pollàn M et al. Identification of genes involved in imatinib resistance in CML: a gene-expression profiling approach. Leukemia 2006; 20: 1047–54.
70. Frank O, Brors B, Li L et al. Gene expression signature of primary imatinib-resistant chronic myeloid leukemia patients. Leukemia 2006; 20: 1400–7.
71. Hughes T, Deininger M, Hochhaus A et al. Monitoring CML patients responding to treatment with tyrosine kinase inhibitors: review and recommendations for harmonizing current methodology for detecting BCR-ABL transcript and kinase domain mutations and for expressing results. Blood 2006; 108: 28–37.
72. Branford S, Cross NCP, Hochhaus A et al. Rationale for the recommendations for harmonizing current methodology for detecting BCR-ABL transcripts in patients with chronic myeloid leukemia. Leukemia 2006; 20: 1925–30.
73. Merx K, Müller MC, Kreil S et al. Early reduction of BCR-ABL mRNA transcript levels predicts cytogenetic response in chronic phase CML patients treated with imatinib after failure of interferon alpha. Leukemia 2002; 16: 1579–83.
74. Wang L, Pearson K, Ferguson JE et al. The early molecular response to imatinib predicts cytogenetic and clinical outcome in chronic myeloid leukaemia. Br J Haematol 2003; 120: 990–9.
75. Cortes J, Talpaz M, O'Brien S et al. Molecular responses in patients with chronic myelogenous leukemia in chronic phase treated with imatinib mesylate. Clin Cancer Res 2005; 11: 3425–32.
76. Press RD, Love Z, Tronnes AA et al. BCR-ABL mRNA levels at and after the time of a complete cytogenetic response (CCR) predict the duration of CCR in imatinib mesylate-treated patients with CML. Blood 2006; 107: 4250–6.
77. Iacobucci I, Sagio G, Rosti G et al. Achieving a major molecular response at the time of a complete cytogenetic response (CCR) predicts a better duration of CCgR in imatinib-treated chronic myeloid leukemia patients. Clin Cancer Res 2006; 12: 3037–42.
78. Martinelli G, Iacobucci I, Rosti G et al. Prediction of response to imatinib by prospective quantitation of BCR-ABL transcript in late chronic phase chronic myeloid leukemia patients. Ann Oncol 2006; 17: 495–502.
79. Iacobucci I, Rosti G, Amabile M et al. Comparison between patients with Philadelphia-positive chronic phase chronic myeloid leukemia who obtained a complete cytogenetic response within 1 year of imatinib therapy and those who achieved such a response after 12 months of treatment. J Clin Oncol 2006; 24: 454–9.
80. Deininger M, Buchdunger E, Druker BJ. The development of imatinib as a therapeutic agent for chronic myeloid leukemia. Blood 2005; 105: 2640–53.
81. Ross DM, Branford S, Moore S et al. Limited clinical value of regular bone marrow cytogenetic analysis in imatinib-treated chronic phase CML patients monitored by RQ-PCR for BCR-ABL. Leukemia 2006; 20: 664–70.
82. Reed SD, Anstrom KJ, Ludmer JA et al. Cost-effectiveness of imatinib versus interferon-alpha plus low-dose cytarabine for patients with newly diagnosed chronic-phase chronic myeloid leukemia. Cancer 2004; 101: 2574–83.
83. Larson RA, Druker BJ, Guilhot F et al. Correlation of pharmacokinetic data with cytogenetic and molecular response in newly diagnosed patients with chronic myeloid leukemia in chronic phase (CML-CP) treated with imatinib. Blood 2006; 108: 131a, abstract 429.
84. Picard S, Titier K, Etienne G et al. Trough imatinib plasma levels are associated with both cytogenetic and molecular responses to standard dose imatinib in chronic myeloid leukemia. Blood 2007; 109: 3496–9.

Clinical aspects of chronic myeloid leukemia

4

Tariq I Mughal, John M Goldman

INTRODUCTION

Patients with chronic myeloid leukemia (CML) have been served well by clinical and laboratory research, particularly over the past two decades, and the unraveling of some of the molecular mechanisms which underlie the indolent or chronic phase (CP) of the disease has paved the way to defining potential specific targets for treatment. Patients with CML have in their leukemia cells a chromosomal translocation [t(9;22)] giving rise to the Philadelphia (Ph) chromosome (22q−), that results in a fusion gene, *BCR-ABL1*.[1–4] This gene encodes a BCR-ABL oncoprotein with enhanced tyrosine kinase activity, which is generally considered to be the 'initiating event' in the leukemia, though there remains some debate as to whether it really is the initial molecular event in all cases.[5,6]

The incidence of CML is about 1.0–2.0 per 100 000 of population per annum and is remarkably constant worldwide, at least in parts where national cancer registries have been maintained. In the Western world it represents approximately 15% of all adult leukemias and <5% of all childhood leukemias but the percentage is probably higher in the East, for example India, where chronic lymphocytic leukemia is very rare. The median age of onset is about 50 years and there is slight male excess. There appear to be no obvious predisposing factors other than following exposure to high doses of irradiation, as occurred in survivors of Hiroshima and Nagasaki atomic bombs in 1945.[7] Even then, the actual risk of developing CML was only marginally increased. A small number of families with a high incidence of the disease have been reported. One convincing case has been reported of CML recurring in cells of donor origin following related allogeneic stem cell transplantation.[8]

NATURAL HISTORY

CML is a remarkably heterogeneous disease. Before the introduction of imatinib mesylate it typically ran a biphasic or triphasic course. It was usually diagnosed in CP and this lasted typically 3–6 years; the leukemia then spontaneously progressed to blast transformation. About 70–80% of patients had a myeloid blast transformation, and they usually survived between 2 and 6 months; patients entering a lymphoid blast transformation had a slightly better survival. About half of the patients in the CP transformed directly into blast transformation and the remainder did so following a period of accelerated phase.[9]

The advent of imatinib mesylate, the first ABL tyrosine kinase inhibitor, has radically changed this natural history for the majority of patients who receive this drug as initial therapy, especially if they remain in complete cytogenetic response beyond the 4th year of therapy.[10,11] The recent 6-year follow-up of the phase III prospective trial (IRIS) which compared imatinib mesylate with the previous best non-transplant therapy, interferon alfa (IFNα) and cytarabine, showed that no patient in complete cytogenetic response

Table 4.1 IRIS study following a 6-year follow-up: annual events in patients who are in complete cytogenetic response (CCyR). Adapted from reference 12, with permission

Year after achieving CCyR	*All events**	*AP/BC*
1st	5.5%	2.1%
2nd	2.3%	0.8%
3rd	1.1%	0.3%
4th	0.4%	0%
5th	0.4%	0%

*All deaths or loss of response including progression to accelerated phase/blast crisis (AP/BC).

continuing beyond the 4th and 5th year of treatment had subsequently entered the advanced phase[12] (Table 4.1). At the time of this landmark analysis, about 60% of the original cohort randomized to receive imatinib mesylate remained in complete cytogenetic response. Most, if not all, of this cohort were in early CP. Patients presenting in late CP appear to fare less well; the Italian collaborative group (GIMEMA) recently demonstrated a complete cytogenetic response rate of 50–60% in a prospective analysis of 277 late CP patients.[13]

For patients subjected to an allogeneic stem cell transplant, the vast majority remain in a complete cytogenetic and molecular remission for 10 years or more. Some of these patients do become intermittently positive for BCR-ABL transcripts, albeit at low levels, but the rare patient with a persisting high transcript level is at a high risk of relapse.[14,15] A very small minority appear to relapse directly into the advanced phases of the disease.

CLINICAL PRESENTATION

The median age of patients at diagnosis appears to be 50 years in the West. However, the median age at diagnosis seems to be considerably lower, perhaps around 36 years, in some countries, such as India (Aggarwal, personal communication). In the West one-third to one-half of patients with CML are diagnosed in CP following a routine blood test and the remainder present with signs and symptoms related to anemia, platelet dysfunction, and splenomegaly. In about 95% of patients the diagnosis is typically made by the examination of a peripheral blood film and the demonstration of the Ph chromosome by conventional marrow cytogenetics; the remainder are diagnosed by the presence of a *BCR-ABL1* gene, though the use of fluorescence *in situ* hybridization (FISH) results in occasional false negative results. It is useful to obtain a baseline real-time quantitative polymerase chain reaction (RQ-PCR) analysis of peripheral blood or marrow to confirm the presence of a *BCR-ABL1* transcript and characterize the BCR-ABL junction.[16,17]

Most patients will have leukocytosis owing to increased numbers of myelocytes and segmented neutrophils; basophilia is almost universal and some patients have eosinophilia. The percentage of blast cells increases in parallel with the leukocyte count and may reach 10% without indicating disease progression. The anemia tends to be mild and normochromic normocytic in nature. Many patients have a minor degree of thrombocytosis, including some who might have it as the sole presenting blood count abnormality at diagnosis. The bone marrow trephine is hypercellular with complete or near complete loss of fat spaces; there is a high myeloid : erythroid ratio. The blast cell count is 5–10% of nucleated cells (Figure 4.1).

Up to half of all CP patients are asymptomatic at diagnosis, which is usually made on a full blood count carried out for some other purpose. When present, typical clinical features may include sweats, weight loss, hemorrhagic manifestations such as spontaneous bruising and retinal hemorrhages, abdominal discomfort owing to splenomegaly, fatigue often, but not always, related to anemia and fever (Table 4.2). The median duration of symptoms prior to diagnosis is about 3 months. Most patients diagnosed in

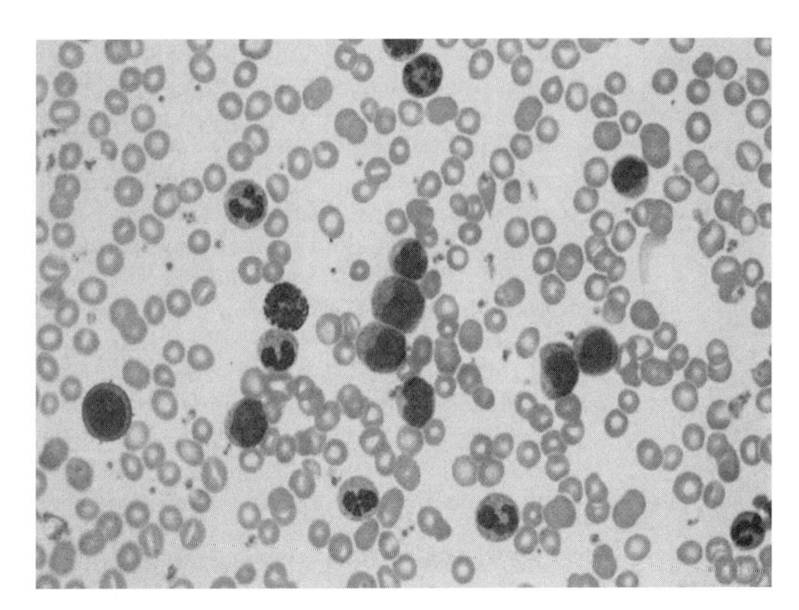

Figure 4.1 A peripheral blood film from a patient with CML in CP.

Table 4.2 Clinical features of patients with chronic phase CML seen at the Hammersmith Hospital London. Adapted from reference 18, with permission

Clinical feature	%
Fatigue	33.5
Bleeding	21.3
Weight loss	20.0
Abdominal discomfort (left upper quadrant)	18.6
Sweats	14.6
Bone pain	7.4
Splenomegaly	75.8
Hepatomegaly	2.2

the advanced phases of CML tend to be symptomatic.

Remarkably the early descriptions of the clinical features, in particular those which appeared to influence survival in the 166 patients studied over a 10-year period by Minot and colleagues in 1926, remain of some use.[19] Various subsequent studies, all in the pre-imatinib mesylate era, have reported the presence of fatigue in about 60% of symptomatic patients, followed by weight loss in 30%, fever and sweats in 25%, bleeding in 20%, and bone pains in <10%.[18,20–22] The most comprehensive recent descriptions have been those from the German CML-1 trialists assessing features in a cohort treated with various antileukemia agents (busulfan, hydroxyurea (hydroxycarbamide), and IFNα), and the Hammersmith Hospital (London) experience assessing 430 patients being considered for allogeneic stem cell transplantation between 1981 and 1997. Despite the fact that the Hammersmith series had a considerably lower median age (34 years), by virtue of patients being referred for possible transplantation, the findings, with the exception of the prevalence of hepatomegaly, were remarkably similar in the two patient populations. The German series reported hepatomegaly in about half of all symptomatic patients, whilst the Hammersmith series noted it in only 2.2% of the patients.

The Hammersmith series reported various laboratory parameters in detail (Table 4.3). The presenting total leukocyte count was $>100\times10^9/l$ in over 70% and $>350\times10^9/l$ in 19% of all patients. The presenting platelet counts were $>450\times10^9/l$ in 50% and just over

Table 4.3 Hematological variables in patients with chronic phase CML seen at the Hammersmith Hospital, London. Adapted from reference 18, with permission

	%
White blood count ($\times 10^9/l$)	
<20	4.5
20–99	23.0
100–249	36.2
250–350	17.2
>350	19.0
Hemoglobin (g/dl)	
<7.5	11.0
7.6–9.4	23.5
9.5–11.4	27.6
>11.5	37.8
Platelets ($\times 10^9/l$)	
<50	6.9
50–149	3.6
150–449	46.0
450–999	38.0
>1000	11.6

10% of all patients had platelet counts of $<150\times10^9/l$. Remarkably <7% of the study cohort had platelet counts of $<50\times10^9/l$, though bleeding was noted in over 20% of patients. Anemia was noted in about 60% of the patients, with 11% having a hemoglobin of <7.5 g/dl and a further 23.5% having hemoglobin between 7.6 and 9.4 g/dl. The authors did not specifically report the prevalence of platelet dysfunction in this series, which might have shed light on the cause of the bleeding manifestation in almost one-fifth of the patients studied.

CLONAL EVOLUTION

It is likely that the acquisition of a *BCR-ABL* fusion gene by a hematopoietic stem cell and the ensuing expansion of the Ph-positive clone set the scene for acquisition and expansion of one or more Ph-positive *subclones* that are genetically more aggressive than the original Ph-positive population. The propensity of the Ph-positive clone to acquire such additional genetic changes is an example of 'genomic instability', but the molecular mechanisms underlying this instability are poorly defined.[23] Such new events may occur in the *BCR-ABL* fusion gene or indeed in other genes in the Ph-positive population of cells.

In about 10% of all chronic phase CML patients, and perhaps up to 50% of those in the advanced phases, additional chromosomal abnormalities are observed at diagnosis.[24,25] The most common abnormalities described include trisomy 8, double Ph, and isochromosome 17 either alone or in combination. The precise significance of these clonal events remains an enigma, with those with an isolated trisomy 8 or a second Ph chromosome faring quite well, in contrast to those with multiple or complex chromosomal abnormalities who fare quite poorly. Studies including patients with clonal evolution who otherwise remain in CP suggest a poorer outcome compared with those without clonal evolution and in CP, particularly in those who do not achieve at least a partial cytogenetic response by 6 months on imatinib mesylate.[26,27]

RISK STRATIFICATION

Various efforts have been made to establish criteria definable at diagnosis, both prognostic (disease-related) and predictive (treatment-related), that may help to predict survival for individual patients.[28,29] The most frequently used method is that proposed by Sokal, whereby patients can be divided into various risk categories based on a mathematical formula that takes into account the patient's age, blast cell count, spleen size, and platelet count at diagnosis. Stratifying patients into good-, intermediate-, and poor-risk categories may assist in the decision-making process regarding appropriate treatment options. Clinically, however, the best prognostic indicators seemed until recently to be the response to initial treatment with IFNα, with those achieving hematological control of their disease having the best survival. The recently introduced Euro or Hasford system is an updated Sokal index, which includes consideration of basophil and eosinophil numbers.[30]

Other possible prognostic factors are the presence or absence of deletions in the region of the reciprocal *ABL-BCR* fusion gene on the derivative 9q+ chromosome and the rate of shortening of telomeres in the leukemia clone.[31–33] Such 9q+ deletions are quite large and associated with a poor prognosis, notably resistance to IFNα therapy. It is, however, possible that the adverse effect of this poor-risk feature is lost in patients treated with imatinib mesylate.[34]

More recently gene expression changes associated with progression and response in CML have been introduced.[35–37] Molecular profiling of CD34+ cells has been noted to identify low expression of CD7, concomitantly with high expression of proteinase 3 or elastase, as potential predictors of longer survival in patients with CML. By using oligonucleotide microarray screening investigators were able to separate gene expression profiling of two subsets of patients: 'aggressive', defined as those who developed blast transformation within 3 years of diagnosis, and 'indolent' defined as those who entered blast transformation at least 7 years following their initial diagnosis (Figure 4.2).

Another recent potential biomarker for risk stratification related to disease heterogeneity appears to be the polycomb group *BMI1* gene, which regulates both normal and leukemic stem cells. Mohty and colleagues demonstrated that the levels of BMI1 RNA were significantly higher in patients with advanced phase of CML, compared with those in CP.[38]

Following the introduction of imatinib mesylate into the clinic more than 10 years ago, and the realization that this agent is indeed the best treatment for almost all patients presenting in CP, efforts were made to assess the continued value of the updated Sokal index.[39] From the update of results of the IRIS study, it appeared that about 63% of previously untreated CP patients remained in complete cytogenetic response on imatinib mesylate therapy at 6 years and there were three distinct progression-free survival probabilities, with patients in the high-risk Sokal category faring the worst (Figure 4.3). It is also of interest that older age, a feature of the Sokal index, might not be of major prognostic relevance in imatinib mesylate-treated patients. Investigators from the MD Anderson Cancer Center (Houston) observed that among a cohort of 187 patients with CML in

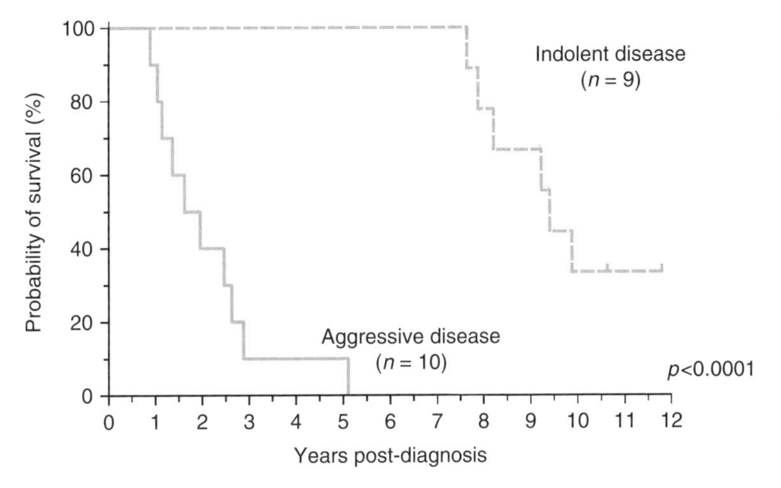

Figure 4.2 Risk stratification of patients with CML in CP by molecular profiling of CD34+ cells. Adapted from reference 36, with permission.

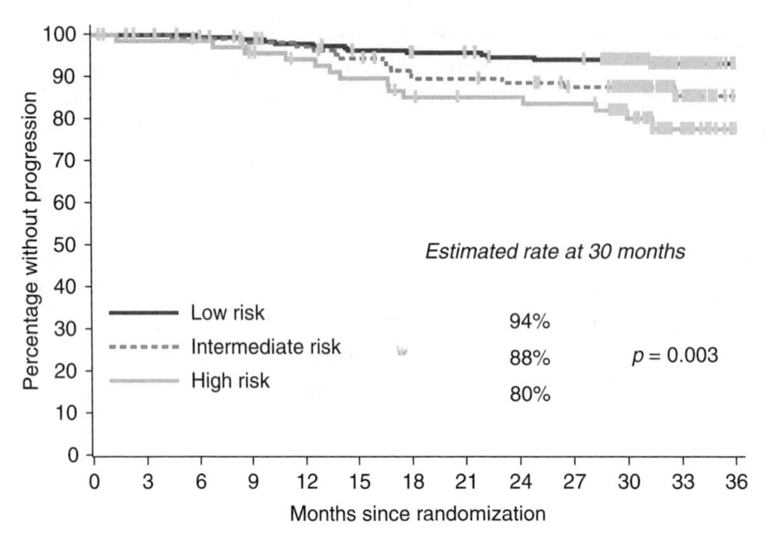

Figure 4.3 Correlation of long-term outcome with Sokal index in patients with newly diagnosed CML in CP treated with imatinib mesylate. Adapted from reference 39, with permission.

early CP, 87% of patients aged >60 years achieved a complete cytogenetic response compared with 79% of patients <60 years when treated with imatinib mesylate.[40] This supports the notion that age *per se* does not influence the biology of the disease – instead the emergence of a potential co-morbid condition in the older patient might increase the probability of treatment-related adverse effects.

Prior to the recent 6-year follow-up of the IRIS cohort, most single-center studies supported the conclusion that the time to achieve a complete cytogenetic response was important, with patients who achieve a complete cytogenetic response within the first 12 months faring the best.[41] The IRIS analysis, however, suggested that patients who achieved a complete cytogenetic response at 18 months or later fared just as well, or just as badly, as patients who achieved a complete cytogenetic response earlier[42] (Table 4.4). This analysis, however, has been criticized on a number of grounds. Nonetheless, the best outcome appears to be for the cohort who achieve a complete cytogenetic response and at least a 3-log or greater reduction of the *BCR-ABL* transcripts, compared with the baseline.[43]

There is also evidence from clinical trials that the depth and quality of the cytogenetic and molecular responses may be influenced by the actual dose of imatinib mesylate. Patients who receive higher doses of imatinib mesylate, particularly 800 mg/day, appear to achieve complete cytogenetic response and major molecular response much earlier than those treated with 400 mg, and there is a trend for improved event-free survival.[44] Interestingly achieving a major molecular response by 12 months has been shown by several workers to be associated with a low imatinib IC_{50}. There also appears to be no correlation between imatinib mesylate plasma trough levels and body weight or body surface area, but high variability between patients, and a correlation of response with imatinib mesylate plasma levels on day 29 following the initiation of therapy.[45] Larson and colleagues determined plasma concentrations of imatinib mesylate and its metabolite, CGP74588, by liquid chromatography/mass spectrometry, on day 29 and observed that high imatinib mesylate trough levels were predictive of higher complete cytogenetic response independent of Sokal risk group. Adverse effects were similar among the imatinib mesylate quartile categories, except

Table 4.4 Time to complete cytogenetic response (CCyR) does not affect long-term outcomes for patients (n=509) with CML-CP on imatinib therapy. Adapted from reference 42, with permission

Time to achieve a CCyR	*n (%)*	*OS at 6 years (%)*	*EFS at 6 years (%)*	*PFS at 6 years (%)*
≤6 months	265(52)	94	93	97
>6 months – ≤12 months	99(19)	95	90	97
>12 months – ≤18 months	34(7)	91	87	97
>18 months	49(10)	98	89	98
No CCyR achieved	62(12)	63	33	63

*For overall survival (OS), event-free survival (EFS), and progression-free survival (PFS) p<0.001 for patients with no CCyR versus CCyR irrespective of time.

for fluid retention, rash, myalgia, and anemia, which were more common at higher imatinib mesylate concentrations.[44]

Amongst other parameters which appear to have some use as prognostic and predictive tools in the imatinib mesylate era, the degree of myelosuppression which an individual patient experiences may be important.[46] There is one multivariant analysis which supports the notion that patients who experience persistent grade 3 and 4 myelosuppression fare relatively badly with the lowest rates of complete cytogenetic response.[47] Similarly Marin and colleagues have shown that a low neutrophil count and poor cytogenetic response to imatinib mesylate at 3 months comprise a poor risk significance, but a similar analysis from another center did not support this conclusion.[48,49] The inferior survival seen in some patients with myelosuppression might be a consequence of a reduced number of Ph-negative, and presumably largely normal, progenitors in such patients.

RESISTANCE TO IMATINIB MESYLATE

Defining responses to imatinib mesylate therapy and monitoring of patients have been a challenge for some time and are discussed in Chapter 5. Various efforts to define failure and suboptimal responses have resulted in two prinicipal consensus panels[50,51] (Table 4.5). Primary resistance or refractoriness to imatinib mesylate appears to be very rare and when seen may be related to poor compliance, abnormal drug efflux and influx, poor gastrointestinal absorption, p450 cytochrome polymorphism, and interactions with other medications.[52] In a small cohort of patients a correlation of human OCT1 expression and response has been observed: the higher the levels of OCT1 the better the molecular responses (Figure 4.4).[53,54]

Table 4.5 Criteria for failure and suboptimal response to imatinib. Adapted from reference 50, with permission

Time (months)	*Response*	
	Failure	*Suboptimal*
3	No HR	No CHR
6	No CHR 100% Ph+	≥35% Ph+
12	≥35% Ph+	≥5% Ph+
18	≥5% Ph+	No MMR (<3-log reduction BCR-ABL/ABL)
Any	Loss of CHR	Clonal evolution
	Loss of CCyR	Loss of MMR
	Mutation	Mutation

HR, hematological response; CHR, complete HR;
MMR, major molecular response;
CCyR, complete cytogenetic response.

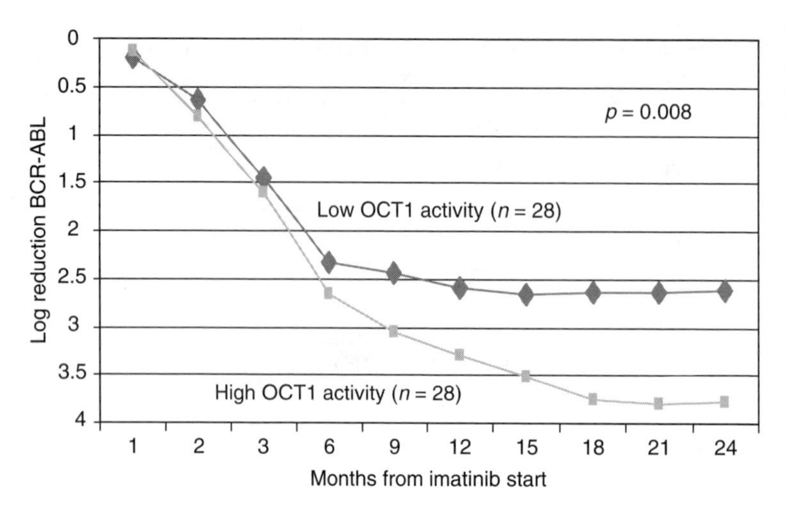

Figure 4.4 Correlation of molecular response with levels of OCT1 activity in CML. Adapted from reference 54, with permission.

A somewhat larger proportion of patients, about 20% in the CP, respond initially to imatinib mesylate and then lose their response. Some of these patients show evidence of expansion of subclones with point mutations in the *BCR-ABL* kinase domain (KD), which code for amino acid substitutions that may impede binding of imatinib mesylate but do not impair phosphorylation of downstream substrates that mediate the leukemia signal.[55,56] The precise position of the mutation appears to dictate the degree of resistance to imatinib mesylate; some mutations are associated with minor degrees of imatinib mesylate resistance whereas one notorious mutation, the replacement of threonine by isoleucine at position 315 (T315I), is associated with near total non-responsiveness to imatinib mesylate as well as with resistance to the newer tyrosine kinase inhibitors, namely dasatinib, nilotinib, and bosutinib.[57,58] The precise significance and indeed the kinetics of the over 70 currently well-characterized mutations remain largely unelucidated.

CONCLUSIONS

The past decade has witnessed an increasing proportion of patients with CML being diagnosed following a routine blood test and prior to the emergence of any clinical features. Many of these patients, though not all, are in early stage CP. The introduction of the original ABL tyrosine kinase inhibitor, imatinib mesylate, in 1998 for the treatment of CML appears to have changed not only the treatment paradigm, but also the natural history of the disease. The recent 6-year follow-up of the IRIS trail has confirmed a robust reduction of all events in patients who remain on imatinib mesylate treatment beyond 4 years and for the cohort who have achieved and remain in complete cytogenetic response, none progressed to the advanced phases of CML (Table 4.1). *Pari passu*, methods to stratify patients in accordance with the risks associated with disease and treatment-related parameters have improved. Notably prognostic scores in use during the pre-imatinib mesylate era have also been validated for current use. We can anticipate further advances in the gene microarray applications and the identification and use of more candidate genes in the near future.

REFERENCES

1. Nowell PC, Hungerford DA. A minute chromosome in human granulocytic leukemia. Science 1960; 132: 1497–501.
2. Sawyers CL. Chronic myeloid leukemia. N Engl J Med 1999; 340: 1330–40.

3. Daley GQ, Van Etten RA, Baltimore D. Induction of chronic myelogenous leukemia in mice by the p210 bcr/abl gene of the Philadelphia chromosome. Science 1990; 24: 824–30.
4. Mughal TI, Goldman JM. Chronic myeloid leukaemia: STI571 magnifies the therapeutic dilemma. Eur J Cancer 2001; 37: 561–8.
5. Goldman JM, Melo JV. Chronic myeloid leukemia – advances in biology and new approaches to treatment. N Engl J Med 2003; 349: 1451–64.
6. Zaccaria A, Valenti AM, Donti E et al. Persistence of chromosomal abnormalities additional to the Philadelphia chromosome after Philadelphia chromosome disappearance during imatinib therapy for chronic myeloid leukemia. Haematologica 2007; 4: 564–5.
7. Ichimaru M, Ichimaru T, Belsky JL. Incidence of leukemia in atomic bomb survivors belonging to a fixed cohort on Hiroshima and Nagasaki, 1950–71. Radiation dose, years after exposure, age at exposure, and type of leukemia. J Radiat Res (Tokyo) 1978; 3: 262–82.
8. Marmont A, Frassoni F, Bacigalupo A et al. Recurrence of Ph[1]-positive leukemia in donor cells after marrow transplantation for chronic granulocytic leukemia. N Engl J Med 1984; 310: 903–6.
9. Mughal TI, Goldman JM. Molecularly targeted treatment of chronic myeloid leukemia: beyond the imatinib era. Front Biosci 2006; 1: 209–20.
10. Druker BJ, Tamura S, Buchdunger E et al. Effects of a selective inhibitor of the Abl tyrosine kinase on the growth of the BCR-ABL positive cells. Nat Med 2000; 2: 561–66.
11. Druker BJ, Guilhot F, O'Brien SG et al. Five-year follow-up of patients receiving imatinib for chronic myeloid leukemia. N Engl J Med 2006; 355: 2408–17.
12. Hochhaus A, on behalf of the IRIS investigators. Outcomes post imatinib for patients on the IRIS trial: a 6 year follow-up. Blood 2007; 110, abstract 25.
13. Palandri F, Iacobucci I, Martinelli G et al. Long-term outcome of complete cytogenetic responders after imatinib 400mg in late chronic phase, Philadelphia-positive chronic myeloid leukemia: the GIMEMA Working Party on CML. J Clin Oncol 2008; 26: 106–11.
14. Mughal TI, Yong A, Szydlo R et al. The probability of long-term leukaemia free survival for patients in molecular remission 5 years after allogeneic stem cell transplantation for chronic myeloid leukaemia in chronic phase. Br J Haematol 2001; 115: 569–74.
15. Kaeda JS, O'Shea D, Szydlo R et al. Serial measurements BCR-ABL transcripts in the peripheral blood after allogeneic stem cell transplant for chronic myeloid leukaemia: An attempt to define patients who may not require further therapy. Blood 2006; 102: 4121–6.
16. Goldman JM. How I treat chronic myeloid leukemia in the imatinib era. Blood 2007; 110: 2828–37.
17. Schiffer CA. BCR-ABL tyrosine kinase inhibitors for chronic myelogenous leukemia. N Engl J Med 2007; 357: 258–65.
18. Savage D, Szydlo R, Goldman JM et al. Clinical features at diagnosis of 430 patients with chronic myeloid leukemia seen at a referral centre over a 16-year period. Br J Haematol 1997; 96: 111–16.
19. Minot GR, Buckman TE, Isaacs R. Chronic myelogenous leukemia: age, incidence, duration and benefit derived from irradiation. JAMA 1924; 82: 1489–94.
20. Faderl S, Talpaz M, Estrov Z et al. Chronic myelogenous leukaemia: biology and therapy. Ann Intern Med 131: 207–19.
21. Hasford J, Ansari H, Pfirrman M et al. Analysis and validation of prognostic factors for CML. German CML study group. Bone Marrow Transplant 1996; 17: 549–54.
22. Hehlmann R, Heimpel H, Hasford J et al. Randomized comparison of interferon-alfa with busulfan and hydroxyurea in chronic myelogenous leukemia. Blood 1994; 84: 4064–77.
23. Mughal TI, Goldman JM. A perspective on the molecular evolution of chronic myeloid leukemia from chronic phase to blast transformation. Clin Leuk 2006; 1: 101–07.
24. Kantarjian H, Keating MJ, Smith TL et al. Proposal for a simple synthesis prognostic staging system in chronic myelogenous leukemia. Am J Med 1990; 88: 1–8.
25. Majlis A, Smith TL, Talpaz M et al. Significance of cytogenetic clonal evolution in chronic myelogenous leukemia. J Clin Oncol 1996; 14: 1 96–203.
26. Cortes J, Talpaz M, Giles F et al. Prognostic significance of cytogenetic clonal evolution in patients with chronic myelogenous leukemia on imatinib mesylate therapy. Blood 2003; 101: 3794–800.
27. O'Dwyer ME, Mauro M, Blasdel C et al. Clonal evolution and lack of cytogenetic response are adverse prognostic factors for hematologic relapse of chronic phase CML patients treated with imatinib mesylate. Blood 2004; 103: 451–5.
28. Sokal JE, Cox EB, Baccarani M et al. Prognostic discrimination in good-risk chronic granulocytic leukemia. Blood 1984; 63: 789–99.
29. Gratwohl A, Hermans J, Goldman JM et al. Risk assessment for patients with chronic myeloid leukaemia before allogeneic bone marrow transplantation. Lancet 1998; 352: 1087–92.
30. Hasford J, Pfirmann M, Hehlmann R et al. A new prognostic score for survival of patients with chronic

myeloid leukemia treated with interferon-alpha. J Natl Cancer Inst 1998; 90: 850–8.
31. Sinclair PB, Nacheva EP, Leversha M et al. Large deletions at the t(9;22) breakpoint are common and may identify a poor prognosis subgroup of patients with chronic myeloid leukemia. Blood 2000; 95: 738–43.
32. Cohen N, Rozenfeld-Granot G, Hardan I et al. Subgroup of patients with Philadelphia-positive chronic myeloid leukemia characterised by a deletion of 9q proximal to Abl gene: expression profiling, resistance to interferon therapy and poor prognosis. Cancer Genet Cytogenet 2001; 128: 114–19.
33. Huntly BJP, Bench A, Green AR. Double jeopardy from a single translocation: deletions of the derivative chromosome 9 in chronic myeloid leukemia. Blood 2003; 102: 1160–8.
34. Quintas-Cardama A, Kantarjian H, Talpaz M et al. Imatinib mesylate therapy may overcome the poor prognostic significance of deletions of derivative chromosome 9 in patients with chronic myelogenous leukemia. Blood 2005; 105: 2281–6.
35. Radich J, Dai H, Mao M et al. Gene expression changes associated with progression and response in CML. Proc Natl Acad Sci U S A 2006; 103: 2794–9.
36. Yong A, Szydlo R, Goldman JM et al. Molecular profiling of CD38+ cells identifies low expression of CD7, along with high expression of proteinase 3 or elastase, as predictors of longer survival in patients with CML. Blood 2006; 107: 205–12.
37. Brazma D, Grace C, Howard J et al. Genomic profile of chronic myelogenous leukemia: imbalances associate with disease progression. Genes Chromosomes Cancer 2007; 46: 1039–50.
38. Mohty M, Yong A, Szydlo R et al. The polycomb BMI1 gene is a molecular marker for predicting prognosis of CML. Blood 2007; 110: 380–3.
39. Simonsson B, on behalf of the IRIS Study Group. Beneficial effects of cytogenetic and molecular response on long-term outcome in patients with newly diagnosed chronic myeloid leukemia in chronic phase (CML-CP) treated with imatinib (IM): update from the IRIS Study. Blood 2005; 106: abstract 52a.
40. Cortes J, Talpaz M, O'Brien et al. Effects of age on prognosis with imatinib mesylate therapy for patients with Philadelphia-positive chronic myelogenous leukemia. Cancer 2003; 98: 1105–3.
41. O'Brien S, Guilhot F, Larson R et al. Imatinib compared with interferon and low dose cytarabine for newly diagnosed chronic phase chronic myeloid leukemia. N Engl J Med 2003; 348: 994–1004.
42. Guilhot F, on behalf of the IRIS investigators. Time to complete cytogenetic response does not affect long term outcomes for patients with CML-CP on imatinib therapy. Blood 2007; 110: abstract 27.
43. Hughes T, Branford S. Molecular monitoring of BCR-ABL as a guide to clinical management in chronic myeloid leukaemia. Blood Rev 2006; 20: 29–41.
44. Larson RA, Druker BJ, Guihot FA et al. Imatinib pharmacokinetics and its correlation with response and safety in chronic phase CML: a subanalysis of the IRIS study. Blood 2008; 111: 4022–8.
45. Kantarjian H, Talpaz M, O'Brien S et al. High-dose imatinib mesylate therapy in newly diagnosed Philadelphia chromosome-positive chronic phase chronic myeloid leukemia. Blood 2004; 103: 2873–8.
46. Kantarjian H, Sawyers C, Hochhaus A et al. Hematological and cytogenetic responses to imatinib mesylate in chronic myelogenous leukemia. N Engl J Med 2002; 346: 645–52.
47. Sneed TB, Kantarjian H, Talpaz M et al. The significance of myelosuppression during therapy with imatinib mesylate in patients with chronic myelogenous leukemia. Cancer 2004; 100: 116–21.
48. Marin D, Marktel S, Bua M et al. Prognostic factors for patients with chronic myeloid leukemia in chronic phase treated with imatinib mesylate after failure of interferon-alfa. Leukemia 2003; 17: 1448–53.
49. Kantarjian H, Cortes J. Testing the prognostic model of Marin et al in an independent chronic myelogenous leukemia study group. Leukemia 2004; 18: 650.
50. Baccarani M, Saglio G, Goldman JM et al. Evolving concepts in the management of chronic myeloid leukemia: recommendations from an expert panel on behalf of the European LeukemiaNet. Blood 2006; 108: 1809–20.
51. Kantarjian H, Schiffer CA, Jones D, Cortes JI. Monitoring the response and course of chronic myeloid leukemia in the era of Bcr-Abl tyrosine kinase inhibitors: practical advice on the use and interpretation of monitoring methods. Blood 2008; 111: 1774–80.
52. Apperley J. Part I: Mechanisms of resistance to imatinib in chronic myeloid leukemia. Lancet Oncol 2007; 8: 1018–29.
53. Thomas J, Wang L, Clark RE, Pirmohamed M. Active transport of imatinib into and out of cells: implications for drug resistance. Blood 2004; 104: 3739–45.
54. White DL, Saunders VA, Dang P et al. OCT-1 mediated influx is a key determinant of the intracellular uptake of imatinib but not nilotinib (AMN107): reduced OCT-1 activity is the cause of low in vitro sensitivity to imatinib. Blood 2006; 108: 697–704.
55. Druker BJ. Circumventing resistance to kinase-inhibitor therapy. N Engl J Med 2006; 354: 2594–6.

56. Deininger M, Buchdunger E, Druker BJ. The development of imatinib as a therapeutic agent for chronic myeloid leukemia. Blood 2005; 105: 2640–53.
57. Mughal TI, Goldman JM. Emerging strategies for the treatment of mutant Bcr-Abl T315I myeloid leukemias. Clin Lymph Myeloma 2007; 7: S81–4.
58. Soverini S, Iacobucci I, Baccarani M, Martinelli M. Targeted therapy and the T315I mutation in Philadelphia-positive leukemias. Haematologica 2007; 4: 437–9.

Chronic myeloid leukemia: current first-line treatment options

5

Elias Jabbour, Hagop Kantarjian, Jorge Cortes

INTRODUCTION

Chronic myeloid leukemia (CML) is an uncommon disease. Its incidence is low, but its prevalence is increasing. In the US, approximately 4500 new cases of CML are diagnosed annually.[1] The median age at diagnosis is 55 years. With an estimated survival rate of 90% at 5 years, and an annual mortality rate of 2%, the prevalence of CML in 20 years may reach 200 000–300 000 cases in the US.

CML is associated with a specific chromosomal abnormality, the Philadelphia chromosome (Ph), that results from a balanced reciprocal translocation between chromosomes 9 and 22.[2] This translocation, designated t(9;22)(q34;q11.2), creates an aberrant fusion gene derived from the *ABL* gene encoded on chromosome 9 and the *BCR* (breakpoint cluster region) gene encoded on chromosome 22. The product of this fusion *BCR-ABL* gene, is a constitutively active protein-tyrosine kinase, p210 *BCR-ABL*, that promotes cellular proliferation and suppresses apoptosis. BCR-ABL kinase activity is critical to the development of CML.

Historically, CML was treated with busulfan or hydroxyurea, and was associated with a poor prognosis.[2,3] These agents controlled the hematological manifestations of the disease, but did not delay disease progression. Treatment with interferon alfa (IFNα) produced complete cytogenetic responses in 5–25% of patients with CML in chronic phase (CP), and improved survival compared with previous treatments.[4] Combining IFNα with cytarabine produced additional benefits.[5,6] Allogeneic stem cell transplantation (alloSCT) may be curative in CML, but it is applicable to only a fraction of CML patients and carries a significant risk of morbidity and mortality. In one recent study, the 5-year survival with IFNα (in most instances followed by imatinib) was significantly superior to that with alloSCT.[7]

Imatinib mesylate, a potent and selective BCR-ABL tyrosine kinase inhibitor, is now established first-line standard therapy in CML. A complete cytogenetic response can be achieved in 50–60% of patients treated in chronic phase after failure with IFNα[8,9] and in over 80% of those receiving imatinib as first-line therapy.[10,11] Responses are durable in most patients treated in early chronic phase, particularly among those who achieve major molecular responses (e.g. ≥3-log reduction in transcript levels).[12,13]

Here we review the most current information regarding first-line therapy in CML, and briefly summarize the status of previous drugs such as IFNα and cytotoxic agents.

CYTOTOXIC AGENTS

Busulfan (1,4-dimethane-sulfonyl-oxybutane) was the first alkylating agent to demonstrate activity in CML.[14] Busulfan therapy was associated with significant toxicities, including severe and prolonged myelosuppression. Busulfan should be used today only as part of some conditioning regimens in alloSCT, and must be avoided in patients awaiting alloSCT because its use prior to alloSCT has been associated with an adverse outcome.

Hydroxyurea, a ribonucleotide reductase inhibitor, is a well-tolerated oral cytotoxic agent that can control blood counts rapidly in most patients with CML. Rare side-effects include nausea, rash, mouth ulcers, and hand or leg ulcers. Hydroxyurea is usually given at a daily dose of 1–10 g, depending on the degree of leukocytosis, and the dose adjusted to keep the WBC count between 2 and 10×10^9/l. Hydroxyurea may be used for initial cytoreduction, as a temporary measure to control counts in between definitive therapies. Although it is not necessary to use hydroxyurea or any other agent to decrease the WBC prior to the start of imatinib therapy, hydroxyurea may be used in patients in whom CML is suspected while the confirmatory detection of the Ph chromosome is under way. It should not be used alone as a definitive treatment in CML since it rarely suppresses Ph-positive cells.

INTERFERON ALFA

IFNα showed anti-CML activity in the 1980s, and was the standard of care in CML until the advent of imatinib. IFNα induced a complete hematological response in 50–80% of patients with previously untreated chronic phase CML, and cytogenetic response in 40–60% (major in 10–40%; complete in 5–30%).[4] A meta-analysis of randomized studies of IFNα versus hydroxyurea or busulfan, showed that IFNα therapy was associated with better survival than cytotoxic agents (5-year survival rates 57% versus 42%, $p < 0.00001$).[4] The addition of cytarabine to IFNα increased the probability of achieving a complete cytogenetic response to up to 35%.[5] IFNα, however, has minimal activity in the accelerated (AP) or blastic (BP) phases of CML. Administration of IFNα is associated with significant side-effects including flu-like symptoms, fever, chills, myalgias, fatigue, depression, neuropathy, diarrhea, memory loss, immune-mediated complications, myelosuppression, and others.[15]

Probably the most important lesson learnt from the IFNα era was the recognition of the significance of achieving a complete cytogenetic response. Those patients achieving this level of response had a 78% probability of survival at 10 years, compared with only 39% for those who achieve a partial cytogenetic response, and 25% for those with minor or no cytogenetic response.[16] Furthermore, approximately 30% of patients who achieved a complete cytogenetic response had undetectable BCR-ABL transcripts by polymerase chain reaction (PCR); none of them relapsed after a median follow-up of 10 years and they were therefore probably cured.[16,17] Interestingly, 40–60% of those in complete cytogenetic response with presence of minimal residual disease at the molecular level did not relapse after 10 years. This has been attributed to IFNα-induced immune modulation, such as the presence of cytotoxic T lymphocytes specific for PR1, a peptide derived from proteinase 3 which is over-expressed in CML cells. This phenomenon has been demonstrated in patients in complete remission after IFNα therapy and autologous stem cell transplantation (auto-SCT) but not in those who fail to achieve complete cytogenetic response or those treated with chemotherapy.[18]

New formulations of IFNα attached to polyethylene glycol (PEG) prolong its half-life, allow weekly administration, reduce toxicity, and may also improve results.[19]

IMATINIB: THE STANDARD OF CARE IN CHRONIC MYELOID LEUKEMIA

The introduction of the orally administered 2-phenylaminopyrimidine derivative imatinib (STI571; Gleevec™/Glivec®) has dramatically improved the outcome of patients with CML. Preclinical studies established that imatinib inhibits ABL and the related protein-tyrosine kinase ABL-related gene (ARG) as well as the kinase activity of members of the class III family of receptor tyrosine kinases including KIT, PDGFR, and the macrophage colony-stimulating factor receptor CSF-1R (cFMS).[20–24] Inhibition of BCR-ABL protein-tyrosine kinase activity with imatinib blocks intracellular oncogenic signal transduction pathways.[25,26]

Imatinib was established as first-line therapy for CML by the phase III International Randomized Study of Interferon versus STI571 (IRIS) in which 1106 patients with newly diagnosed CML in chronic phase were randomized to receive imatinib (400 mg/day) or IFNα (target dose 5 million U/m^2/day) plus cytarabine (20 mg/m^2/day for 10 days every month).[10] After a median follow-up of 18 months, 95% of patients in the imatinib group achieved a complete hematological response, compared with 56% in the IFNα plus cytarabine group (p <0.001). The rates of complete cytogenetic response were 68% and 5%, respectively (p <0.001). More importantly, the molecular response rates were also significantly better, with estimated 12-month major molecular response rates of 40% for imatinib-treated patients versus 2% for those treated with IFNα.[13]

A 5-year follow-up to the IRIS study provided evidence of the continued benefit with imatinib.[27] The rate of survival free from transformation to AP or BP was 93% and the event-free survival rate 83%. Excluding deaths unrelated to CML, the survival rate was 95% and the overall survival rate was 89%. An important observation was that the probability of losing a response or progression to AP or BP decreased significantly over time. The rate of progression was less than 1% during the 5th year of treatment for patients originally randomized to imatinib, compared with rates during the previous 4 years of 1.5%, 2.8%, 1.6%, and 0.9%. The depth of the cytogenetic response after 12 and 18 months of imatinib therapy correlated with survival without transformation. The estimated 5-year survival rate without transformation in patients not achieving a major cytogenetic response at 12 months was significantly less (81%) than in those who achieved major cytogenetic response (complete 97%, partial 93%; p <0.001). Based on the response at 18 months, the estimated 5-year rate of survival without transformation for patients not achieving a complete cytogenetic response was significantly lower than in those who achieved complete cytogenetic response (99% versus 90%; p <0.001).[27] In addition a significant number of patients without a complete cytogenetic response by 12 months were lost by 18 months, presumably from progression emphasizing the importance of achieving optimal response early during the course of therapy. This is emphasized in the criteria for optimal response to imatinib recently proposed by the European LeukemiaNet (Table 5.1).[28]

Similarly, molecular responses correlate with outcome. Patients with a complete cytogenetic response and at least a 3-log reduction in transcript levels after 12 months of therapy have a projected survival rate free from transformation at 60 months of 100%, compared with 95% for those with a complete cytogenetic response but less than a 3-log reduction in transcript levels and 88% for those without a complete cytogenetic response. There was a continuous improvement in the rate of molecular response: the rate of major molecular

Table 5.1 Imatinib therapy: thresholds for optimal response, suboptimal response, and failure

Time from initiation	*Optimal response*	*Suboptimal response*	*Failure*
3 months	CHR, some cytogenetic response	Less than CHR	No hematological response
6 months	MCyR	Less than MCyR	Less than CHR
			No CyR
12 months	CCyR	MCyR	Less than MCyR
	MMR	Less than MMR	
18 months	CMR/MMR	Less than MMR	Less than CCyR

CHR, complete hematological response; MCyR, major cytogenetic response; CCyR, complete cytogenetic response; MMR, major molecular response; CMR, complete molecular response.

response improved from 53% at 1 year to 80% at 4 years of therapy (p <0.001).[27] These results, however, represent a subset of 124 patients with available data and it is possible that they overrepresented the actual rates. However, other studies have also suggested an increase in the percentage of patients achieving a major molecular response until approximately 3 years after which the rate reaches a plateau where approximately one-third of patients will not achieve a major molecular response.

SURVIVAL ADVANTAGE

The IRIS trial did not initially document a survival advantage for patients treated with imatinib. This was probably owing to the crossover design and the approval of imatinib while the study was still young. This resulted in over 90% of patients crossing over from the IFNα arm to imatinib. Since imatinib effectively rescues patients who fail IFNα, this negated any possible survival benefit. Still, the recent 5-year follow-up has now shown a survival benefit for those who initiated therapy with imatinib from the onset.

Comparisons with historical cohorts treated with IFNα-based therapy have confirmed the long-term survival superiority of first-line imatinib therapy in newly diagnosed CML. In a retrospective study, the estimated 5-year survival rate for imatinib was 88%, compared with 63% for IFN-based therapies (p = 0.00001).[29] A second study compared long-term survival rates among patients originally randomized to imatinib in the IRIS trial with patients treated with IFNα and cytarabine.[30] The estimated 3-year survival rate with imatinib in the IRIS trial was 92% compared with 84% with IFNα plus cytarabine. Figure 5.1 shows the survival of patients treated at our institution since 1965 by year of therapy. Imatinib has also demonstrated a survival advantage in patients with more advanced phases of CML treated with imatinib. For example, in accelerated phase, the median survival following treatment with imatinib has not yet been reached at 4 years; the historical median survival is 2 years. This benefit was seen even when comparing with patients treated with alloSCT, mostly owing to the early mortality of the latter.[31]

IMATINIB DOSE SCHEDULES

The standard dose of imatinib is 400 mg daily. However, the phase I study of imatinib in CML evaluated doses ranging from 25 to 1000 mg/day. The selection of 400 mg as the

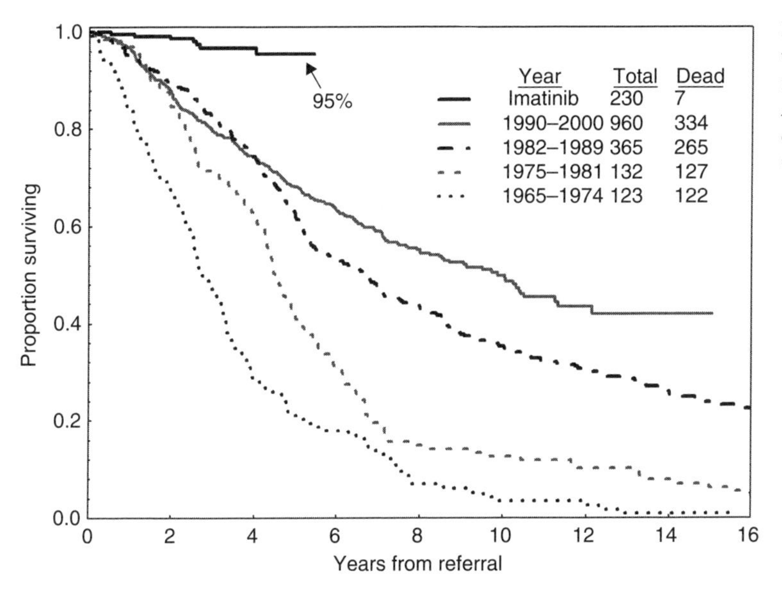

Figure 5.1 Survival of patients with early chronic phase chronic myeloid leukemia treated at MD Anderson Cancer Center in different eras compared with those treated with imatinib.

dose to use in subsequent studies was based on results from patients who received ≥300 mg/day, among whom the complete hematological response rate was 98% and cytogenetic response rate was 54%.[32] Also, the blood concentration of imatinib at 400 mg daily was consistently higher than that required to inhibit 50% of BCR-ABL tyrosine kinase activity *in vitro*.[33,34] However, no dose limiting toxicity was identified, and a maximal tolerated dose was not defined. In addition, imatinib 600 mg daily was more effective than 400 mg for patients in AP or BP disease.[35–37] Furthermore, among patients who had primary or secondary failure to standard-dose imatinib after dose escalation to 800 mg/day (600 mg/day if previously reduced to 300 mg/day) 38% of those with cytogenetic resistance or relapse achieved a major cytogenetic response.[38]

Thus, there has been interest to explore higher doses of imatinib to determine whether outcome may be further improved. This was first investigated among patients with CML in late chronic phase post-IFNα. Patients received imatinib 400 mg twice daily and a complete cytogenetic response rate of 90% was achieved compared with 48% in historical controls treated with standard-dose therapy. In addition, 56% of patients had a major molecular response, including 41% with undetectable levels.[39]

Several phase II studies using high-dose imatinib as first-line therapy in patients with previously untreated CML in chronic phase, have documented high rates of complete cytogenetic (up to 95%) and major molecular responses, as well as a high proportion of patients reaching undetectable BCR-ABL transcript levels.[29,40–42] When compared with historical experience in similar patients treated with standard-dose imatinib, those treated with high dose had higher rates of complete cytogenetic response (91% versus 76%, $p = 0.002$) and these occurred earlier, with 88% achieving this response by 6 months of therapy compared with 56% with standard dose ($p < 0.00001$). The cumulative rates of major molecular response and 'complete' molecular response (i.e. undetectable transcript levels) were significantly better with high-dose imatinib.[43] More importantly, progression-free and transformation-free survival were significantly better for the high-dose group ($p = 0.02$ and 0.005). Other studies have shown nearly identical results, confirming the high rate of cytogenetic and molecular responses with high-dose imatinib.[42,44,45] Higher doses are well tolerated in most patients. There is no difference in the frequency of non-hematological toxicity grade 3–4, but some studies have suggested a higher rate of hematological toxicity compared with what is seen with standard-dose imatinib. This translates into approximately 85% of patients continuing to receive >400 mg imatinib 12 months after the start of therapy. Results from ongoing randomized studies will determine whether high-dose imatinib should be considered a standard approach.

LONG-TERM SAFETY AND CARDIOTOXICITY

Most adverse events with imatinib therapy are mild to moderate in severity, and usually occur early during the course of therapy, with the incidence decreasing over time. Treatment is eventually discontinued for adverse events in only 3–5% of patients.[10,30,32,33] Grade 3–4 hematological toxicities are also moderate, with neutropenia occurring in up to 48%, thrombocytopenia in up to 42%, and anemia in up to 42%. Myelosuppression is usually transient and mostly seen during the first 3 months of therapy. Persistent or recurrent myelosuppression can be managed with hematopoietic growth factors in most instances.[46–48] Recently, it was reported that imatinib therapy could be associated with congestive heart failure possibly mediated by inhibition of ABL. This came from a report of ten selected patients with this condition, while receiving imatinib.[49] However, this toxicity is very rare. Among 1276 patients treated at a single institution, 22 (1.8%) patients (median age of 70 years) were identified as having symptoms that could be attributed to congestive heart failure,[50] and only eight were considered possibly or probably related to imatinib. Eleven of the 22 patients continued imatinib therapy with dose adjustments and management for the congestive heart failure symptoms with no further complications. Thus, at the present time there is no indication for increased cardiac screening for patients receiving imatinib. However, those who develop symptoms that may suggest this condition should be adequately investigated.

MONITORING RESPONSE TO IMATINIB THERAPY AND MINIMAL RESIDUAL DISEASE

With most patients achieving complete cytogenetic response with imatinib, achievement of molecular response has become the therapeutic goal in CML. The IRIS trial showed that a reduction of BCR-ABL transcript level by at least 3 logs below a standardized baseline value correlated with an improved progression-free survival.[13] In addition, achieving a major molecular response within the first 12 months of therapy is predictive of durable cytogenetic remission.[12] The lack of consistency in reporting BCR-ABL transcript levels has been a source of confusion and debate. A recent consensual proposal suggests harmonizing the differing methodologies for measuring BCR-ABL transcripts by using a conversion factor whereby individual laboratories can express BCR-ABL transcript levels on internationally agreed scales: results will be converted by comparing analysis of standardized reference samples with the corresponding laboratories. It is suggested that after such adjustment, a value of 0.1% would correspond to a major molecular response in all laboratories.[51] However, a uniform source of standards for harmonization of all laboratories is not yet available.

Current recommendations are to monitor patients by real-time PCR every 3–6 months. A routine cytogenetic analysis should be performed every 3–6 months, and every 12 months once a complete cytogenetic response is achieved.

DISCONTINUATION OF IMATINIB THERAPY

The optimal duration of imatinib therapy is unknown. The current recommendation is to continue treatment indefinitely unless there is unacceptable toxicity or treatment failure. There is no evidence to support the concept that imatinib can safely be discontinued even after transcript levels become undetectable. Most patients who have discontinued imatinib therapy even after having sustained undetectable levels of BCR-ABL for significant periods of time have experienced molecular or cytogenetic relapse usually shortly after discontinuation.[52–54] Rousselot *et al.* reported on 12 patients who discontinued imatinib after maintaining undetectable BCR-ABL levels for 24 months or longer. Six patients were still PCR negative after a median follow-up of 18 months (range 9–24 months).[55] Although all six patients with sustained response had been previously treated with IFNα, four out of the six who relapsed had also received IFNα previously. Thus, although it has been suggested that the effects of IFNα may contribute to the patient's ability to achieve a sustained and prolonged molecular response, this is still debatable. It has been suggested that the earliest, probably quiescent, progenitor cells in CML are insensitive to imatinib *in vitro.* It is conceivable that these progenitors might trigger proliferation of CML once the inhibitory pressure of imatinib is eliminated.

SIGNIFICANCE OF OTHER CYTOGENETIC ABNORMALITIES

Approximately 5–15% of patients who obtain a cytogenetic response develop karyotypic abnormalities in Ph-negative cells. These do not represent clonal evolution as they occur in cells without the Ph and should not be considered as part of the definition of accelerated phase. The significance of these events is currently unknown.[56] The most common such cytogenetic abnormalities include trisomy 8, monosomy 5 or 7, and deletion 20q.[57–60] These abnormalities frequently regress spontaneously, and patients with these abnormalities have similar long-term outcome to patients without such abnormalities. However, occasional cases of progression to acute myeloid leukemia or myelodysplastic syndrome have been reported,[61] mainly in patients with a deletion of chromosome 7 and/or other complex abnormalities, but also in occasional patients with isolated trisomy 8, warranting a careful follow-up.

IMATINIB RESISTANCE AND MONITORING OF MUTATIONS

Despite the benefit of imatinib over prior treatments, some patients may develop resistance,[62] with a reported annual relapse rate of 1–4% in newly diagnosed patients in chronic phase with the incidence decreasing over time.[63] In fact, during the 4th and the 5th year of follow-up on the IRIS trial, less than 1% of patients lost response per year. Multiple mechanisms of resistance to imatinib, BCR-ABL dependent and BCR-ABL independent, have been identified; one of the best characterized is owing to mutations in the BCR-ABL kinase domain. Mutations have been detected in 30–50% of patients who develop imatinib resistance.[64] Clinically relevant mutations disrupt critical contact points between imatinib and BCR-ABL or may favor the active conformation of BCR-ABL, to which imatinib is unable to bind.[62,65] Numerous BCR-ABL mutations have been identified. Not all mutations have the same biochemical and clinical properties: some BCR-ABL mutations result in a highly resistant phenotype *in vitro*; others are still relatively sensitive to imatinib and resistance may potentially be overcome by an increase in dose of imatinib.[64,66–69] The T315I mutation and some mutations affecting the so-called P-loop of BCR-ABL confer a greater level of resistance to imatinib and to the novel tyrosine kinase inhibitors.[51,70] Kinase domain mutation screening for patients in chronic phase is indicated in cases of hematological or cytogenetic resistance/relapse,[51] or if there is an increase in BCR-ABL : ABL transcript ratio of at least 0.5–1 log.[71] Kinase domain mutations should be investigated in any patients presenting in advanced phase disease. Although mutations have been detected in occasional patients with advanced phases prior to therapy with imatinib, they have never been found in patients with chronic phase at the time of diagnosis.

NOVEL APPROACHES TO OVERCOME RESISTANCE

Novel more potent tyrosine kinase inhibitors have been developed to overcome imatinib resistance.[72] Dasatinib, an orally bioavailable dual BCR-ABL and SRC inhibitor, is now approved for the treatment of CML and Ph-positive acute lymphoblastic leukemia after imatinib failure.[73] Nilotinib is an oral potent and selective BCR-ABL inhibitor in advanced clinical trials.[74] Both of these agents have shown significant activity in patients who have failed imatinib therapy and studies in early chronic phase have been initiated (Table 5.2). Preliminary results in 14 patients with newly diagnosed CML treated with nilotinib 400 mg twice daily as first-line of therapy were recently reported.[75] Major cytogenetic response was observed in all patients at 3 months (complete in 13 and partial in one), and all seven

Table 5.2 Response to therapy in patients with newly diagnosed chronic myeloid leukemia in chronic phase

Response at 3 months	*Imatinib 400 mg/day (n = 49)*	*Imatinib 800 mg/day (n = 202)*	*Nilotinib (n = 14)*	*Dasatinib (n = 27)*
MCyR (%)	73	90	100	81
CCyR (%)	37	61	93	73

MCyR, major cytogenetic response; CCyR, complete cytogenetic response.

evaluable patients were in complete cytogenetic response at 6 months. Major molecular response rates at 6 and 9 months were significantly higher with nilotinib compared with historical data with standard-dose imatinib.[75] In another phase II study in newly diagnosed CML-CP, 24 patients received dasatinib 100 mg once daily or 50 mg twice daily. The complete cytogenetic response rates at 6 and 9 months were 73% and 95%, respectively, which are significantly better than results with historical data in patients treated with standard-dose imatinib.[76]

These studies are still ongoing, and others including randomized trials comparing these agents with imatinib, and studies of yet another new agent, bosutinib as first line of therapy are being initiated.

IMMUNOTHERAPY AND RESIDUAL DISEASE

The observation of a graft versus leukemia effect following alloSCT suggests that immunotherapy aimed at CML is an approach worth investigating. An effective immune modulation approach could potentially eliminate the leukemic stem cell, and could be a strategy that might be pursued in order to allow safe discontinuation of therapy with imatinib if such immune modulation could prevent the disease from recurring.

Because the BCR-ABL fusion protein represents a unique tumor-specific antigen, vaccination using peptides based on the BCR-ABL junction point may be useful, especially in reducing residual disease levels after maximal responses to imatinib have been achieved.[77,78] Two recent clinical studies of vaccination, using peptides derived from the BCR-ABL fusion region, have demonstrated that patients develop a functional immune response to these peptides.[79,80] In one study, vaccination of nine patients who had achieved stable but incomplete cytogenetic responses (median Ph-positive level 10%) on imatinib resulted in improved cytogenetic response, including complete cytogenetic response, in five patients. Three patients also achieved complete molecular response. Additional studies with this vaccine are ongoing. Other vaccines have also shown promising results. These include PR1, a nonapeptide derived from proteinase 3 and able to induce immunological, and in some instances clinical responses.[81] Also, a K562 cell genetically engineered to secrete granulocyte-macrophage colony-stimulating factor (GM-CSF) has also shown early encouraging results. Polyethylene glycolated interferon has also been used as a means of non-specific immune stimulation with little success to date.[82,83] The role of these and other immune modulating approaches in eliminating residual disease and potentially allowing permanent treatment discontinuation is still debatable.

CONCLUSION

The introduction of imatinib has marked an important and revolutionary step in the management of CML. The long-term outcomes after 5 years of follow-up are very favorable, and suggest a major change in the history of the disease. Current and future studies are exploring the role of high-dose imatinib and the new tyrosine kinase inhibitors as first-line therapy in CML to further improve the long-term outcome. Long-term treatment of CML may require a combination of tyrosine kinase inhibitors, and possibly compounds with other mechanisms of action, both conventional and targeted. Vaccines to stimulate patient immunity may control and eliminate residual disease. With these strategies, the treatment prospects of patients with CML are very hopeful.

REFERENCES

1. Jemal A, Siegel R, Ward E et al. Cancer statistics, 2006. CA Cancer J Clin 2006; 56: 106–30.
2. Faderl S, Talpaz M, Estrov Z et al. The biology of chronic myeloid leukemia. N Engl J Med 1999; 341: 164–72.
3. Faderl S, Kantarjian HM, Talpaz M. Chronic myelogenous leukemia: update on biology and treatment. Oncology (Williston Park) 1999; 13: 169–80.
4. Chronic Myeloid Leukemia Trialists' Collaborative Group. Interferon alfa versus chemotherapy for

chronic myeloid leukemia: a meta-analysis of seven randomized trials. J Natl Cancer Inst 1997; 89: 1616–20.
5. Guilhot F, Chastang C, Michallet M et al. Interferon alfa-2b combined with cytarabine versus interferon alone in chronic myelogenous leukemia. French Chronic Myeloid Leukemia Study Group. N Engl J Med 1997; 337: 223–9.
6. Kantarjian HM, O'Brien S, Smith TL et al. Treatment of Philadelphia chromosome-positive early chronic phase chronic myelogenous leukemia with daily doses of interferon alpha and low-dose cytarabine. J Clin Oncol 1999; 17: 284–92.
7. Hehlmann R, Berger U, Pfirrmann M et al. Drug treatment is superior to allografting as first-line therapy in chronic myeloid leukemia. Blood 2007; 109: 4686–92.
8. Kantarjian H, Sawyers C, Hochhaus A et al. Hematologic and cytogenetic responses to imatinib mesylate in chronic myelogenous leukemia. N Engl J Med 2002; 346: 645–52.
9. Kantarjian HM, Cortes JE, O'Brien S et al. Long-term survival benefit and improved complete cytogenetic and molecular response rates with imatinib mesylate in Philadelphia chromosome-positive chronic-phase chronic myeloid leukemia after failure of interferon-alpha. Blood 2004; 104: 1979–88.
10. O'Brien SG, Guilhot F, Larson RA et al. Imatinib compared with interferon and low-dose cytarabine for newly diagnosed chronic-phase chronic myeloid leukemia. N Engl J Med 2003; 348: 994–1004.
11. Kantarjian H, Talpaz M, O'Brien S et al. High-dose imatinib mesylate therapy in newly diagnosed Philadelphia chromosome-positive chronic phase chronic myeloid leukemia. Blood 2004; 103: 2873–78.
12. Cortes J, Talpaz M, O'Brien S et al. Molecular responses in patients with chronic myelogenous leukemia in chronic phase treated with imatinib mesylate. Clin Cancer Res 2005; 11: 3425–32.
13. Hughes TP, Kaeda J, Branford S et al. Frequency of major molecular responses to imatinib or interferon alfa plus cytarabine in newly diagnosed chronic myeloid leukemia. N Engl J Med 2003; 349: 1423–32.
14. Sokal JE, Cox EB, Baccarani M et al. Prognostic discrimination in "good-risk" chronic granulocytic leukemia. Blood 1984; 63: 789–99.
15. O'Brien S, Kantarjian H, Talpaz M. Practical guidelines for the management of chronic myelogenous leukemia with interferon alpha. Leuk Lymphoma 1996; 23: 247.
16. Kantarjian HM, O'Brien S, Cortes JE et al. Complete cytogenetic and molecular responses to interferon-alpha-based therapy for chronic myelogenous leukemia are associated with excellent long-term prognosis. Cancer 2003; 97: 1033–41.
17. Hochhaus A, Reiter A, Saussele S et al. Molecular heterogeneity in complete cytogenetic responders after interferon-alpha therapy for chronic myelogenous leukemia: low levels of minimal residual disease are associated with continuing remission. German CML Study Group and the UK MRC CML Study Group. Blood 2000; 95: 62–6.
18. Molldrem JJ, Lee PP, Wang C et al. Evidence that specific T lymphocytes may participate in the elimination of chronic myelogenous leukemia. Nat Med 2000; 6: 1018–23.
19. Michallet M, Maloisel F, Delain M et al. PEG-Intron CML Study Group. Pegylated recombinant interferon alpha-2b vs recombinant interferon alpha-2b for the initial treatment of chronic-phase chronic myelogenous leukemia: a phase III study. Leukemia 2004; 18: 309–15.
20. Buchdunger E, Zimmermann J, Mett H et al. Inhibition of the Abl protein-tyrosine kinase in vitro and in vivo by a 2-phenylaminopyrimidine derivative. Cancer Res 1996; 56: 100–4.
21. Buchdunger E, Cioffi CL, Law N et al. Abl protein-tyrosine kinase inhibitor STI571 inhibits in vitro signal transduction mediated by c-kit and platelet-derived growth factor receptors. J Pharmacol Exp Ther 2000; 295: 139–45.
22. Okuda K, Weisberg E, Gilliland DG, Griffin JD. ARG tyrosine kinase activity is inhibited by STI571. Blood 2001; 97: 2440–8.
23. Heinrich MC, Blanke CD, Druker BJ, Corless CL. Inhibition of KIT tyrosine kinase activity: a novel molecular approach to the treatment of KIT-positive malignancies. J Clin Oncol 2002; 20: 1692–703.
24. Dewar AL, Cambareri AC, Zannettino AC et al. Macrophage colony-stimulating factor receptor c-fms is a novel target of imatinib. Blood 2005; 105: 3127–32.
25. Goldman JM, Melo JV. Chronic myeloid leukemia–advances in biology and new approaches to treatment. N Engl J Med 2003; 349: 1451–64.
26. Ren R. Mechanisms of BCR-ABL in the pathogenesis of chronic myelogenous leukaemia. Nat Rev Cancer 2005; 5: 172–83.
27. Druker BJ, Guilhot F, O'Brien S et al. Five-year follow-up of patients receiving imatinib for chronic myeloid leukemia. N Engl J Med 2006; 355: 2408–17.
28. Baccarani M, Saglio G, Goldman J et al. Evolving concepts in the management of chronic myeloid leukemia: recommendations from an expert panel on behalf of the European LeukemiaNet. Blood 2006; 108: 1809–20.
29. Kantarjian HM, Talpaz M, O'Brien S et al. Survival benefit with imatinib mesylate versus interferon-α-based regimens in newly diagnosed chronic-phase chronic myelogenous leukemia. Blood 2006; 108: 1835–40.

30. Roy L, Guilhot J, Krahnke T et al. Survival advantage from imatinib compared with the combination interferon-α plus cytarabine in chronic-phase chronic myelogenous leukemia: historical comparison between two phase 3 trials. Blood 2006; 108: 1478–84.
31. Kantarjian H, Talpaz M, O'Brien S et al. Survival benefit with imatinib mesylate therapy in patients with accelerated-phase chronic myelogenous leukemia—comparison with historic experience. Cancer 2005; 103: 2099–108.
32. Druker BJ, Talpaz M, Resta DJ et al. Efficacy and safety of a specific inhibitor of the BCR-ABL tyrosine kinase in chronic myeloid leukemia. N Engl J Med 2001; 344: 1031–7.
33. Peng B, Hayes M, Resta D et al. Pharmacokinetics and pharmacodynamics of imatinib in a phase I trial with chronic myeloid leukemia patients. J Clin Oncol 2004; 22: 935–42.
34. Schmidli H, Peng B, Riviere GJ et al. Population pharmacokinetics of imatinib mesylate in patients with chronic-phase chronic myeloid leukaemia: results of a phase III study. Br J Clin Pharmacol 2005; 60: 35–44.
35. Sawyers CL, Hochhaus A, Feldman E et al. Imatinib induces hematologic and cytogenetic responses in patients with chronic myelogenous leukemia in myeloid blast crisis: results of a phase II study. Blood 2002; 99: 3530–9.
36. Talpaz M, Silver RT, Druker BJ et al. Imatinib induces durable hematologic and cytogenetic responses in patients with accelerated phase chronic myeloid leukemia: results of a phase 2 study. Blood 2002; 99: 1928–37.
37. Silver RT, Talpaz M, Sawyers CL et al. Four years of follow-up of 1027 patients with late chronic phase (L-CP), accelerated phase (AP), or blast crisis (BC) chronic myeloid leukemia (CML) treated with imatinib in three large phase II trials. Blood 2004; 104: 11a.
38. Kantarjian H, Talpaz M, O'Brien S et al. Dose escalation of imatinib mesylate can overcome resistance to standard-dose therapy in patients with chronic myelogenous leukemia. Blood 2003; 101: 473–5.
39. Cortes J, Giles F, O'Brien S et al. Result of high-dose imatinib mesylate in patients with Philadelphia chromosome-positive chronic myeloid leukemia after failure of interferon-α. Blood 2003; 102: 83–6.
40. Hughes TP, Branford S, Matthews J et al. Trial of higher dose imatinib with selective intensification in newly diagnosed CML patients in chronic phase. Blood 2003; 102: 31a.
41. Cortes J, Giles F, Salvado A et al. High-dose (HD) imatinib in patients with previously untreated chronic myeloid leukemia (CML) in early chronic phase (CP): preliminary results of a multicenter community based trial. J Clin Oncol 2005; 23: 564a.
42. Rosti G, Martinelli G, Castagnetti F et al. Imatinib 800 mg: preliminary results of a phase II trial of the GIMEMA CML working party in intermediate Sokal risk patients and status-of-the-art of an ongoing multinational, prospective randomized trial of imatinib standard dose (400 mg daily) vs high dose (800 mg daily) in high Sokal risk patients. Blood 2005; 106: 320a.
43. Aoki E, Kantarjian H, O'Brien S et al. High-dose (HD) imatinib provides better responses in patients with untreated early chronic phase (CP) chronic myeloid leukemia (CML). Blood 2006; 108: 608a.
44. Cortes J, Giles F, Salvado A et al. High-dose (HD) imatinib in patients with previously untreated chronic myeloid leukemia (CML) in early chronic phase (CP): preliminary results of a multicenter community based trial. J Clin Oncol 2005; 23: 564a.
45. Hughes TP, Deininger MW, Hochhaus A et al. Monitoring CML patients responding to treatment with tyrosine kinase inhibitors: review and recommendations for harmonizing current methodology for detecting BCR-ABL transcripts and kinase domain mutations and for expressing results. Blood 2006; 108: 28–37.
46. Quintas-Cardama A, Kantarjian H, O'Brien S et al. Granulocyte-colony-stimulating factor (filgrastim) may overcome imatinib-induced neutropenia in patients with chronic-phase chronic myelogenous leukemia. Cancer 2004; 100: 2592–7.
47. Ault P, Kantarjian H, Welch MA et al. Interleukin 11 may improve thrombocytopenia associated with imatinib mesylate therapy in chronic myelogenous leukemia. Leuk Res 2004; 28: 613–18.
48. Cortes J, O'Brien S, Quintas A et al. Erythropoietin is effective in improving the anemia induced by imatinib mesylate therapy in patients with chronic myeloid leukemia in chronic phase. Cancer 2004; 100: 2396–402.
49. Kerkela R, Grazette L, Yacobi R et al. Cardiotoxicity of the cancer therapeutic agent imatinib mesylate. Nat Med 2006; 12: 908–16.
50. Atallah E, Durand JB, Kantarjian H, Cortes J. Congestive heart failure is a rare event in patients receiving imatinib therapy. Blood 2007; 110: 1233–7.
51. Hughes TP, Deininger MW, Hochhaus A et al. Monitoring CML patients responding to treatment with tyrosine kinase inhibitors: review and recommendations for harmonizing current methodology for detecting BCR-ABL transcripts and kinase domain mutations and for expressing results. Blood 2006; 108: 28–37.
52. Cortes J, O'Brien S, Kantarjian H. Discontinuation of imatinib therapy after achieving a molecular response. Blood 2004; 104: 2204–5.
53. Mauro MJ, Druker BJ, Maziarz RT. Divergent clinical outcome in two CML patients who discontinued

imatinib therapy after achieving a molecular remission. Leuk Res 2004; 28: 71–3.
54. Ghanima W, Kahrs J, Dahl TG 3rd, Tjonnfjord GE. Sustained cytogenetic response after discontinuation of imatinib mesylate in a patient with chronic myeloid leukaemia. Eur J Haematol 2004; 72: 441–3.
55. Rousselot P, Huguet F, Rea D et al. Imatinib mesylate discontinuation in patients with chronic myelogenous leukaemia in complete molecular remission for more than two years. Blood 2007; 109: 61–4.
56. Loriaux M, Deininger M. Clonal cytogenetic abnormalities in Philadelphia chromosome negative cells in chronic myeloid leukemia patients treated with imatinib. Leuk Lymphoma 2004; 45: 2197–203.
57. Fayad L, Kantarjian H, O'Brien S et al. Emergence of new clonal abnormalities following interferon-alpha induced complete cytogenetic response in patients with chronic myeloid leukemia: report of three cases. Leukemia 1997; 11: 767–71.
58. Medina J, Kantarjian H, Talpaz M et al. Chromosomal abnormalities in Philadelphia chromosome-negative metaphases appearing during imatinib mesylate therapy in patients with Philadelphia chromosome-positive chronic myelogenous leukemia in chronic phase. Cancer 2003; 98: 1905–11.
59. Bumm T, Muller C, Al-Ali HK et al. Emergence of clonal cytogenetic abnormalities in Ph- cells in some CML patients in cytogenetic remission to imatinib but restoration of polyclonal hematopoiesis in the majority. Blood 2003; 101: 1941–9.
60. Jabbour E, Kantarjian H, O'Brien S et al. Chromosomal abnormalities in Philadelphia chromosome (Ph)-negative metaphases appearing during imatinib mesylate therapy in patients with newly diagnosed chronic myeloid leukemia in chronic phase. Blood 2007; 110: 2991–5.
61. Kovitz C, Kantarjian H, Garcia-Manero G, Abruzzo LV, Cortes J. Myelodysplastic syndromes and acute leukemia developing after imatinib mesylate therapy for chronic myeloid leukemia. Blood 2006; 108: 2811–3.
62. Shah NP. Loss of response to imatinib: mechanisms and management. Hematology Am Soc Hematol Educ Program 2005: 183–7.
63. Hochhaus A, Hughes T. Clinical resistance to imatinib: mechanisms and implications. Hematol Oncol Clin North Am 2004; 18: 641–56.
64. Hochhaus A, Kreil S, Corbin AS et al. Molecular and chromosomal mechanisms of resistance to imatinib (STI571) therapy. Leukemia 2002; 16: 2190–6.
65. Deininger M, Buchdunger E, Druker BJ. The development of imatinib as a therapeutic agent for chronic myeloid leukemia. Blood 2005; 105: 2640–53.
66. Shah NP, Nicoll JM, Nagar B et al. Multiple BCR-ABL kinase domain mutations confer polyclonal resistance to the tyrosine kinase inhibitor imatinib (STI571) in chronic phase and blast crisis chronic myeloid leukemia. Cancer Cell 2002; 2: 117–25.
67. von Bubnoff N, Schneller F, Peschel C, Duyster J. BCR-ABL gene mutations in relation to clinical resistance of Philadelphia-chromosome-positive leukaemia to STI571: a prospective study. Lancet 2002; 359: 487–91.
68. Corbin AS, Buchdunger E, Pascal F, Druker BJ. Analysis of the structural basis of specificity of inhibition of the Abl kinase by STI571. J Biol Chem 2002; 277: 32214–19.
69. Azam M, Latek RR, Daley GQ et al. Mechanisms of autoinhibition and STI-571/imatinib resistance revealed by mutagenesis of BCR-ABL. Cell 2003; 112: 831–43.
70. Jabbour E, Kantarjian H, Jones D et al. Frequency and clinical significance of BCR-ABL mutations in patients with chronic myeloid leukemia treated with imatinib mesylate. Leukemia 2006; 20: 1767–73.
71. Branford S, Rudzki Z, Parkinson I et al. Real-time quantitative PCR analysis can be used as a primary screen to identify patients with CML treated with imatinib who have BCR-ABL kinase domain mutations. Blood 2004; 104: 2926–32.
72. Jabbour E, Cortes JE, Giles FJ, O'Brien S, Kantarjian HM. Current and emerging treatment options in chronic myeloid leukemia. Cancer 2007; 109: 2171–81.
73. Talpaz M, Shah NP, Kantarjian H et al. Dasatinib in imatinib-resistant Philadelphia chromosome-positive leukemias. N Engl J Med 2006; 354: 2531–41.
74. Kantarjian H, Giles F, Wunderle L et al. Nilotinib in imatinib-resistant CML and Philadelphia chromosome-positive ALL. N Engl J Med 2006; 354: 2542–51.
75. Jabbour E, Cortes J, Giles F et al. Preliminary activity of AMN107, a novel potent oral selective BCR-ABL tyrosine kinase inhibitor, in newly diagnosed Philadelphia chromosome (Ph)-positive chronic phase chronic myelogenous leukaemia (CML-CP). Blood 2006; 108: 616a.
76. Cortes J, O'Brien S, Jones D et al. Dasatinib in patients with previously untreated chronic myeloid leukemia in chronic phase. Blood 2006; 108: 613a.
77. Pinilla-Ibarz J, Cathcart K, Scheinberg DA. CML vaccines as a paradigm of the specific immunotherapy of cancer. Blood Rev 2000; 14: 111–20.
78. Quintas-Cardama A, Cortes J. Chronic myeloid leukemia: diagnosis and treatment. Mayo Clin Proc 2006; 81: 973–88.

79. Cathcart K, Pinilla-Ibarz J, Korontsvit T et al. A multivalent bcr-abl fusion peptide vaccination trial in patients with chronic myeloid leukemia. Blood 2004; 103: 1037–42.
80. Bocchia M, Gentili S, Abruzzese E et al. Effect of a p210 multipeptide vaccine associated with imatinib or interferon in patients with chronic myeloid leukaemia and persistent residual disease: a multicenter observational trial. Lancet 2005; 365: 657–62.
81. Qazilbash MH, Thall PF, Wang X et al. PR1 peptide vaccination for patients with myeloid leukemias. J Clin Oncol 2007; 25(18s): 361, abstract 7017.
82. Smith BD, Kasamon YL, Miller CB et al. K562/GM-CSF Vaccination reduces tumor burden, including achieving molecular remissions, in chronic myeloid leukemia (CML) patients with residual disease on imatinib mesylate (IM). Blood 2005; 106: 801a.
83. Quintas-Cardama A, Kantarjian HM, Ravandi F et al. Immune modulation of minimal residual disease (MRD) in patients (pts) with chronic myelogenous leukemia (CML) in early chronic phase (CP): a randomized trial of first-line high-dose (HS) imatinib mesylate (IM) with or without pegylated-Interferon (PEG-IFN) and GM-CSF. Blood 2006; 108: 626a.

Chronic myeloid leukemia: new targeted therapies

6

Elias Jabbour, Jorge Cortes, Hagop M Kantarjian

INTRODUCTION

Chronic myeloid leukemia (CML) is a progressive, often fatal, hematopoietic neoplasm characterized by the malignant expansion of pluripotent stem cells in the bone marrow. The disease comprises three clinically recognized phases – chronic, accelerated, and blastic – although not all patients follow the classic three-phase course described.[1] The initial chronic phase is typically indolent and often asymptomatic; in half of patients the disease progresses directly from the chronic to the blastic phase.[1] The biology of CML has been extensively reviewed.[2–5]

CML was the first neoplastic disease for which a direct chromosomal link was found. CML represents an important model for the development of targeted therapies in cancer, because a single oncogene is responsible for initiating the disease process.[4] Cytogenetically, CML is characterized in 95% of patients by the presence of the Philadelphia chromosome (Ph), a truncated derivative of chromosome 22 that arises following translocation of genetic material between this chromosome and chromosome 9 (t[9;22][q34;q11]).[6] The resulting fusion gene, *BCR-ABL* (breakpoint cluster region–Abelson murine leukemia viral proto-oncogene) codes for an abnormal, non-membrane-bound oncoprotein (p210 *BCR-ABL*). The oncoprotein is a constitutively active tyrosine kinase that perturbs numerous signal transduction pathways, resulting in uncontrolled cell proliferation and reduced apoptosis, or programmed cell death.[1,7] Signal transduction pathways activated by BCR-ABL may be important targets for new therapies and include Ras/Raf/mitogen activated protein kinase (MAPK),[8–13] phosphatidylinositol 3 kinase,[14–18] STAT5/Janus kinase,[19–24] and Myc.[25–28] Activation of specific signaling pathways by BCR-ABL is mediated via SRC family kinases, which may also represent a therapeutic target.[8,29] The pathogenesis of evolution from chronic phase to advanced phases of CML is not fully understood.[1] Acquisition of the *BCR-ABL* fusion gene increases the propensity of the Ph-positive clone to acquire additional genetic changes. Moreover, the *BCR-ABL* gene may acquire new mutations that allow an already genetically unstable phenotype to acquire further changes. Common gene mutations in the evolution from chronic phase to blastic phase involve the p53 gene,[30] loss of p16, INK41/arf EXON 2,[31,32] and RB.[33] Mutations can also be critical in the development of treatment resistance. Acquisition and expansion of CML clones with mutations in the ATP phosphate-binding loop (P-loop) of the kinase domain may be associated with an increased risk of disease progression and early mortality in patients treated with imatinib mesylate.[34–36] This review describes the novel treatment strategies for patients who cannot obtain benefit from imatinib because of resistance or intolerance.

IMATINIB RESISTANCE

Incidence

The incidence of primary resistance (patients who never respond to imatinib) and secondary resistance (patients who become resistant after an initial response) increases with more advanced phases of CML. For example, in a 4.5-year follow-up of patients with chronic, accelerated, or blastic phase CML (total n = 300),[37] primary resistance occurred in 3%, 9%, and 51% of patients (failure to achieve a complete hematological response), respectively. Secondary resistance (hematological recurrence) was noted in 22%, 32%, and 41% of patients, respectively.[37]

The recent IRIS trial update described the discontinuation of treatment with imatinib in patients with CML.[38] At 5 years, 171 out of 553 patients (31%) had discontinued treatment with first-line imatinib. Treatment was discontinued for the following reasons: side-effects (i.e. imatinib intolerance)/non-CML related deaths 6% (n = 32); lack of efficacy/progression (i.e. imatinib resistance) 11% (n = 60); crossed-over to interferon alfa/cytarabine then discontinued 3% (n = 14); and 'other' reasons 12% (n = 65). Recently, imatinib failure has been defined based on hematological and cytogenetic responses at set time points as well as on progression and signs of warning.[39] Thus, there is a need to overcome imatinib resistance in CML.

Mechanisms of imatinib resistance

Several mechanisms of resistance to imatinib, BCR-ABL dependent and BCR-ABL independent, have been identified and are discussed below.

BCR-ABL-dependent mechanisms of resistance

Gene amplification resulting in increased expression of *BCR-ABL* may account for a small proportion of cases resistant to imatinib.[40,41] *BCR-ABL* gene mutations are noted in 30–50% of patients with imatinib resistance. Clinically relevant mutations disrupt critical contact points between imatinib and BCR-ABL or induce a transition from the inactive to the active configuration, to which imatinib is unable to bind.[27,30] Numerous *BCR-ABL* mutations have been identified. Not all mutations have the same biochemical and clinical properties: some result in a highly resistant phenotype *in vitro*; others are relatively sensitive; and resistance may be overcome by imatinib dose increase.[8,31–34] The T315I mutation and some mutations affecting the so-called P-loop of BCR-ABL confer a greater level of resistance to imatinib and to the novel tyrosine kinase inhibitors.[35,36,42]

BCR-ABL-independent mechanisms of resistance

Resistance to imatinib may result from decreased intracellular drug concentrations, either caused by drug efflux proteins,[43,44] or by binding to plasma proteins.[45,46] Clonal evolution might also contribute to imatinib resistance.[41] The exact contribution of such mechanisms to resistance is unclear at present.

Recently, the role of SRC family kinases has attracted particular interest in understanding imatinib resistance in CML.[47–49] BCR-ABL activates multiple signal transduction pathways normally associated with growth, survival, and differentiation of hematopoietic cells. Tyrosine phosphorylation is a critical step in this activation. BCR-ABL itself has a constitutively active tyrosine kinase domain. It may also initiate signaling by activating other non-receptor tyrosine kinases, including members of the SRC family.[50–53]

Overexpression and activation of the SRC family kinases (LYN) have been reported in imatinib-resistant CML cell lines.[48,49] Blood cell lysates from imatinib-resistant patients also contained high levels of LYN protein.[48]

Overcoming imatinib resistance

Several approaches have been investigated to overcome or prevent the development of resistance to imatinib. These include (1) high-dose imatinib, (2) new more potent tyrosine kinase inhibitors, which would also be less susceptible to mutation-induced mechanisms of resistance, (3) imatinib combinations, and (4) non-tyrosine kinase inhibitors. The first of the newer-generation tyrosine kinase inhibitors, dasatinib (Sprycel®; BMS-354825), an orally bioavailable dual BCR-ABL and SRC inhibitor, has been recently approved by the Food and Drug Administration (FDA) for the treatment of CML post-imatinib failure. Nilotinib (Tasigna®; AMN-107) is another oral more potent and selective BCR-ABL inhibitor awaiting approval. Bosutinib and others are in advanced clinical trials. Other strategies include vaccines and investigational approaches.

High-dose imatinib

As the phase I clinical study of imatinib did not identify a maximum tolerated dose for imatinib, dose escalation beyond the standard 400 mg/day is a potential strategy for addressing some forms of suboptimal response or secondary resistance to imatinib.[54] In a study of 54 patients whose CML had met criteria for non-responsiveness to standard-dose imatinib or had relapsed after a course of imatinib, treatment was initiated with imatinib at 600 or 800 mg/day. Among 20 patients unresponsive to standard-dose imatinib, 13 (65%) achieved a hematological response (nine achieved a complete hematological response); however, only one achieved a major cytogenetic response. Among 34 patients with cytogenetic resistance or relapse, 13 (38%) achieved a major cytogenetic response (six complete).

The ability of higher doses of imatinib to improve responses in patients with primary or secondary imatinib resistance raises the question of whether imatinib should be initiated at a higher dose in newly diagnosed CML. Investigators from our institution compared outcome of patients with newly diagnosed CML treated high-dose imatinib with historical matched cohorts of patients treated with standard dose.[55] Patients treated with high-dose imatinib had higher rates of complete cytogenetic response (91% versus 76%, $p = 0.002$); these occurred earlier, with 88% achieving this response after 6 months of therapy versus 56% with standard dose ($p < 0.00001$). The cumulative incidences of major molecular response and complete molecular response were significantly better with high-dose imatinib.[40] Progression-free and transformation-free survival were also better in the high-dose group ($p = 0.02$ and $p = 0.005$).[55]

The ability of higher doses of imatinib to elicit responses in patients refractory to or relapsed from previous therapy suggests that dose escalation represents a feasible second-line alternative. Dose escalation is likely to be effective in a subset of patients in whom imatinib resistance is mainly owing to either BCR-ABL overexpression or BCR-ABL mutations resulting in only partial resistance,[56] and in patients who previously achieved a prior cytogenetic response and lost it. Thus, alternative treatment options are still required.

DASATINIB

Dasatinib is a newly approved, potent, oral multitargeted kinase inhibitor of five critical oncogenic enzymes, BCR-ABL, SRC, c-KIT, platelet-derived growth factor receptor, and ephrin A receptor kinases.[57] It has 325-fold greater potency compared with imatinib against cells expressing wild-type BCR-ABL, and was effective against all imatinib-resistant kinase domain mutations, with the exception of T315I.[58,59] In preclinical studies, dasatinib prolonged survival of mice with BCR-ABL-driven disease, and inhibited proliferation of BCR-ABL-positive marrow progenitor cells from patients with imatinib-sensitive and -resistant CML.[58]

Phase I study

In a phase I dose finding study, dasatinib showed efficacy in all phases of CML.[60] In chronic phase, 35 of the 40 patients (88%) treated achieved a complete hematological response, and 16 (40%) had a major cytogenetic response (33% complete). In advanced phases, the major hematological response (bone marrow blasts <5%) rate was 80% (8/10) in accelerated phase (complete 50%),

Table 6.1 Results of dasatinib phase II studies in chronic myeloid leukemia and Philadelphia chromosome (Ph)-positive acute lymphoblastic leukemia (ALL) after imatinib failure

		Hematological response (%)		*Cytogenetic response (%)*	
Disease phase	*n*	*Major*	*Complete*	*Major*	*Complete*
Chronic	387	91		58	49
Accelerated	174	64	45	37	28
Blastic	157	50	27	38	31
Ph-positive ALL	46	51	35	57	54
Chronic-randomized					
dasatinib	101	92		48	35
high-dose imatinib	49	82		33	16

77% (17/22) in myeloid blastic phase (complete 18%), and 60% (6/10) in lymphoid blastic phase/Ph-positive acute lymphoblastic leukemia (ALL). The overall rates of major and complete cytogenetic responses in advanced disease were 36% (15/42) and 21% (9/42), respectively.

Phase II studies

The phase II studies (SRC-ABL Tyrosine kinase inhibition Activity Research Trials (START)) included four trials evaluating the effects of single-agent dasatinib 70 mg twice daily in imatinib-resistant/-intolerant patients with chronic phase CML (START C),[61] accelerated phase CML (START A),[62] myeloid and lymphoid blastic phase CML (START B),[63] and Ph-positive ALL (START L).[64]

In all 387 patients with chronic phase CML who had either imatinib resistance (n = 288) or intolerance (n = 99) were evaluable. After a median follow-up of 15 months, 80% of patients intolerant of imatinib achieved a major cytogenetic response (75% complete), and 52% of patients resistant to imatinib achieved a major cytogenetic response (40% complete).[61] In another phase II study, patients with chronic phase CML after resistance to standard dose imatinib (400–600 mg/day) were randomized (2 : 1) to dasatinib 70 mg twice daily (n = 101) or high-dose imatinib (n = 49).[65] With a median follow-up of 15 months, 35% of patients treated with dasatinib achieved a complete cytogenetic response compared with 16% of patients treated with imatinib. The difference in response rates was most evident after failure on imatinib 600 mg daily (major cytogenetic response rates 49% versus 24%) but after failure on imatinib 400 mg/day the major cytogenetic response rates were 58% versus 53%, respectively. Progression-free survival was better with dasatinib (estimated 12-month rates 94% versus 70%; p <0.0001). Dasatinib has also shown activity in patients with accelerated and blastic phase CML after imatinib failure. Preliminary results from the first 174 patients treated in accelerated phase showed a major hematological response in 64% of patients (complete in 45%); major cytogenetic response was achieved in 48% of patients.[62] The complete hematological response rates in patients with blastic phase CML and Ph-positive ALL were 27% and 35%, respectively; the major cytogenetic response rates were 38% (31% complete) and 57% (54% complete), respectively (Table 6.1).[63,64]

Safety data

Pooled safety analysis of all six studies showed that dasatinib was well tolerated. Most drug-related serious adverse events were managed with dose interruptions or reductions. Myelosuppression was the most common reason for dose reductions or interruptions. Grade 3–4 thrombocytopenia, neutropenia, and anemia were reported in 50–60% of patients in chronic phase. Non-hematological adverse events were mild to moderate. Pleural effusions were observed in 5–35%; they were severe in 3–15%. These were managed with treatment interruptions/dose reductions, steroids, and diuretics.

Optimizing dose and schedule

The initial phase I trial of dasatinib suggested similar response rates at total daily doses of 100 mg daily or above given in twice daily and once daily schedules. Side-effects appeared to be lower with lower doses and with single dose daily schedules. Based on these observations, 662 patients with CML chronic phase after imatinib failure were randomized to four treatment arms: dasatinib 100 mg once daily ($n = 166$), dasatinib 50 mg twice daily ($n = 166$), dasatinib 140 mg once daily ($n = 163$), or dasatinib 70 mg twice daily ($n = 167$).[66] With a minimum follow-up of 6 months, there was no difference in efficacy in the four arms: complete hematological response rates varied between 87% and 93%, major cytogenetic response rates between 54% and 59%, and complete cytogenetic response rates between 42% and 45%. However, patients receiving dasatinib 100 mg once daily had less pleural effusions ($p = 0.028$), anemia ($p = 0.032$), neutropenia ($p = 0.035$), and thrombocytopenia ($p = 0.001$) than those receiving the other three dose schedules.[66] In patients with advanced stage disease, dasatinib 140 mg once daily was equivalent in activity to 70 mg twice daily, and was associated with a significantly lower incidence of pleural effusion ($p = 0.024$).[67]

First-line therapy

In a phase II study in newly diagnosed CML chronic phase, 24 patients received dasatinib 100 mg once daily or 50 mg twice daily. The complete cytogenetic response rates at 6 and 9 months were 73% and 95%, respectively, and were better than the results with historical data in patients treated with standard- and high-dose imatinib.[68]

NILOTINIB

Nilotinib (AMN107, Novartis, Basel, Switzerland) is an orally administered derivative of imatinib that inhibits BCR-ABL with a 30- to 50-fold greater potency than imatinib.[59] Replacement of the methylpiperazinyl group of imatinib and further rational design to optimize drug-like properties led to the discovery of nilotinib, which has substantially increased binding affinity and selectivity for the ABL kinase compared with imatinib.[69] Similar to imatinib, nilotinib binds BCR-ABL in its inactive conformation. Nilotinib has demonstrated activity against nearly all BCR-ABL mutants tested, although similar to dasatinib (and imatinib), nilotinib is unable to inhibit the T315I mutation.[59,70] Nilotinib inhibits PDGFR and KIT, but to a lower extent than dasatinib. Unlike dasatinib, it does not inhibit the SRC family of kinases.

Phase I study

In a phase I dose escalation study, nilotinib showed anti-CML activity in 119 patients (17 chronic phase, 56 accelerated phase (ten with clonal evolution only), 24 myeloid blastic phase, and 22 lymphoid blastic phase/Ph-positive ALL) with imatinib-resistant CML.[71] Patients received nilotinib at dosages ranging from 50 to 1200 mg/day. Hematological responses were seen in 72% of patients in accelerated phase and in 38% of patients in blastic phase. Cytogenetic response rates ranged from 27% in lymphoid and myeloid blastic phase, to 48% in accelerated phase, and 53% in chronic phase. Nilotinib dosage was escalated up to 1200 mg/day with good tolerance, and the maximum tolerated dose was estimated at 600 mg twice daily. Hematological and cytogenetic responses were similar in patients with or without mutations, and in patients with P-loop or other mutations. The two patients with a T315I mutation did not respond to nilotinib.[71]

Table 6.2 Results of nilotinib phase II studies in chronic myeloid leukemia (CML) and Philadelphia chromosome (Ph)-positive acute lymphoblastic leukemia (ALL) after imatinib failure

			Cytogenetic response	
Disease	*n*	*CHR (%)*	*Major (%)*	*Complete (%)*
CML chronic	280	74	52	34
CML accelerated	64	25	36	22
CML blastic	120	21	NR	NR
Ph-positive ALL	41	24	NR	NR

CHR, complete hematological response.

Phase II studies

The efficacy of nilotinib was confirmed in three ongoing phase II studies in imatinib-resistant or -intolerant patients with CML in chronic, accelerated, and blastic phases. In all 282 patients with chronic phase after imatinib failure were treated with nilotinib 400 mg twice daily. The complete hematological response rate was 74%, the major cytogenetic response rate 52%, and the complete cytogenetic response rate 34%. The estimated 1-year survival rate was 95%. Side-effects were modest, including grade 3–4 myelosuppression in 20–30%; no pleural effusions were observed. Response rates were similar in patients with imatinib resistance versus intolerance and in patients with or without mutations.[72] The activity of nilotinib in CML accelerated and blastic phase after imatinib failure was also encouraging, although response rates were lower and response durations shorter (Table 6.2).[73,74] Among 64 patients in accelerated phase, the hematological response rate was 59% and the major cytogenetic rate 36%. Among 161 patients in blastic phase, the hematological response rate was 33% (complete 21%). Among 41 patients with Ph-positive ALL, the complete hematological response rate was 24%.[74]

Safety data

In all three phase II studies, nilotinib was well tolerated. The rate of grade 3–4 neutropenia was 28% and of thrombocytopenia 29% in chronic phase. Non-hematological side-effects were infrequent and usually grade 1–2. These included fatigue, pruritus, headache, muscle spasms, and gastrointestinal disturbances. Nilotinib was not associated with the common toxic effects seen with imatinib such as fluid retention, edema, cramps, and weight gain, or with pleural effusions. Nilotinib prolonged the QTcF interval in rare patients.

First-line therapy

In preliminary results from 14 patients with newly diagnosed CML treated with nilotinib 400 mg twice daily,[75] a major cytogenetic response was observed in all patients at 3 months (complete in 13 and partial in one); the complete cytogenetic response rate was 100% in all evaluable patients at 6 months ($n = 13$) and 9 months ($n = 11$). Major molecular response rates at 6 and 9 months were significantly higher with nilotinib compared with historical data with standard-dose and high-dose imatinib.[73]

BOSUTINIB

Bosutinib (SKI606), an orally available dual SRC/ABL inhibitor, is 30–200 times more potent than imatinib. It has minimal inhibitory activity against c-KIT and PDGFR (therefore it is expected to produce less myelosuppression and pleural effusions). In a phase I/II study of 69 patients with CML treated after imatinib failure, the complete hematological response rate among 48 patients in chronic phase was

Table 6.3 Results of bosutinib phase I/II study in chronic phase chronic myeloid leukemia after imatinib failure

Response in chronic phase (n = 48)	*Percentage*
Complete hematological response	84
Cytogenetic response	81
major	52
complete	33

84%, and the cytogenetic response rate 81% (major 52%, complete 33%) (Table 6.3).[76] The median follow-up on study was short. Grade 3–4 toxicities were minimal including skin rashes in 6% and thrombocytopenia in 6%. Mild to moderate diarrhea was common at the phase II dose of 500 mg orally daily.

INNO-406

INNO-406 is an orally available, dual ABL/LYN kinase inhibitor that is up to 55 times more potent than imatinib in BCR-ABL cell lines. INNO-406 demonstrated specific SRC kinase activity against LYN kinase. In an ongoing phase I study, INNO-406 was well tolerated in patients at dose ranges of 60 mg daily to 240 mg twice daily. Encouraging activity was noted in imatinib-resistant and nilotinib-intolerant patients, with six out of 14 patients (43%) showing evidence of response.[77]

NON-ATP BINDING TYROSINE KINASE INHIBITORS

MK0457 (Merck) is an aurora kinase inhibitor with selective inhibitory activity against T315I mutant CML. In a preliminary experience involving 11 patients with CML advanced phases and T315I mutations, MK0457 given by intravenous infusion at 8–32 mg/m^2 hourly for 5 days induced responses in five patients: two complete cytogenetic responses, and three partial minor cytogenetic responses.[78] Other aurora kinase inhibitors with potential activity against T315I mutant CML include AT9283 and KW2449.

OTHER THERAPEUTIC APPROACHES

Other approaches are being developed for patients who develop resistance to imatinib. Two orally administered farnesyl transferase inhibitors (tipifarnib, R115777; and lonafarnib, SCH66336) have shown clinical activity both as single agents and in combinations with imatinib in heavily pretreated patients with advanced phase disease.[79–82] Decitabine (5-aza-2′-deoxycytidine) administered to 35 patients with imatinib-resistant CML induced hematological response in 23 patients (66%; 34% complete hematological response) and cytogenetic response in 16 (46%).[83,84] Homoharringtonine may have an additive or synergistic effect with imatinib. In preliminary data of a study administering subcutaneous homoharringtonine to five evaluable patients with CML in chronic phase who had failed imatinib therapy, all achieved a hematological response, and three patients achieved a cytogenetic response.[85]

CONCLUSION

For patients with CML, imatinib represented a significant breakthrough in first-line treatment. Resistance to imatinib monotherapy has emerged as an important clinical challenge. The recent availability of highly potent tyrosine kinase inhibitors, dasatinib and nilotinib, has further broadened the treatment armamentarium against CML. With the advent of novel agents and the combination of tyrosine kinase inhibitors, farnesyl transferase inhibitors, and possibly compounds with other mechanisms of actions, both conventional and targeted, the treatment prospects of patients with CML are very hopeful.

REFERENCES

1. Mughal TI, Goldman JM. Chronic myeloid leukemia: why does it evolve from chronic phase to blast transformation? Front Biosci 2006; 11: 198–208.
2. Hill JM, Meehan KR. Chronic myelogenous leukemia. Curable with early diagnosis and treatment. Postgrad Med 1999; 106: 149–52, 157–9.

3. Faderl S, Talpaz M, Estrov Z, Kantarjian HM. Chronic myelogenous leukemia: biology and therapy. Ann Intern Med 1999; 131: 207–19.
4. Faderl S, Kantarjian HM, Talpaz M. Chronic myelogenous leukemia: update on biology and treatment. Oncology (Williston Park) 1999; 13: 169–80.
5. Pasternak G, Hochhaus A, Schultheis B, Hehlmann R. Chronic myelogenous leukemia: molecular and cellular aspects. J Cancer Res Clin Oncol 1998; 124: 643–60.
6. Barnes DJ, Melo JV. Cytogenetic and molecular genetic aspects of chronic myeloid leukaemia. Acta Haematol 2002; 108: 180–202.
7. Melo JV, Hughes TP, Apperley JF. Chronic myeloid leukemia. Hematology Am Soc Hematol Educ Program 2003: 132–52.
8. Pendergast AM, Quilliam LA, Cripe LD et al. BCR-ABL-induced oncogenesis is mediated by direct interaction with the SH2 domain of the GRB-2 adaptor protein. Cell 1993; 75: 175–85.
9. Puil L, Liu J, Gish G et al. Bcr-Abl oncoproteins bind directly to activators of the Ras signalling pathway. EMBO J 1994; 13: 764–73.
10. Pelicci G, Lanfrancone L, Salcini AE et al. Constitutive phosphorylation of Shc proteins in human tumors. Oncogene 1995; 11: 899–907.
11. Oda T, Heaney C, Hagopian JR et al. Crkl is the major tyrosine-phosphorylated protein in neutrophils from patients with chronic myelogenous leukemia. J Biol Chem 1994; 269: 22925–8.
12. Bhat A, Kolibaba K, Oda T et al. Interactions of CBL with BCR-ABL and CRKL in BCR-ABL-transformed myeloid cells. J Biol Chem 1997; 272: 16170–5.
13. Marais R, Light Y, Paterson HF, Marshall CJ. Ras recruits Raf-1 to the plasma membrane for activation by tyrosine phosphorylation. EMBO J 1995; 14: 3136–45.
14. Skorski T, Kanakaraj P, Nieborowska-Skorska M et al. Phosphatidylinositol-3 kinase activity is regulated by BCR/ABL and is required for the growth of Philadelphia chromosome-positive cells. Blood 1995; 86: 726–36.
15. Skorski T, Bellacosa A, Nieborowska-Skorska M et al. Transformation of hematopoietic cells by BCR/ABL requires activation of a PI-3k/Akt-dependent pathway. EMBO J 1997; 16: 6151–61.
16. Jonuleit T, van der Kuip H, Miething C et al. Bcr-Abl kinase down-regulates cyclin-dependent kinase inhibitor p27 in human and murine cell lines. Blood 2000; 96: 1933–9.
17. Franke TF, Kaplan DR, Cantley LC. PI3K: downstream AKTion blocks apoptosis. Cell 1997; 88: 435–7.
18. Komatsu N, Watanabe T, Uchida M et al. A member of Forkhead transcription factor FKHRL1 is a downstream effector of STI571-induced cell cycle arrest in BCR-ABL-expressing cells. J Biol Chem 2003; 278: 6411–19.
19. Shuai K, Halpern J, ten Hoeve J et al. Constitutive activation of STAT5 by the Bcr-Abl oncogene in chronic myelogenous leukemia. Oncogene 1996; 13: 247–54.
20. Ilaria RL Jr, Van Etten RA. P210 and P190 (BCR/ABL) induce the tyrosine phosphorylation and DNA binding activity of multiple specific STAT family members. J Biol Chem 1996; 271: 31704–10.
21. Frank DA, Varticovski L. BCR/abl leads to the constitutive activation of Stat proteins, and shares an epitope with tyrosine phosphorylated Stats. Leukemia 1996; 10: 1724–30.
22. Klejman A, Schreiner SJ, Nieborowska-Skorska M et al. The Src family kinase Hck couples BCR/ABL to STAT5 activation in myeloid leukemia cells. EMBO J 2002; 21: 5766–74.
23. Horita M, Andreu EJ, Benito A et al. Blockade of the Bcr-Abl kinase activity induces apoptosis of chronic myelogenous leukemia cells by suppressing signal transducer and activator of transcription 5-dependent expression of Bcl-xL. J Exp Med 2000; 191: 977–84.
24. Nieborowska-Skorska M, Hoser G, Kossev P, Wasik MA, Skorski T. Complementary functions of the antiapoptotic protein A1 and serine/threonine kinase pim-1 in the BCR/ABL-mediated leukemogenesis. Blood 2002; 99: 4531–9.
25. Menssen A, Hermeking H. Characterization of the c-MYC-regulated transcriptome by SAGE: identification and analysis of c-MYC target genes. Proc Natl Acad Sci U S A 2002; 99: 6274–9.
26. Sawyers CL, Callahan W, Witte ON. Dominant negative MYC blocks transformation by ABL oncogenes. Cell 1992; 70: 901–10.
27. Afar DE, Goga A, McLaughlin J, Witte ON, Sawyers CL. Differential complementation of Bcr-Abl point mutants with c-Myc. Science 1994; 264: 424–6.
28. Xie S, Wang Y, Liu J et al. Involvement of Jak2 tyrosine phosphorylation in Bcr-Abl transformation. Oncogene 2001; 20: 6188–95.
29. Pendergast AM, Muller AJ, Havlik MH, Maru Y, Witte ON. BCR sequences essential for transformation by the BCR-ABL oncogene bind to the ABL SH2 regulatory domain in a non-phosphotyrosine-dependent manner. Cell 1991; 66: 161–71.
30. Skorski T, Nieborowska-Skorska M, Wlodarski P et al. Blastic transformation of p53-deficient bone marrow cells by p210bcr/abl tyrosine kinase. Proc Natl Acad Sci U S A 1996; 93: 13137–42.
31. Hernandez-Boluda JC, Cervantes F, Colomer D et al. Genomic p16 abnormalities in the progression of chronic myeloid leukemia into blast crisis: a sequential study in 42 patients. Exp Hematol 2003; 31: 204–10.
32. Serrano M, Lee H, Chin L et al. Role of the INK4a locus in tumor suppression and cell mortality. Cell 1996; 85: 27–37.

33. Beck Z, Kiss A, Toth FD et al. Alterations of P53 and RB genes and the evolution of the accelerated phase of chronic myeloid leukemia. Leuk Lymphoma 2000; 38: 587–97.
34. Branford S, Rudzki Z, Walsh S et al. Detection of BCR-ABL mutations in patients with CML treated with imatinib is virtually always accompanied by clinical resistance, and mutations in the ATP phosphate-binding loop (P-loop) are associated with a poor prognosis. Blood 2003; 102: 276–83.
35. Jabbour E, Kantarjian H, Jones D et al. Frequency and clinical significance of BCR-ABL mutations in patients with chronic myeloid leukemia treated with imatinib mesylate. Leukemia 2006; 20: 1767–73.
36. Nicolini FE, Corm S, Le QH et al. Mutation status and clinical outcome of 89 imatinib mesylate-resistant chronic myelogenous leukemia patients: a retrospective analysis from the French intergroup of CML (Fi(phi)-LMC GROUP). Leukemia 2006; 20: 1061–6.
37. Lahaye T, Riehm B, Berger U et al. Response and resistance in 300 patients with BCR-ABL-positive leukemias treated with imatinib in a single center: a 4.5-year follow-up. Cancer 2005; 103: 1659–69.
38. Druker BJ, Guilhot F, O'Brien S et al. Five-year follow-up of patients receiving imatinib for chronic myeloid leukemia. N Engl J Med 2006; 355: 2408–17.
39. Baccarani M, Saglio G, Goldman J et al. Evolving concepts in the management of chronic myeloid leukemia: recommendations from an expert panel on behalf of the European LeukemiaNet. Blood 2006; 108: 1809–20.
40. Gorre ME, Mohammed M, Ellwood K et al. Clinical resistance to STI-571 cancer therapy caused by BCR-ABL gene mutation or amplification. Science 2001; 293: 876–80.
41. Hochhaus A, Kreil S, Corbin AS et al. Molecular and chromosomal mechanisms of resistance to imatinib (STI571) therapy. Leukemia 2002; 16: 2190–6.
42. Soverini S, Martinelli G, Rosti G et al. ABL mutations in late chronic phase chronic myeloid leukemia patients with up-front cytogenetic resistance to imatinib are associated with a greater likelihood of progression to blast crisis and shorter survival: a study by the GIMEMA Working Party on Chronic Myeloid Leukemia. J Clin Oncol 2005; 23: 4100–9.
43. Illmer T, Schaich M, Platzbecker U et al. P-glycoprotein-mediated drug efflux is a resistance mechanism of chronic myelogenous leukemia cells to treatment with imatinib mesylate. Leukemia 2004; 18: 401–8.
44. Thomas J, Wang L, Clark RE, Pirmohamed M. Active transport of imatinib into and out of cells: implications for drug resistance. Blood 2004; 104: 3739–45.
45. Larghero J, Leguay T, Mourah S et al. Relationship between elevated levels of the alpha 1 acid glycoprotein in chronic myelogenous leukemia in blast crisis and pharmacological resistance to imatinib (Gleevec) in vitro and in vivo. Biochem Pharmacol 2003; 66: 1907–13.
46. le Coutre P, Kreuzer KA, Na IK et al. Determination of alpha-1 acid glycoprotein in patients with Ph+ chronic myeloid leukemia during the first 13 weeks of therapy with STI571. Blood Cells Mol Dis 2002; 28: 75–85.
47. Lionberger JM, Wilson MB, Smithgall TE. Transformation of myeloid leukemia cells to cytokine independence by Bcr-Abl is suppressed by kinase-defective Hck. J Biol Chem 2000; 275: 18581–5.
48. Donato NJ, Wu JY, Stapley J et al. BCR-ABL independence and LYN kinase overexpression in chronic myelogenous leukemia cells selected for resistance to STI571. Blood 2003; 101: 690–8.
49. Dai Y, Rahmani M, Corey SJ, Dent P, Grant S. A Bcr/Abl-independent, Lyn-dependent form of imatinib mesylate (STI-571) resistance is associated with altered expression of Bcl-2. J Biol Chem 2004; 279: 34227–39.
50. Danhauser-Riedl S, Warmuth M, Druker BJ, Emmerich B, Hallek M. Activation of Src kinases p53/56lyn and p59hck by p210bcr/abl in myeloid cells. Cancer Res 1996; 56: 3589–96.
51. Warmuth M, Bergmann M, Priess A, Hauslmann K, Emmerich B, Hallek M. The Src family kinase Hck interacts with Bcr-Abl by a kinase-dependent mechanism and phosphorylates the Grb2-binding site of Bcr. J Biol Chem 1997; 272: 33260–70.
52. Ernst TJ, Slattery KE, Griffin JD. p210Bcr/Abl and p160v-Abl induce an increase in the tyrosine phosphorylation of p93c-Fes. J Biol Chem 1994; 269: 5764–9.
53. Lionberger JM, Smithgall TE. The c-FES protein-tyrosine kinase suppresses cytokine-independent outgrowth of myeloid leukaemia cells induced by Bcr-Abl. Cancer Res 2000; 60: 1097–103.
54. Kantarjian HM, Talpaz M, O'Brien S et al. Dose escalation of imatinib mesylate can overcome resistance to standard-dose therapy in patients with chronic myelogenous leukemia. Blood 2003; 101: 473–5.
55. Aoki E, Kantarjian H, O'Brien S et al. High-dose (HD) imatinib provides better responses in patients with untreated early chronic phase (CP) chronic myeloid leukemia (CML). Blood 2006; 108: 605a.
56. Shah NP. Loss of response to imatinib: mechanisms and management. Hematology Am Soc Hematol Educ Program 2005; 183–7.
57. Tokarski JS, Newitt JA, Chang CY et al. The structure of Dasatinib (BMS-354825) bound to activated ABL kinase domain elucidates its inhibitory activity

against imatinib-resistant ABL mutants. Cancer Res 2006; 66: 5790–7.

58. Shah NP, Tran C, Lee FY et al. Overriding imatinib resistance with a novel ABL kinase inhibitor. Science 2004; 305: 399–401.
59. O'Hare T, Walters DK, Stoffregen EP et al. In vitro activity of Bcr-Abl inhibitors AMN107 and BMS-354825 against clinically relevant imatinib-resistant Abl kinase domain mutants. Cancer Res 2005; 65: 4500–5.
60. Talpaz M, Shah NP, Kantarjian H et al. Dasatinib in imatinib-resistant Philadelphia chromosome-positive leukemias. N Engl J Med 2006; 354: 2531–41.
61. Baccarani M, Kantarjian HM, Apperley JF et al. Efficacy of dasatinib (SPRYCEL) in patients (pts) with chronic phase chronic myelogenous leukemia (CP-CML) resistant to or intolerant of imatinib: updated results of the CA180013 START-C phase II study. Blood (ASH Annual Meeting Abstracts) 2006; 108: 53a.
62. Cortes J, Kim DW, Guilhot F et al. Dasatinib (SPRYCEL) in patients (pts) with chronic myelogenous leukemia in accelerated phase (AP-CML) that is imatinib-resistant (im-r) or -intolerant (im-i): updated results of the CA180-005 START-A phase II study. Blood (ASH Annual Meeting Abstracts) 2006; 108: 613a.
63. Martinelli G, Hochhaus A, Coutre S et al. Dasatinib (SPRYCEL) efficacy and safety in patients (pts) with chronic myelogenous leukemia in lymphoid (CML-LB) or myeloid blast (CML-MB) phase who are imatinib-resistant (im-r) or -intolerant (im-i). Blood (ASH Annual Meeting Abstracts) 2006; 108: 224a.
64. Dombret H, Ottman OG, Rosti G et al. Dasatinib (SPRYCEL) in patients (pts) with Philadelphia chromosome-positive acute lymphoblastic leukemia who are imatinib-resistant (im-r) or -intolerant (im-i): updated results from the CA180-015 START-L study. Blood (ASH Annual Meeting Abstracts) 2006; 108: 88a, abstract 286.
65. Kantarjian H, Pasquini R, Hamerschlak N et al. Dasatinib or high-dose imatinib for chronic-phase chronic myeloid leukemia after failure of first-line imatinib: a randomized phase-II trial. Blood 2007; 109: 5143–50.
66. Hochhaus A, Kim DW, Rousselot P et al. Dasatinib (SPRYCEL®) 50 mg or 70 mg BID versus 100 mg or 140mg QD in patients with chronic myeloid leukemia in chronic phase (CML-CP) resistant or intolerant to imatinib: results of the CA180-034 study. Blood (ASH Annual Meeting Abstracts) 2006; 108: 166.
67. Kantarjian H, Ottmann O, Pasquini R et al. Dasatinib (SPRYCEL®) 140 mg once daily (QD) vs 70 mg twice daily (BID) in patients (pts) with advanced phase chonic myeloid leukemia (ABP-CML) or Ph(+) ALL who are resistant or intolerant to imatinib (im): results of the CA180-035 study. Blood (ASH Annual Meeting Abstracts) 2006; 108: 746.
68. Cortes J, O'Brien S, Jones D et al. Dasatinib in patients with previously untreated chronic myeloid leukemia in chronic phase. Blood 2006; 108: 613a.
69. Weisberg E, Manley PW, Breitenstein W et al. Characterization of AMN107, a selective inhibitor of native and mutant Bcr-Abl. Cancer Cell 2005; 7: 129–41.
70. Weisberg E, Manley P, Mestan J et al. AMN107 (nilotinib): a novel and selective inhibitor of BCR-ABL. Br J Cancer 2006; 94: 1765–9.
71. Kantarjian H, Giles F, Wunderle L et al. Nilotinib in imatinib-resistant CML and Philadelphia chromosome-positive ALL. N Engl J Med 2006; 354: 2542–51.
72. Coutre P, Bhalla K, Giles F et al. A phase II study of nilotinib, a novel tyrosine kinase inhibitor administered to imatinib-resistant and -intolerant patients with chronic myelogenous leukemia (CML) in chronic phase (CP). Blood (ASH Annual Meeting Abstracts) 2006; 108: 53a.
73. Kantarjian HM, Gattermann N, Hochhaus A et al. A phase II study of nilotinib a novel tyrosine kinase inhibitor administered to imatinib-resistant or intolerant patients with chronic myelogenous leukemia (CML) in accelerated phase (AP). Blood (ASH Annual Meeting Abstracts) 2006; 108: 615a.
74. Larson R, Ottmann O, Kantarjian H et al. A phase II study of nilotinib administered to imatinib resistant or intolerant patients with chronic myelogenous leukemia (CML) in blast crisis (BC) or relapsed/refractory Ph+ acute lymphoblastic leukemia (ALL). J Clin Oncol 2007; 25: 367s, abstract 7040.
75. Jabbour E, Cortes J, Giles F et al. Preliminary activity of AMN107, a novel potent oral selective Bcr-Abl tyrosine kinase inhibitor, in newly diagnosed Philadelphia chromosome (Ph)-positive chronic phase chronic myelogenous leukaemia (CML-CP). Blood 2006; 108: 616a.
76. Cortes J, Kantarjian HM, Baccarani M et al. A phase 1/2 study of SKI-606, a dual inhibitor of Src and Abl kinases, in adult patients with Philadelphia chromosome positive (Ph+) chronic myelogenous leukemia (CML) or acute lymphocytic leukemia (ALL) relapsed, refractory or intolerant of imatinib. Blood (ASH Annual Meeting Abstracts) 2006; 108: 54a.
77. Craig AR, Kantarjian HM, Cortes JE et al. Phase I study of INNO-406, a dual inhibitor of Abl and Lyn kinases, in adult patients with Philadelphia chromosome positive (Ph+) chronic myelogenous leukemia (CML) or acute lymphocytic leukemia (ALL) relapsed, refractory, or intolerant of imatinib. J Clin Oncol 2007; 25: 368s, abstract 7046.

78. Giles FJ, Cortes JE, Jones D et al. MK-0457, a novel kinase inhibitor, is active in patients with chronic myeloid leukemia or acute lymphocytic leukemia with the T315I BCR-ABL mutation. Blood 2007; 109: 500–2.
79. Cortes J, Albitar M, Thomas D et al. Efficacy of the farnesyl transferase inhibitor R115777 in chronic myeloid leukemia and other hematologic malignancies. Blood 2003; 101: 1692–7.
80. Peters DG, Hoover RR, Gerlash MJ et al. Activity of the farnesyl protein transferase inhibitor SCH66336 against BCR/ABL-induced murine leukemia and primary cells from patients with chronic myeloid leukemia. Blood 2001; 97: 1404–12.
81. Hoover RR, Mahon FX, Melo JV, Daley GQ. Overcoming STI571 resistance with the farnesyl transferase inhibitor SCH66336. Blood 2002; 100: 1068–71.
82. Reichert A, Heisterkamp N, Daley GQ, Groffen J. Treatment of Bcr/Abl-positive acute lymphoblastic leukemia in P190 transgenic mice with the farnesyl transferase inhibitor SCH66336. Blood 2001; 97: 1399–403.
83. Issa JP, Gharibyan V, Cortes J et al. Phase II study of low-dose decitabine in patients with chronic myelogenous leukemia resistant to imatinib mesylate. J Clin Oncol 2005; 23: 3948–56.
84. Kantarjian HM, O'Brien S, Cortes J et al. Results of decitabine (5-aza-2'deoxycytidine) therapy in 130 patients with chronic myelogenous leukemia. Cancer 2003; 98: 522–8.
85. Quintas-Cardama A, Cortes J, Verstovsek S et al. Subcutaneous (SC) homoharringtonine (HHT) for patients (pts) with chronic myelogenous leukemia (CML) in chronic phase (CP) after imatinib mesylate failure. Blood 2005; 106: 4839.

Hematopoietic cell transplantation for chronic myeloid leukemia and myelofibrosis

7

Uday Popat, Sergio Giralt

INTRODUCTION

Myeloproliferative disorders (MPD) are clonal stem cell diseases, which typically include Philadelphia (Ph) chromosome/*BCR-ABL*-positive chronic myeloid leukemia (CML), polycythemia vera, idiopathic myelofibrosis, and essential thrombocytosis. Recently, the World Health Organization proposed that chronic myelomonocytic leukemia (CMML) and atypical CML (CML without evidence of Ph chromosome or BCR-ABL translocation) should also be considered as MPD.[1] Many of these disorders have been shown to arise from chromosomal abnormalities leading to mutations that result in proteins with abnormal tyrosine kinase activity. Ph-positive CML has been the prototype of these disorders, and treatment with specific inhibitors has dramatically altered the natural history of the disease.[2,3] The identification of JAK2 mutations as an important molecular event in the development of other MPD could similarly revolutionize treatment of JAK2+ MPD.[4] Nevertheless, many patients with CML and other MPD will fail to respond to tyrosine kinase inhibitors. For these patients allogeneic hematopoietic stem cell transplantation (HSCT) remains the most effective curative therapy. In this chapter we review the results of HSCT in CML and other MPD, and their current and future role in the treatment of these disorders in the era of tyrosine kinase inhibitors.

ALLOGENEIC TRANSPLANT FOR CHRONIC MYELOID LEUKEMIA

Imatinib has revolutionized the treatment of CML[2,3] and has changed the role of hematopoietic stem cell transplantation, which was once the only curative treatment for CML. Since the advent of imatinib the number of transplants performed for CML has declined.[5,6] Imatinib has now become the first-line therapy for patients with CML, both because of its effectiveness as an orally administered drug and because of its limited side-effects. The best complete cytogenetic response in patients receiving imatinib was 69% at 12 months and 89% at 60 months with overall survival and progression-free survival rates of 89% and 83%, respectively.[7] Thus, the role of HSCT in the treatment of CML needs to be defined in this context.

Allogeneic transplant is a highly efficacious and potentially curative therapy for patients with CML. Its efficacy is as a result of both the graft-versus-leukemia effect and the effect of conditioning chemotherapy. Since the beginning of allogeneic transplant in the early 1980s, stem cells from a variety of sources have been used and the results of transplant have significantly improved.[2,8]

Transplant outcomes have improved over time. The most recent analysis from the European Group for Blood and Marrow Transplantation (EBMT) registry showed that, for all patients, the 2-year overall survival rate improved from 53% to 61% in the most recent years (2000–2003) compared with the years 1980–1990. This improvement was mainly owing to a reduction in transplant-related mortality of from 41% to 30% in all patients and from 31% to 17% in patients with low-risk disease (EBMT risk score of 0–1). These patients with low-risk disease have a 2-year overall survival rate of 80%.[8] Likewise, a recent study from Seattle has shown an 86%

3-year survival rate in young patients (median age, 43 years) with CML in the chronic phase receiving transplants from matched siblings with targeted busulfan and cyclophosphamide (Bu/Cy) conditioning.[9]

In the pre-imatinib era, the outcome after allogeneic transplant was compared with the outcome after interferon-based therapy. In these early studies higher transplant-related mortality negated the benefit of transplant. A retrospective registry study comparing the outcome of patients treated with a HLA-identical sibling transplant and a cohort of patients treated with hydroxyurea or interferon showed a survival advantage for drug therapy in the first 4 years after transplantation. An advantage for transplant was seen only in the 6th year after diagnosis. This benefit was even delayed for patients with low-risk disease.[10] A randomized trial comparing the best-available drug therapy (interferon based) with allogeneic transplant, performed to confirm these earlier results, showed significantly superior survival for patients treated with drug therapy after a median follow-up of 8.9 years. In particular, the overall survival rates at 5 years in the transplant group and interferon-based drug therapy group were 62% and 73%, respectively. This was most pronounced in low-risk patients. However, overall survival at 10 years was similar in both groups, at 53% and 52%, respectively.[11] With advances in transplant technology and more importantly with availability of imatinib, these data are largely of historical interest.

The outcome of patients in the accelerated phase and of patients in blast crisis is much worse, with only a 41% and 18% leukemia-free survival rate, respectively, compared with 57% in patients in the chronic phase, in a registry study of patients who received transplants between 1987 and 1994. This was due in large part to a high risk of relapse of 26% and 58%, respectively,[12] in these two groups of patients. Similar results were noted in a study from Seattle, with a 43% event-free survival rate in patients with accelerated phase disease.[13] However, the survival was better for patients who had accelerated phase disease solely based on cytogenetics criteria than for patients who had accelerated disease based on other criteria (66% versus 34%, respectively).[13] Unfortunately unlike the outcome from transplant in patients with chronic phase CML, the outcome from transplant in patients in the accelerated phase or in blast crisis has changed little in recent years, with the recent EBMT data for patients treated between 2000 and 2003 showing a 47% and 16% 2-year survival rate for patients in the accelerated phase and blast phase, respectively.[2]

For patients without a matched related donor, a matched unrelated-donor (MUD) transplant is an alternative.[14] Early reports of 196 consecutive patients who received transplants procured by the National Marrow Donor Program (NMDP) confirmed the feasibility and efficacy of this approach: the 2-year disease-free survival rates were 45%, 36%, 27%, and 0% in patients who received their transplants in the chronic phase within 1 year of diagnosis, more than 1 year after diagnosis, in the accelerated phase, and in the blast phase, respectively.[15] A further update of NMDP data, in this case for 1423 patients treated over a period of 8.5 years, showed an improved outcome over that reported earlier: the 3-year disease-free survival rate in patients who received their transplants within 1 year of diagnosis had risen to 63%.[16] Subsequently, better results were reported from single centers. For example, in a series of 198 patients who underwent transplantation between May 1985 and December 1994, the overall survival rate was 57% at a median follow-up of 5 years. Factors found in this study to adversely affect survival were an interval from diagnosis to transplant of ≥ 1 year, HLA DRB1 mismatch, and age >50 years. The survival rate was 74% in those with more favorable characteristics, in particular age younger than 50 years and interval from diagnosis to transplant <1 year.[17] With modern HLA typing techniques some single-institution studies have shown similar outcomes in both groups of patients in contrast to earlier studies which in general showed inferior outcomes for unrelated donor recipients.[16–21]

For patients who do not have a HLA-identical related or unrelated donor, a transplant from a haploidentical related donor or from cord blood is an alternative. However, these approaches are associated with a higher treatment-related mortality, but some patients do survive long-term leukemia free.[22–24]

SOURCE OF STEM CELLS: PERIPHERAL BLOOD OR BONE MARROW

In randomized trials and a meta-analysis, peripheral blood stem cell grafts were found to improve disease-free survival and overall survival compared with bone marrow, though at the expense of a higher incidence of chronic graft versus host disease (GVHD) disease in patients receiving transplants from HLA-identical siblings; therefore, it is a preferred stem cell source in this setting.[25,26] The benefit is not so clear in patients receiving a transplant from a matched unrelated donor. In particular, use of a peripheral blood stem cell graft from such donors was associated with earlier engraftment, no difference in the incidence of acute GVHD or risk of relapse, a higher incidence of chronic GVHD, and a better leukemia-free survival rate in patients with advanced CML (33% versus 25%) but lower leukemia-free survival rate in patients in the first chronic phase (41% versus 61%) compared with use of bone marrow.[27,28]

CONDITIONING REGIMEN

The most commonly used myeloablative conditioning regimens used in HSCT for CML are the combination of cyclophosphamide with total body irradiation (Cy/TBI) or Bu/Cy.[29,30] These regimens have been compared in four randomized trials. Both regimens were found to be equally effective in early disease, but Bu/Cy was better tolerated and was thought to be an acceptable alternative to Cy/TBI.[31,32]

To overcome the eratic oral absorption of oral busulfan some investigators have used pharmacologic monitoring and dose adjustment to a target steady-state level of 900–1200 ng/ml, which showed an impressive 86% 3-year overall survival rate in patients in the chronic phase.[33] In summary, Bu/Cy and Cy/TBI remain the two most commonly used conditioning regimens for patients with CML.

NON-ABLATIVE TRANSPLANTATION

The graft-versus-leukemia effect is particularly potent in patients with CML making it particularly susceptible to the immune effect of transplant. Several studies[34–41] (Table 7.1) of non-ablative transplantation have demonstrated the safety and efficacy of this approach. It is therefore a suitable option for patients who cannot tolerate myeloablative transplantation because of age or co-morbidity.

Crawley *et al.* reported on the outcomes of 186 patients who underwent non-ablative transplantation recorded in the EBMT registry. These authors found a 2-year non-relapse mortality (NRM) rate of 23%, a 3-year overall survival rate of 58%, and a disease-free survival rate of 37% in this group of patients. However, outcomes varied according to the phase of the disease. Specifically, the overall survival rates were 69%, 57%, 24%, and 8%, and the progression-free survival rates were 44%, 30%, 10%, and 0% in patients in the first chronic phase, second chronic phase, advanced phase, and blast phase, respectively.[35]

GVHD is the major cause of NRM in this group of patients. The overall incidence of GVHD is increased in these patients as a result of the early withdrawal of immunosuppressive treatment and/or the increased use of donor lymphocyte infusions (DLI) to promote full donor engraftment and prevent relapse. NRM is higher in patients in the advanced phase of disease than in patients in the chronic phase (20.3% versus 11.6%).[35] The incidences of both acute and chronic GVHD are lower in patients who receive antithymocyte globulin (ATG) or alemtuzumab, but this is at the expense of a higher incidence of relapse. The highest risk of relapse, 76% at 2 years, is seen after alemtuzumab use.[35]

Although there are no randomized trials comparing different conditioning regimens for non-ablative transplantation, the best reported outcome has been seen for the combination

Table 7.1 Non-ablative hematopoietic cell transplantation for chronic myeloid leukemia

	No. of patients	*Conditioning regimen*	*Median age (years)*	*Interval from diagnosis (months)*	*Disease phase (CP1/CP2/AP/BC)*	*Related/MUD*	*Median follow-up (months)*	*NRM (%)*	*DFS (%)*	*OS (%)*
Or *et al.*[38]	24	Flu/Bu/ATG	35	9		19/5	42	13	85	85
Crawley *et al.*[35]	186	Multiple*	50	13.5		133/52	35	23.3	37	58
Baron *et al.*[34]	21	TBI/Flu	54	26	12/2/5/1	0/21	867 days	2/21	7/21	14/21
Weisser *et al.*[40]	35	Flu/Cy/TBI/ATG	51		26/9	19/16	30	28.5	49	63
Kerbauy *et al.*[37]	24	TBI/Flu or TBI	58	28	14/4/6/0	24/0	36	21	54	54
Ruiz-Arguelles *et al.*[39]	24	Flu/Bu/Cy	41	19	24/0	24/0	17	8	92	92
Kebriaei *et al.*[41]	64	Flu/Mel or Flu/Ara/Ida	64	31	13/17/29/5	34/30	84	48	20	33

*Largest number ($n = 95$) Flu/Bu. CP1, first chronic phase; CP2, second chronic phase; AP, accelerated phase; BC, blast crisis; MUD, matched unrelated donor; GVHD, graft versus host disease; NRM, non-relapse mortality; DFS, disease-free survival; OS, overall survival; ATG, antithymocyte globulin; TBI, total body irradiation; Flu, fludarabine; Bu, busulfan; Mel, melphalan; Cy, cyclophosphamide; Ara, Ara C; Ida, idarubicin.

of busulfan, fludarabine (Flu), and ATG.[35] In contrast, a high incidence of rejection (45%) was seen in patients who received a low-dose TBI-based regimen, particularly in MUD transplant recipients, probably owing to the highly proliferative nature of the disease and the lack of previous aggressive chemotherapy.[36] Marrow grafts in patients who undergo non-ablative transplantation were found to be associated with a higher risk of graft failure than was the case for recipients of peripheral blood stem cell grafts.[42] Sloand *et al.* found that the majority of patients who underwent Flu/Cy conditioning failed to achieve remission and required further intervention (DLI, imatinib, or a second transplant) for disease eradication.[43]

Molecular remission is achievable but occurs more slowly or is delayed in patients who receive non-ablative as opposed to conventional transplants. This occurs usually with or after conversion to full donor T-cell chimerism, which is delayed compared with the timing of conversion in recipients of ablative transplants,[44] although complete donor chimerism is not necessary for response. A persistently high level of BCR-ABL transcripts 28–56 days after transplant predicts for relapse in patients who undergo 2-Gy TBI-based conditioning.[45] The kinetics of the molecular clearance of disease are similar between patients undergoing non-ablative transplantation and those receiving DLI: the maximal response often occurs only after a delay of up to 1 year after the therapy.[46]

PROGNOSTIC FACTORS

The outcome after transplantation depends on the disease biology and the health of the recipient. The most important prognostic factor is the phase of the disease, with the outcome in patients in the chronic phase being better than that in patients with more advanced disease, either in the accelerated phase or blast phase.[47] Even among patients with chronic phase disease, the outcome is better for those who receive transplants early, within 1 year of diagnosis, as opposed to later.[10,47]

The EBMT registry developed a prognostic index that could be used to predict survival after transplant, help make treatment decisions, and counsel patients.[48] This index was subsequently validated.[49] The EBMT score is based on five variables: donor type (HLA-identical sibling donor versus MUD), age (<20, 20–40, and >40 years), disease phase (first chronic, accelerated, and blast), donor–recipient sex combination (female donor–male recipient, other), and interval from diagnosis to transplant (<1 year versus >1 year). Survival rates at 5 years were shown to be 72%, 70%, 62%, 48%, 40%, 18%, and 22% for risk scores of 0, 1, 2, 3, 4, 5, and 6 or 7, respectively.

IMPACT OF PRETRANSPLANT IMATINIB ON OUTCOME

The use of imatinib prior to transplant does not impair engraftment, increase non-relapse-related mortality, or lead to inferior overall or event-free survival.[50] Even patients with a mutation in the ABL tyrosine kinase domain, which confers imatinib resistance, can be successfully salvaged with transplant.[51,52] Although relatively small retrospective studies found a higher incidence of liver toxicity[53] in patients in whom this approach was used, three larger studies did not find an increased incidence of liver toxicity in such patients.[53,54] Likewise, reports on the incidence and severity of GVHD have been mixed, with a higher incidence of GVHD seen in some studies but not others.[53,54]

In patients with advanced phase CML, imatinib pretreatment before transplant did improve the outcome particularly in patients who converted to a second chronic phase with <35% Ph-positive cells; the 3-year overall survival rate in these latter patients was 81%,[55] but no such improvement was seen in another study.[56]

RELAPSE AFTER ALLOGENEIC TRANSPLANT

Relapse continues to occur after allogeneic transplant, with an incidence of up to 20% in patients who undergo transplantation in the chronic phase and up to 60% in patients who undergo the procedure in the advanced phase of disease.[8–10] Survival after relapse is limited and is worse for patients in the advanced phase of disease at the time of relapse or at the time of transplant, for patients who undergo transplantation in the late chronic phase more than 2 years after diagnosis, and for patients who receive transplants from an unrelated donor.[57]

Relapse post-transplant can be successfully treated with DLI,[58–64] with approximately 70% of patients in the chronic phase responding and achieving a prolonged durable remission. The response rate is low (10–20%) in patients with advanced disease but high in patients with molecular or cytogenetic relapse. DLI can sometimes be complicated by fatal GVHD or aplasia. A higher incidence of GVHD and treatment-related mortality has been noted after higher doses of DLI. The first dose of DLI should not exceed 0.2×10^8 T cells/kg.[61] To prevent or reduce incidence of GVHD, escalating doses of DLI have been used, using the least possible cell dose that will result in a therapeutic response.[62] Alternatively CD8 depletion of donor lymphocytes has also been successfully used for this purpose.[63,64]

Relapsed CML after allogeneic transplantation also responds to imatinib.[65] Imatinib treatment in patients who suffered relapse following allogeneic transplant was observed to result in a complete hematological response in 100%, 83%, and 43% of patients in the chronic phase, accelerated phase, and blast phase, respectively. The main side-effects were GVHD and myelosuppression.[65,66] Interferon alfa (IFNα) is also effective in some patients, but its use has been superseded by more effective drugs such as imatinib.[67]

Despite the high rate of response to imatinib, most patients are not cured of their disease and the responses are not as durable as those that have been seen with DLI. For example, in a small study of patients treated with imatinib following allogeneic transplant, nine of ten patients who suffered relapse after allogeneic transplant responded to imatinib. However, six of these nine patients suffered relapse while being treated with imatinib and the other three suffered relapse when imatinib treatment was stopped.[68–70]

The use of polymerase chain reaction (PCR) to monitor for minimal residual disease may allow relapse to be predicted, which will permit early intervention. The finding of three consecutive BCR-ABL : ABL ratios of >0.02% or two consecutive values of >0.05% 6 months after transplantation is considered to signify molecular relapse; the relapse rate in this group is 70%.[71] However, these results cannot be considered as standard, as PCR assays are different at different laboratories. Standardization of these assays among centers will go a long way to resolving this problem.[72]

In summary, with the advances in modern drug therapy for CML, allogeneic transplant cannot be recommended as a first-line therapy for patients in the early chronic phase,[73] but only at the first sign of an inadequate response. An international expert panel has recommended that allogeneic transplant should be considered at the first sign of drug therapy failure.[73] Based on data from the IRIS trial, this has been defined as a lack of hematological response by 3 months to first-line imatinib therapy at a dose of 400 mg daily, no cytogenetic response (Ph-positive cells >95%) by 6 months, less than a partial cytogenetic response (Ph-positive cells >35%) by 12 months, and a complete cytogenetic response not reached until 18 months. In patients failing to achieve the stated response by the said time, the likelihood of eventual response is small and alternative therapy is very reasonable.[74] Allogeneic transplant, with its long track record, is an appropriate second-line therapy for such patients who have an available donor.

ALLOGENEIC TRANSPLANT FOR PHILADELPHIA-NEGATIVE CHRONIC MYELOPROLIFERATIVE DISORDERS

Primary myelofibrosis and myelofibrosis secondary to polycythemia vera and essential thrombocythemia are disorders severe enough to warrant hematopoietic cell transplantation. The challenge is to identify the patients who will respond poorly with standard measures. The annual incidence of primary myelofibrosis ranges from 0.5 to 1.5 per 100 000, and the median age at diagnosis is 67 years,[75,76] factors that account for the limited data on the role of HCT in these diseases. This is likely to change with exciting recent data on the efficacy of allogeneic transplantation with reduced intensity regimens in older patients with these disorders.[77,78]

These clonal myeloproliferative disorders are caused by an acquired somatic mutation of a hematopoietic progenitor cell, resulting in clonal erythrocytes, platelets, granulocytes, monocytes, and their precursors. These malignant megakaryocytes and monocytes secrete fibrogenic cytokines (transforming growth factor (TGF), platelet-derived growth factor (PDGF), and fibroblast growth factor (FGF)), which cause polyclonal fibroblast proliferation, collagen and reticulin deposition, and eventual bone marrow fibrosis, the hallmark of the disease. Most patients with primary myelofibrosis present with anemia, marked splenomegaly, early satiety, and constitutional symptoms. During the clinical course, most patients experience progressive anemia requiring frequent blood transfusions, and death occurs eventually owing to bone marrow failure or leukemic transformation.[75] Current treatment of primary myelofibrosis is palliative, consisting of supportive care with blood transfusions, erythropoietin, splenectomy, splenic radiation, hydroxyurea, and more recently thalidomide as well as lenalidomide.[79–84] None of these therapies alters the natural history of this disease.

In patients with primary myelofibrosis, the median survival is 5 years from diagnosis, but survival can vary from 2 years to greater than

10 years depending on the presence or absence of well-defined prognostic indicators.[85–91] These indicators include anemia (Hb <10 g/dl), advanced age (>64 years), constitutional symptoms (fever, night sweats, weight loss), leukocytosis ($>30\times10^9$/l) or leukopenia ($<4.0\times10^9$/l), circulating blasts (>1%), and high-risk cytogenetic abnormalities (+8, 12p−). A simple but widely accepted scoring system using two of these factors, namely Hb <10 g/dl and WBC $>30\times10^9$/l or $<4.0\times10^9$/l, separates patients into three groups with low (no factors), intermediate (one factor), and high (two factors) risks, associated with median survivals of 93, 26, and 13 months, respectively.[90] Allogeneic transplantation would therefore be justifiable for patients with intermediate-risk and high-risk disease. However, for patients with low-risk disease (median survival of more than 7–10 years), the risk of transplant-related mortality outweighs the potential benefit from transplant. These prognostic factors were derived from patients with primary myelofibrosis and may have limited applicability to patients with post-polycythemia vera and post-essential thrombocythemia myelofibrosis. In a study from the Mayo Clinic, cytogenetic abnormalities other than del 20q and del 13q were identified as adverse factors indicating poor survival. In the same study, when cytogenetic abnormality was excluded from analysis, multivariate analysis identified age >45 years, anemia (Hb <10 g/dl), and polycythemia vera to be independent risk factors for shortened survival.[92] All the above-mentioned risk factors for primary and secondary myelofibrosis should be taken into account to select patients with significantly shortened life expectancy for allogeneic transplantation.

MYELOABLATIVE ALLOGENEIC STEM CELL TRANSPLANTATION

By eradicating the malignant clone and restoring normal hematopoiesis, allogeneic hematopoietic cell transplantation would be expected to alter the natural history of primary myelofibrosis. Owing to intuitive concern about engraftment in the hostile microenvironment and to the uncommon occurrence of this disease and older age at disease onset, very few studies with more than 20 patients have been reported in the literature, and all but one are multicenter/registry studies (Table 7.2). Several reports in the 1990s demonstrated the feasibility of alloHCT in myelofibrosis.[94–101] Overall survival, disease-free survival, and transplant-related mortality were 47%, 39%, and 27%, respectively. Osteosclerosis, low hemoglobin (<10 g/dl), older age, and abnormal karyotype were associated with adverse outcome. In an update of this series,[100] Guardiola *et al.* published data on 66 patients, demonstrating inferior results for older patients: 5-year survival was 14% in patients older than 45 years and 62% in younger patients.[97] In the largest single center study,[98] from the Fred Hutchinson Cancer Center in Seattle, 56 patients with a median age of 43 years were transplanted from HLA-matched donors for myelofibrosis. At a median follow-up of 34 months, the 5-year survival was 58%, with continuing resolution of fibrosis, reduction in spleen size, transfusion independence, and improvement in blood counts. Six patients either rejected the graft ($n = 3$) or were mixed chimera ($n = 3$). The major reason for treatment failure was transplant-related mortality of 32%. Dupriez score, abnormal karyotype, and degree of marrow fibrosis adversely affected survival; however, the use of targeted busulfan and cyclophosphamide was associated with a higher probability of survival. Interestingly, outcomes were similar for both patients with related donors and those with unrelated donors in this study. An update from the same center with 104 patients confirmed these results, with NRM of 34% and 7-year survival of 61%. In addition to the above-mentioned prognostic factors, a higher comorbidity score was associated with increased mortality.[99] The most representative trials are summarized in Table 7.3.

In summary, with myeloablative transplantation, 40–60% of patients are long-term survivors, but the biggest problem is a high NRM of 27–48%. The best reported results are with a targeted busulfan and cyclophosphamide

Table 7.2 Allogeneic transplantation for myelofibrosis: reduced intensity regimens

Study	*No. of patients*	*Median age (years)*	*Median time from diagnosis to transplantation (months)*	*Non-relapse mortality (%)*	*Median follow-up (months)*	*Overall survival (%)*
Rondelli *et al.*[77]	21	54	11	10	31	85
Kroger *et al.*[78]	21	53	18	16	22	84
Synder *et al.*[93]	9	54	41	44	32	56

Table 7.3 Allogeneic transplantation for myelofibrosis

Study	*No. of patients*	*Median age (years)*	*Median time from diagnosis (months)*	*Non-relapse mortality (%)*	*Median follow-up (months)*	*Overall survival (%)*
Guardiola *et al.*[97]	55	42	21	27	36	47
Daly *et al.*[101]	25	48	10	48	35	41
Kerbauy *et al.*[99]	104	49	15	34	63	61
Ballen *et al.* (related donor)[100]	170	45	—	22*	41	39
Ballen *et al.* (unrelated donor)[100]	117	47	—	42*	48	31

*100-day non-relapse mortality.

conditioning regimen, young age (<45 years), and transplant performed early in the natural history of disease. A special problem area is the treatment of older or debilitated patients, who form the majority of patients with this disease and who require an alternative approach.

REDUCED INTENSITY ALLOGENEIC TRANSPLANT: RECENT DATA

Another approach would be to use a reduced intensity (RIC) or a non-myeloablative conditioning regimen, which have been reported to successfully extend the use of allogeneic transplants to older patients and patients with other co-morbid medical conditions in other hematological malignancies.[102–105] These early reports and demonstration of graft versus myelofibrosis effect set the stage for evaluation of RIC in patients with myelofibrosis.[106,107] In an early report, four patients with a median age of 56 years were treated with fludarabine and melphalan and with stem cells from a HLA-identical sibling. At a median follow-up of 13 months, all four patients were alive with stable full donor chimerism.[108] Further follow-up of these four patients and additional patients treated at multiple institutions with various RIC regimens, for a total of 21 patients, was reported by Rondelli *et al.*[77] Patients had intermediate-risk or high-risk disease per Dupriez criteria, with a median age of 54 years. Of the 21 patients, 18 had a HLA-identical related donor graft. With a median follow-up of 31 months, overall survival and NRM were 85% and 10%, respectively. Snyder *et al.* reported on nine patients with a median age of 54 years undergoing an RIC allogeneic transplant with fludarabine and melphalan from an unrelated donor ($n = 7$) or a related donor ($n = 2$). Five patients were alive at a median follow-up of 32 months.[93]

In the largest prospective study of RIC allogeneic transplantation, which used busulfan

10 mg/kg, fludarabine 180 mg/m^2, and antithymocyte globulin (ATG), 21 patients with a median age of 53 years received grafts from matching related donors (n = 8) or unrelated donors (n = 13). With a median follow-up of 22 months, overall survival was 84%, with the majority of patients having full donor chimerism.[78] Likewise, in a study of RIC allogeneic transplant conducted at The University of Texas MD Anderson Cancer Center, a low early treatment-related mortality (0% at 100 days) was seen in the first 12 patients with a median age of 59 years; the follow-up was too short to draw any other conclusions.[109] A Swedish study of 27 patients found a lower NRM with an RIC regimen compared with a myeloablative regimen (10% compared with 30%, respectively). There were no significant differences in other outcomes.[110]

In summary, RIC allogeneic transplantation results in a low NRM of 10–16% and is an option for older patients and those with co-morbidities, but further larger prospective studies are needed. Several such studies are ongoing in both Europe and America.

ALLOGENEIC TRANSPLANTATION FOR MYELOFIBROSIS: IMPORTANT CONSIDERATIONS

In general, response after transplant is delayed in terms of fibrosis and splenomegaly. These may take a long time to resolve, even in patients who are 100% donor chimera. In one large study, complete resolution of fibrosis occurred between 1 and 23 months (median 6 months).[97] In another study, of 66 patients with intact spleen and splenomegaly, the spleen was normal in size in 50 patients but enlargement persisted in 13 patients at the time of the latest examination (between 6 months and 3 years after transplant).[99] Therefore, histology is not the best marker for assessing disease response early after transplant. Chimerism studies and molecular studies are more helpful in patients who are JAK2 positive. Post-transplant minimal residual disease can be monitored by a sensitive assay for JAK2. This can be used to detect relapse early and therefore allow planning for any immune interventions such as donor lymphocyte infusion.[110]

ROLE OF SPLENECTOMY BEFORE TRANSPLANT

Because of concern about engraftment, splenectomy is frequently performed before a transplant, but available data do not support routine splenectomy before transplant in all patients. Splenomegaly is associated with delayed engraftment,[97,98,110] but no definite data exist documenting increased rejection risk or showing that prophylactic splenectomy prevents this risk. Splenectomy in patients with myelofibrosis entails high rates of morbidity and mortality (33% and 9% of patients, respectively). Bleeding (14%), thrombosis (10%), and infections (10%) are some of the major complications. Leukemic transformation (14%) and increasing hepatomegaly (10%) have also been reported after splenectomy; these latter complications probably reflect advanced disease stage in patients who need to undergo splenectomy.[83,111]

CONCLUSIONS

Allogeneic transplant is a promising therapy for curing myelofibrosis. Ongoing research studies in patients with RIC regimens hold promise for extending this therapy to the majority of patients with this disease.

REFERENCES

1. Harris NL, Jaffe ES, Diebold J et al. World Health Organization classication of neoplastic diseases of the hematopoietic and lymphoid tissues: report of the clinical advisory committee meeting, Airlie house, Virginia, November 1997. J Clin Oncol 1999; 17: 3835–49.
2. Goldman JM, Melo JV. Chronic myeloid leukemia – advances in biology and new approaches to treatment. N Engl J Med 2003; 349: 1451–64.
3. Savage DG, Antman KH. Imatinib mesylate – a new oral targeted therapy. N Engl J Med 2002; 346: 683–93.
4. Tefferi A. JAK and MPL mutations in myeloid malignancies. Leuk Lymphoma 2008; 49: 388–97.
5. Giralt SA, Arora M, Goldman JM et al. Impact of imatinib therapy on the eve of allogeneic hematopoietic

progenitor cell transplatation. Br J Haematol 2007; 137: 461–7.
6. Gratwohl A, Baldomero H, Frauendorfer K, Urbano-Ispizua A. EBMT activity survey 2004 and changes in disease indication over the past 15 years. Bone Marrow Transplant 2006; 37: 1069–85.
7. Druker BJ, Guilhot F, O'Brien SG et al. Five-year follow-up of patients receiving imatinib for chronic myeloid leukemia. N Engl J Med 2006; 355: 2408–17.
8. Weisser M, Ledderose G, Jochem KH. Long-term follow-up of allogeneic HSCT for CML reveals significant improvement in the outcome over the last decade. Ann Hematol 2007; 86: 127–32.
9. Radich JP, Gooley T, Bensinger W et al. HLA-matched related hematopoietic cell transplantation for chronic-phase CML using a targeted busulfan and cyclophosphamide preparative regimen. Blood 2003; 102: 31–5.
10. Gale RP, Hehlmann R, Zhang MJ et al. Survival with bone marrow transplantation versus hydroxyurea or interferon for chronic myelogenous leukemia. The German CML Study Group. Blood 1998; 91: 1810–19.
11. Hehlmann R, Berger U, Pfirrmann M et al. Drug treatment is superior to allografting as first line therapy in chronic myeloid leukemia. Blood 2007; 109: 4686–92.
12. Horowitz MM, Rowlings PA, Passweg JR. Allogeneic bone marrow transplantation for CML: a report from the International Bone Marrow Transplant Registry. Bone Marrow Transplant 1996; 17: S5–6.
13. Clift RA, Buckner CD, Thomas ED et al. Marrow transplantation for patients in accelerated phase of chronic myeloid leukemia. Blood 1994; 84: 4368–73.
14. Kernan NA, Bartsch G, Ash RC et al. Analysis of 462 transplantations from unrelated donors facilitated by the National Marrow Donor Program. N Engl J Med 1993; 328: 593–602.
15. McGlave P, Bartsch G, Anasetti C et al. Unrelated donor marrow transplantation therapy for chronic myelogenous leukemia: initial experience of the National Marrow Donor Program. Blood 1993; 81: 543–50.
16. McGlave PB, Shu XO, Wen W et al. Unrelated donor marrow transplantation for chronic myelogenous leukemia: 9 years' experience of the national marrow donor program. Blood 2000; 95: 2219–25.
17. Hansen JA, Gooley TA, Martin PJ et al. Bone marrow transplants from unrelated donors for patients with chronic myeloid leukemia. N Engl J Med 1998; 338: 962–8.
18. Weisdorf DJ, Anasetti C, Antin JH et al. Allogeneic bone marrow transplantation for chronic myelogenous leukemia: comparative analysis of unrelated versus matched sibling donor transplantation. Blood 2002; 99: 1971–7.
19. Davies SM, DeFor TE, McGlave PB et al. Equivalent outcomes in patients with chronic myelogenous leukemia after early transplantation of phenotypically matched bone marrow from related or unrelated donors. Am J Med 2001; 110: 339–46.
20. Ottinger HD, Ferencik S, Beelen DW et al. Hematopoietic stem cell transplantation: contrasting the outcome of transplantations from HLA-identical siblings, partially HLA-mismatched related donors, and HLA-matched unrelated donors. Blood 2003; 102: 1131–7.
21. Yakoub-Agha I, Mesnil F, Kuentz M et al. Allogeneic marrow stem-cell transplantation from human leukocyte antigen-identical siblings versus human leukocyte antigen-allelic-matched unrelated donors (10/10) in patients with standard-risk hematologic malignancy: a prospective study from the French Society of Bone Marrow Transplantation and Cell Therapy. J Clin Oncol 2006; 24: 5695–702.
22. Bogdanic V, Nemet D, Kastelan A et al. Umbilical cord blood transplantation in a patient with Philadelphia chromosome-positive chronic myeloid leukemia. Transplantation 1993; 56: 477–9.
23. Laporte JP, Gorin NC, Rubinstein P et al. Cord-blood transplantation from an unrelated donor in an adult with chronic myelogenous leukemia. N Engl J Med 1996; 335: 167–70.
24. Aversa F, Tabilio A, Velardi A et al. Treatment of high-risk acute leukemia with T-cell-depleted stem cells from related donors with one fully mismatched HLA haplotype. N Engl J Med 1998; 339: 1186–93.
25. Bensinger WI, Martin PJ, Storer B et al. Transplantation of bone marrow as compared with peripheral-blood cells from HLA-identical relatives in patients with hematologic cancers. N Engl J Med 2001; 344: 175–81.
26. Stem Cell Trialists, Collaborative Group. Allogeneic peripheral blood stem-cell compared with bone marrow transplantation in the management of hematologic malignancies: an individual patient data meta-analysis of nine randomized trials. J Clin Oncol 2005; 23: 5074–87.
27. Schmitz N, Eapen M, Horowitz MM et al. Long-term outcome of patients given transplants of mobilized blood or bone marrow: a report from the International Bone Marrow Transplant Registry and the European Group for Blood and Marrow Transplantation. Blood 2006; 108: 4288–9.
28. Champlin RE, Schmitz N, Horowitz MM et al. Blood stem cells compared with bone marrow as a source of hematopoietic cells for allogeneic transplantation. IBMTR Histocompatibility and Stem Cell Sources Working Committee and the European Group for Blood and Marrow Transplantation (EBMT). Blood 2000; 95: 3702–9.
29. Clift RA, Buckner CD, Appelbaum FR et al. Allogeneic marrow transplantation in patients with chronic myeloid leukemia in the chronic phase: a

randomized trial of two irradiation regimens. Blood 1991; 77: 1660–5.
30. Tutschka PJ, Copelan EA, Klein JP. Bone marrow transplantation for leukemia following a new busulfan and cyclophosphamide regimen. Blood 1987; 70: 1382–8.
31. Socie G, Clift RA, Blaise D et al. Busulfan plus cyclophosphamide compared with total-body irradiation plus cyclophosphamide before marrow transplantation for myeloid leukemia: long-term follow-up of 4 randomized studies. Blood 2001; 98: 3569–74.
32. Clift RA, Radich J, Appelbaum FR et al. Long-term follow-up of a randomized study comparing cyclophosphamide and total body irradiation with busulfan and cyclophosphamide for patients receiving allogenic marrow transplants during chronic phase of chronic myeloid leukemia. Blood 1999; 94: 3960–2.
33. Radich JP, Gooley T, Bensinger W et al. HLA-matched related hematopoietic cell transplantation for chronic-phase CML using a targeted busulfan and cyclophosphamide preparative regimen. Blood 2003; 102: 31–5.
34. Baron F, Maris MB, Storer BE et al. HLA-matched unrelated donor hematopoietic cell transplantation after nonmyeloablative conditioning for patients with chronic myeloid leukemia. Biol Blood Marrow Transplant 2005; 11: 272–9.
35. Crawley C, Szydlo R, Lalancette M et al. Outcomes of reduced-intensity transplantation for chronic myeloid leukemia: an analysis of prognostic factors from the Chronic Leukemia Working Party of the EBMT. Blood 2005; 106: 2969–76.
36. Das M, Saikia TK, Advani SH, Parikh PM, Tawed S. Use of a reduced-intensity conditioning regimen for allogeneic transplantation in patients with chronic myeloid leukemia. Bone Marrow Transplant 2003; 32: 125–9.
37. Kerbauy FR, Storb R, Hegenbart U et al. Hematopoietic cell transplantation from HLA-identical sibling donors after low-dose radiation-based conditioning for treatment of CML. Leukemia 2005; 19: 990–7.
38. Or R, Shapira MY, Resnick I et al. Nonmyeloablative allogeneic stem cell transplantation for the treatment of chronic myeloid leukemia in first chronic phase. Blood 2003; 101: 441–5.
39. Ruiz-Arguelles GJ, Gomez-Almaguer D, Morales-Toquero A et al. The early referral for reduced-intensity stem cell transplantation in patients with Ph1 (+) chronic myelogenous leukemia in chronic phase in the imatinib era: results of the Latin American Cooperative Oncohematology Group (LACOHG) prospective, multicenter study. Bone Marrow Transplant 2005; 36: 1043–7.
40. Weisser M, Schleuning M, Ledderose G et al. Reduced-intensity conditioning using TBI (8 Gy), fludarabine, cyclophosphamide and ATG in elderly CML patients provides excellent results especially when performed in the early course of the disease. Bone Marrow Transplant 2004; 34: 1083–8.
41. Kebriaei P, Detry MA, Giralt S et al. Long-term follow-up of allogeneic hematopoietic stem-cell transplantation with reduced-intensity conditioning for patients with chronic myeloid leukemia. Blood 2007; 110: 3456–62.
42. Maris MB, Niederwieser D, Sandmaier BM et al. HLA-matched unrelated donor hematopoietic cell transplantation after nonmyeloablative conditioning for patients with hematologic malignancies. Blood 2003; 102: 2021–30.
43. Sloand E, Childs RW, Solomon S et al. The graft-versus-leukemia effect of nonmyeloablative stem cell allografts may not be sufficient to cure chronic myelogenous leukemia. Bone Marrow Transplant 2003; 32: 897–901.
44. Uzunel M, Mattsson J, Brune M et al. Kinetics of minimal residual disease and chimerism in patients with chronic myeloid leukemia after nonmyeloablative conditioning and allogeneic stem cell transplantation. Blood 2003; 101: 469–72.
45. Lange T, Deininger M, Brand R et al. BCR-ABL transcripts are early predictors for hematological relapse in chronic myeloid leukemia after hematopoietic cell transplantation with reduced intensity conditioning. Leukemia 2004; 18: 1468–75.
46. Schetelig J, Kiani A, Schmitz M, Ehninger G, Bornhauser M. T cell-mediated graft-versus-leukemia reactions after allogeneic stem cell transplantation. Cancer Immunol Immunother 2005; 54: 1043–58.
47. Bacigalupo A, Gualandi F, Van Lint MT et al. Multivariate analysis of risk factors for survival and relapse in chronic granulocytic leukemia following allogeneic marrow transplantation: impact of disease related variables (Sokal score). Bone Marrow Transplant 1993; 12: 443–8.
48. Gratwohl A. Risk assessment in haematopoietic stem cell transplantation. Best Pract Res Clin Haematol 2007; 20: 119–24.
49. Passweg JR, Walker I, Sobocinski KA et al. Validation and extension of the EBMT Risk Score for patients with chronic myeloid leukaemia (CML) receiving allogeneic haematopoietic stem cell transplants. Br J Haematol 2004; 125: 613–20.
50. Oehler VG, Gooley T, Snyder DS et al. The effects of imatinib mesylate treatment before allogeneic transplantation for chronic myeloid leukemia. Blood 2007; 109: 1782–9.
51. Jabbour E, Cortes J, Kantarjian HM et al. Allogeneic stem cell transplantation for patients with chronic myeloid leukemia and acute lymphocytic leukemia after Bcr-Abl kinase mutation-related imatinib failure. Blood 2006; 108: 1421–3.
52. Shimoni A, Kroger N, Zander AR et al. Imatinib mesylate (STI571) in preparation for allogeneic hematopoietic stem cell transplantation and donor

lymphocyte infusions in patients with Philadelphia-positive acute leukemias. Leukemia 2003; 17: 290–7.
53. Deininger M, Schleuning M, Greinix H et al. The effect of prior exposure to imatinib on transplant-related mortality. Haematologica 2006; 91: 452–9.
54. Zaucha JM, Prejzner W, Giebel S et al. Imatinib therapy prior to myeloablative allogeneic stem cell transplantation. Bone Marrow Transplant 2005; 36: 417–24.
55. Weisser M, Schleuning M, Haferlach C, Schwerdtfeger R. Kolb HJ. Allogeneic stem-cell transplantation provides excellent results in advanced stage chronic myeloid leukemia with major cytogenetic response to pre-transplant imatinib therapy. Leuk Lymphoma 2007; 48: 295–301.
56. Bornhauser M, Kroger N, Schwerdtfeger R et al. Allogeneic haematopoietic cell transplantation for chronic myelogenous leukaemia in the era of imatinib: a retrospective multicentre study. Eur J Haematol 2006; 76: 9–17.
57. Guglielmi C, Arcese W, Hermans J et al. Risk assessment in patients with Ph-positive chronic myelogenous leukemia at first relapse after allogeneic stem cell transplant: an EBMT retrospective analysis. The Chronic Leukemia Working Party of the European Group for Blood and Marrow Transplantation. Blood 2000; 95: 3328–34.
58. Drobyski WR, Keever CA, Roth MS et al. Salvage immunotherapy using donor leukocyte infusions as treatment for relapsed chronic myelogenous leukemia after allogeneic bone marrow transplantation: efficacy and toxicity of a defined T-cell dose. Blood 1993; 82: 2310–18.
59. Kolb HJ, Mittermuller J, Clemm C et al. Donor leukocyte transfusions for treatment of recurrent chronic myelogenous leukemia in marrow transplant patients. Blood 1990; 76: 2462–5.
60. Porter DL, Roth MS, McGarigle C, Ferrara JL, Antin JH. Induction of graft-versus-host disease as immunotherapy for relapsed chronic myeloid leukemia. N Engl J Med 1994; 330: 100–6.
61. Guglielmi C, Arcese W, Dazzi F et al. Donor lymphocyte infusion for relapsed chronic myelogenous leukemia: prognostic relevance of the initial cell dose. Blood 2002; 100: 397–405.
62. Mackinnon S, Papadopoulos EB, Carabasi MH et al. Adoptive immunotherapy evaluating escalating doses of donor leukocytes for relapse of chronic myeloid leukemia after bone marrow transplantation: separation of graft-versus-leukemia responses from graft-versus-host disease. Blood 1995; 86: 1261–8.
63. Alyea EP, Canning C, Neuberg D et al. CD8+ cell depletion of donor lymphocyte infusions using cd8 monoclonal antibody-coated high-density microparticles (CD8-HDM) after allogeneic hematopoietic stem cell transplantation: a pilot study. Bone Marrow Transplant 2004; 34: 123–8.
64. Giralt S, Hester J, Huh Y et al. CD8-depleted donor lymphocyte infusion as treatment for relapsed chronic myelogenous leukemia after allogeneic bone marrow transplantation. Blood 1995; 86: 4337–43.
65. Hess G, Bunjes D, Siegert W et al. Sustained complete molecular remissions after treatment with imatinib-mesylate in patients with failure after allogeneic stem cell transplantation for chronic myelogenous leukemia: results of a prospective phase II open-label multicenter study. J Clin Oncol 2005; 23: 7583–93.
66. Kantarjian HM, O'Brien S, Cortes JE et al. Imatinib mesylate therapy for relapse after allogeneic stem cell transplantation for chronic myelogenous leukemia. Blood 2002; 100: 1590–5.
67. Arcese W, Mauro FR, Alimena G et al. Interferon therapy for Ph1 positive CML patients relapsing after T cell-depleted allogeneic bone marrow transplantation. Bone Marrow Transplant 1990; 5: 309–15.
68. Weisser M, Tischer J, Schnittger S et al. A comparison of donor lymphocyte infusions or imatinib mesylate for patients with chronic myelogenous leukemia who have relapsed after allogeneic stem cell transplantation. Haematologica 2006; 91: 663–6.
69. Cortes J, O'Brien S, Kantarjian H. Discontinuation of imatinib therapy after achieving a molecular response. Blood 2004; 104: 2204–5.
70. Rousselot P, Huguet F, Rea D et al. Imatinib mesylate discontinuation in patients with chronic myelogenous leukemia in complete molecular remission for more than 2 years. Blood 2007; 109: 58–60.
71. Kaeda J, O'Shea D, Szydlo RM et al. Serial measurement of BCR-ABL transcripts in the peripheral blood after allogeneic stem cell transplantation for chronic myeloid leukemia: an attempt to define patients who may not require further therapy. Blood 2006; 107: 4171–6.
72. Hughes T, Deininger M, Hochhaus A et al. Monitoring CML patients responding to treatment with tyrosine kinase inhibitors: review and recommendations for harmonizing current methodology for detecting BCR-ABL transcripts and kinase domain mutations and for expressing results. Blood 2006; 108: 28–37.
73. Baccarani M, Saglio G, Goldman J et al. Evolving concepts in the management of chronic myeloid leukemia: recommendations from an expert panel on behalf of the European LeukemiaNet. Blood 2006; 108: 1809–20.
74. Sawyers CL, Hochhaus A, Feldman E et al. Imatinib induces hematologic and cytogenetic responses in patients with chronic myelogenous leukemia in myeloid blast crisis: results of a phase II study. Blood 2002; 99: 3530–9.
75. Tefferi A. Myelofibrosis with myeloid metaplasia. N Engl J Med 2000; 342: 1255–65.

76. Mesa RA, Silverstein MN, Jacobsen SJ, Wollan PC, Tefferi A. Population-based incidence and survival figures in essential thrombocythemia and agnogenic myeloid metaplasia: an Olmsted County Study, 1976–1995. Am J Hematol 1999; 61: 10–15.
77. Rondelli D, Barosi G, Bacigalupo A et al. Allogeneic hematopoietic stem-cell transplantation with reduced-intensity conditioning in intermediate- or high-risk patients with myelofibrosis with myeloid metaplasia. Blood 2005; 105: 4115–19.
78. Kroger N, Zabelina T, Schieder H et al. Pilot study of reduced-intensity conditioning followed by allogeneic stem cell transplantation from related and unrelated donors in patients with myelofibrosis. Br J Haematol 2005; 128: 690–7.
79. Barosi G, Grossi A, Comotti B et al. Safety and efficacy of thalidomide in patients with myelofibrosis with myeloid metaplasia. Br J Haematol 2001; 114: 78–83.
80. Giovanni B, Michelle E, Letizia C et al. Thalidomide in myelofibrosis with myeloid metaplasia: a pooled-analysis of individual patient data from five studies. Leuk Lymphoma 2002; 43: 2301–7.
81. Mesa RA, Tefferi A. Palliative splenectomy in myelofibrosis with myeloid metaplasia. Leuk Lymphoma 2001; 42: 901–11.
82. Mesa RA, Steensma DP, Pardanani A et al. A phase 2 trial of combination low-dose thalidomide and prednisone for the treatment of myelofibrosis with myeloid metaplasia. Blood 2003; 101: 2534–41.
83. Tefferi A, Mesa RA, Nagorney DM, Schroeder G. Silverstein MN. Splenectomy in myelofibrosis with myeloid metaplasia: a single-institution experience with 223 patients. Blood 2000; 95: 2226–33.
84. Tefferi A. Treatment approaches in myelofibrosis with myeloid metaplasia: the old and the new. Semin Hematol 2003; 40: 18–21.
85. Tefferi A, Cortes J, Verstovsek S et al. Lenalidomide therapy in myelofibrosis with myeloid metaplasia. Blood 2006; 108: 1158–64.
86. Cervantes F, Pereira A, Esteve J et al. Identification of 'short-lived' and 'long-lived' patients at presentation of idiopathic myelofibrosis. Br J Haematol 1997; 97: 635–40.
87. Cervantes F, Barosi G, Demory JL et al. Myelofibrosis with myeloid metaplasia in young individuals: disease characteristics, prognostic factors and identification of risk groups. Br J Haematol 1998; 102: 684–90.
88. Dupriez B, Morel P, Demory JL et al. Prognostic factors in agnogenic myeloid metaplasia: a report on 195 cases with a new scoring system. Blood 1996; 88: 1013–18.
89. Tefferi A, Huang J, Schwager S et al. Validation and comparison of contemporary prognostic models in primary myelofibrosis: analysis based on 334 patients from a single institution. Cancer 2007; 109: 2083–8.
90. Dingli D, Schwager SM, Mesa RA, Li CY, Tefferi A. Prognosis in transplant-eligible patients with agnogenic myeloid metaplasia: a simple CBC-based scoring system. Cancer 2006; 106: 623–30.
91. Tefferi A, Huang J, Schwager S, Li CY, Wu W, Pardanani A. et al. Validation and comparison of contemporary prognostic models in primary myelofibrosis: analysis based on 334 patients from a single institution. Cancer 2007; 109: 2083–8.
92. Dingli D, Schwager SM, Mesa RA et al. Presence of unfavorable cytogenetic abnormalities is the strongest predictor of poor survival in secondary myelofibrosis. Cancer 2006; 106: 1985–9.
93. Snyder DS, Palmer J, Stein AS et al. Allogeneic hematopoietic cell transplantation following reduced intensity conditioning for treatment of myelofibrosis. Biol Blood Marrow Transplant 2006; 12: 1161–8.
94. Singhal S, Powles R, Treleaven J et al. Allogeneic bone marrow transplantation for primary myelofibrosis. Bone Marrow Transplant 1995; 16: 743–6.
95. Przepiorka D, Giralt S, Khouri I, Champlin R, Bueso-Ramos C. Allogeneic marrow transplantation for myeloproliferative disorders other than chronic myelogenous leukemia: review of forty cases. Am J Hematol 1998; 57: 24–8.
96. Anderson JE, Sale G, Appelbaum FR, Chauncey TR, Storb R. Allogeneic marrow transplantation for primary myelofibrosis and myelofibrosis secondary to polycythaemia vera or essential thrombocytosis. Br J Haematol 1997; 98: 1010–16.
97. Guardiola P, Anderson JE, Bandini G et al. Allogeneic stem cell transplantation for agnogenic myeloid metaplasia: a European Group for Blood and Marrow Transplantation, Societe Francaise de Greffe de Moelle, Gruppo Italiano per il Trapianto del Midollo Osseo, and Fred Hutchinson Cancer Research Center Collaborative Study. Blood 1999; 93: 2831–8.
98. Deeg HJ, Gooley TA, Flowers ME et al. Allogeneic hematopoietic stem cell transplantation for myelofibrosis. Blood 2003; 102: 3912–18.
99. Kerbauy DM, Gooley TA, Sale GE et al. Hematopoietic cell transplantation as curative therapy for idiopathic myelofibrosis, advanced polycythemia vera, and essential thrombocythemia. Biol Blood Marrow Transplant 2007; 13: 355–65.
100. Ballen K, Sobocinski KA, Zang M et al. Outcome of Bone Marrow Transplantation for Myelofibrosis. Blood 2005; 106: 53a.
101. Daly A, Song K, Nevill T et al. Stem cell transplantation for myelofibrosis: a report from two Canadian centers. Bone Marrow Transplant 2003; 32: 35–40.
102. Giralt S, Thall PF, Khouri I et al. Melphalan and purine analog-containing preparative regimens: reduced-intensity conditioning for patients with hematologic malignancies undergoing allogeneic progenitor cell transplantation. Blood 2001; 97: 631–7.

103. Khouri IF, Keating M, Korbling M et al. Transplant-lite: induction of graft-versus-malignancy using fludarabine-based nonablative chemotherapy and allogeneic blood progenitor-cell transplantation as treatment for lymphoid malignancies. J Clin Oncol 1998; 16: 2817–24.
104. McSweeney PA, Niederwieser D, Shizuru JA et al. Hematopoietic cell transplantation in older patients with hematologic malignancies: replacing high-dose cytotoxic therapy with graft-versus-tumor effects. Blood 2001; 97: 3390–400.
105. Slavin S, Nagler A, Naparstek E et al. Nonmyeloablative stem cell transplantation and cell therapy as an alternative to conventional bone marrow transplantation with lethal cytoreduction for the treatment of malignant and nonmalignant hematologic diseases. Blood 1998; 91: 756–63.
106. Cervantes F, Rovira M, Urbano-Ispizua A et al. Complete remission of idiopathic myelofibrosis following donor lymphocyte infusion after failure of allogeneic transplantation: demonstration of a graft-versus-myelofibrosis effect. Bone Marrow Transplant 2000; 26: 697–9.
107. Byrne JL, Beshti H, Clark D et al. Induction of remission after donor leucocyte infusion for the treatment of relapsed chronic idiopathic myelofibrosis following allogeneic transplantation: evidence for a 'graft vs. myelofibrosis' effect. Br J Haematol 2000; 108: 430–3.
108. Devine SM, Hoffman R, Verma A et al. Allogeneic blood cell transplantation following reduced-intensity conditioning is effective therapy for older patients with myelofibrosis with myeloid metaplasia. Blood 2002; 99: 2255–8.
109. Popat U, Rondon G, Alousi A, Anderlini P. Myelofibrosis and Reduced Intensity Allogeneic Hematopoietic Stem Cell Transplantation (RISCT). Blood 2007; 110: 3062a.
110. Merup M, Lazarevic V, Nahi H et al. Different outcome of allogeneic transplantation in myelofibrosis using conventional or reduced-intensity conditioning regimens. Br J Haematol 2006; 135: 367–73.
110. Kroger N, Badbaran A, Holler E et al. Monitoring of the JAK2-V617F mutation by highly sensitive quantitative real-time PCR after allogeneic stem cell transplantation in patients with myelofibrosis. Blood 2007; 109: 1316–21.
111. Mesa RA, Nagorney DS, Schwager S, Allred J, Tefferi A. Palliative goals, patient selection, and perioperative platelet management: outcomes and lessons from 3 decades of splenectomy for myelofibrosis with myeloid metaplasia at the Mayo Clinic. Cancer 2006; 107: 361–70.

Monitoring response to therapy for patients with chronic myeloid leukemia

8

Devendra K Hiwase, Timothy Hughes

HISTORY OF MONITORING MINIMAL RESIDUAL DISEASE

Chronic myeloid leukemia (CML) has become a model in cancer medicine for how advances in understanding of the biology of the disease can be translated into the characterization of targets for therapy and how these same targets can be used effectively as molecular markers in the diagnosis and monitoring of the patient's response to therapy. In the 1990s, treatment options available for CML patients were hydroxyurea, busulfan, interferon alfa (IFNα) with or without low-dose cytosine arabinoside, and allogeneic stem cell transplant. Introduction of imatinib mesylate in 1998, revolutionalized treatment of CML. Improvement in treatments necessitates improvement in monitoring of minimal residual disease (MRD) and the past three decades have witnessed significant changes in monitoring of CML patients on therapy.

The degree of tumor load reduction is an important prognostic factor for CML patients on therapy. Response can be expressed in terms of hematological, cytogenetic, and molecular response. Hematological response is defined as the normalization of peripheral blood counts, absence of immature cells from the blood, and normalization of spleen size. Conventional cytogenetics has been considered the 'gold standard' for evaluating response to treatment. Complete cytogenetic response is defined as 0% Philadelphia (Ph)-positive cells, partial cytogenetic response as 1–35% Ph-positive cells in bone marrow metaphase, and major cytogenetic response includes complete cytogenetic response and partial cytogenetic response.[1] Although cytogenetic analysis has been the mainstay of disease monitoring, there are several limitations: (1) it is labor intensive and time consuming, (2) mitotic cells need to be cultured for analysis, and (3) only 20–25 metaphases are generally examinable. This last limitation makes the estimate of the percentage of Ph-positive cells quite imprecise.

Fluorescence *in situ* hybridization (FISH) has been used for monitoring CML patients on treatment. FISH is performed by cohybridization of BCR and ABL probes to denatured metaphase or interphase (I-FISH) chromosomes. I-FISH is relatively insensitive and has a false-positive rate of 1–5%[2] and hence is not suitable for the analysis of MRD. Dual color FISH (D-FISH) utilizes four probes that bind to 5′BCR, 3′ABL, and 3′BCR, 5′ABL spanning breakpoints of both chromosomes 9 and 22. In the presence of the BCR-ABL translocation, D-FISH yields a double fusion signal because the four probes bind to their respective BCR-ABL and ABL-BCR loci.[3] D-FISH provides a much lower level of background positivity (<0.8%), although its sensitivity is still suboptimal. Hypermetaphase FISH provides better sensitivity as well as a low false-positive rate and may be useful for following patients until they achieve complete cytogenetic response.[4] FISH analysis cannot detect other chromosomal abnormality apart from the Ph chromosome and hence cannot replace conventional cytogenetics. FISH may be useful in cases where cytogenetics is not informative.

Patients with leukemia at presentation or relapse usually have a total burden of 10^{11} to 10^{12} malignant cells, and cytogenetics and conventional FISH have a maximum sensitivity of 1%. Thus, a patient with negative results using these assays may harbor as many as

10^9 to 10^{10} residual leukemic cells. In the late 1980s more sensitive methods were assessed to follow patients who achieved complete cytogenetic response following allogeneic stem cell transplant.[5] In 1989, the first encouraging results concerning detection of MRD by polymerase chain reaction (PCR) in CML patients after allogeneic bone marrow transplantation were reported.[6] The leukemia specific BCR-ABL transcript is an excellent target for molecular monitoring by PCR because most CML patients have one of two transcript types (e13a2 or e14a2). Initially qualitative PCR was established which can identify the presence or absence of BCR-ABL transcripts by either single-step amplification or a two-step 'nested' amplification with internal primers to increase sensitivity.[6–8] Nested reverse transcription PCR (RT-PCR) can detect residual CML cells with a sensitivity of up to one in 10^5 or 10^6 cells. This qualitative PCR method has been used to follow patients after allogeneic stem cell transplant. However, patients who are negative by qualitative RT-PCR could have a tumor load up to 10^6 cells,[9] and in patients who are positive the BCR-ABL transcript levels may be declining or increasing. Hence, qualitative PCR has limited value as a predictor of relapse in individual patients.[10]

In view of the limited value of qualitative PCR for monitoring patients who achieved complete cytogenetic response, quantitative PCR methods were developed and used to follow patients after allogeneic stem cell transplant. Low or falling BCR-ABL transcript levels following transplantation were associated with continuous remission, while high or rising BCR-ABL transcript levels predict relapse prior to cytogenetic or hematological relapse.[11–15]

For quantitative RT-PCR, Cross *et al.* used competitive nested PCR strategies that can effectively control for variations in amplification efficiency and reaction kinetics. In general, nested PCR was performed using serial dilutions of a BCR-ABL competitor construct added to the same volume of patients' cDNA. The equivalence point at which the competitor and sample band would be of equal intensity can be determined by densitometry.[11,16] Choosing an appropriate control gene is important for generating reliable and reproducible data. Comparison with control gene results helps not only to identify RNA samples of unacceptable quality but also compensates for variations in transcript levels owing to sample degradation after collection, efficiency of the RT step, and variations in the amount of RNA. The three genes that have been studied extensively and appear most suitable for BCR-ABL quantitation are BCR, ABL, and β-glucuronidase (GUSB). BCR-ABL transcript numbers were expressed per microgram of leukocyte RNA.[11] Hochhaus *et al.* normalized BCR-ABL copy number to control gene transcripts and the value was expressed as a percentage ratio.[16]

However, competitive PCR was time consuming as multiple PCR reactions were required to titrate the sample with competitor and extensive post-PCR manipulation was needed. In the late 1990s, real-time PCR (RQ-PCR) procedures were developed that simplified the quantitation of transcript copy numbers.

CURRENT MONITORING STRATEGIES FOR CHRONIC MYELOID LEUKEMIA-CHRONIC PHASE PATIENTS ON TYROSINE KINASE INHIBITORS

The principal aim of residual disease analysis in patients with CML is to accurately and sensitively determine response to treatment and to enable early diagnosis of relapse.

Baseline investigation

All CML patients should be assessed thoroughly, including detailed history and clinical examination with emphasis on duration of illness and prior treatment, and assessment of liver and spleen span. Sokal[17] and Hasford prognostic scores have some value in predicting response in the imatinib era. In the international randomized trial comparing imatinib with IFNα plus cytosine arabinoside (IRIS) study, Sokal score was predictive of cytogenetic response, complete cytogenetic response at 12 months was 76%, 67%, and 49% in low-, intermediate-, and high-risk patients, respectively.[18] Progression-free survival at 60 months was 97%, 92%, and 83% in low-, intermediate-, and high-Sokal risk patients.[19]

All patients should have a complete blood count, bone marrow biopsy, cytogenetic analysis on bone marrow, and RQ-PCR on peripheral blood. Newer prognostic markers such as intrinsic sensitivity to ABL kinase inhibitors (IC_{50}),[20] OCT1 expression,[21] *in vitro* suppression of Wilms tumor gene (WT1) expression by imatinib,[22] and mRNA expression profile[23,24] may predict cytogenetic or molecular response; however, further evaluation is required.

Patients who are started on imatinib should be followed regularly for hematological, cytogenetic, and molecular response as described below (Figure 8.1).

Hematological response

Complete hematological response is defined as platelet counts $<450 \times 10^9/l$, WBC count $<10 \times 10^9/l$, differential without immature granulocytes, $<5\%$ basophils, and no palpable spleen.[25] In the IRIS study 96% of patients achieved complete hematological response by 12 months and 98% at 60 months.[19] Failure to achieve complete hematological response by 3 months is generally regarded as imatinib failure, indicating the need to consider second-line therapy. Some patients on imatinib develop cytopenia. In the IRIS trial 17%, 9%, and 4% of patients developed grade 3–4 neutropenia, thrombocytopenia, and anemia, respectively.[19] Patients who develop grade 3–4 cytopenia may need temporary cessation or dose reduction of therapy. In the therapeutic intensification in *de novo* leukemia (TIDEL) trial, significant imatinib dose reduction during the first 6 months of therapy reduced the probability of major molecular response (MMR) at 24 months.[26] Hence maintenance of dose intensity is recommended, if at all possible.

The European LeukemiaNet recommendations are that, after starting imatinib, peripheral blood counts should be monitored 2 weekly until complete hematological response is achieved and then 3 monthly unless otherwise required.[25]

Cytogenetic response

Traditionally conventional cytogenetics has been used for monitoring response to treatment. In the IRIS study, 69% of patients achieved complete cytogenetic response by 12 months.[19] Patients who had complete cytogenetic response at 12 months had significantly lower risk of progression at 60 months than patients without complete cytogenetic response ($p < 0.01$).[19] Recently, studies have shown good correlation between cytogenetic response and RQ-PCR results.[27–30] Ross *et al.*[30] reported that in patients who had simultaneous blood RQ-PCR and bone marrow cytogenetics, 98% of patients who achieved 1–2-log reduction from a standardized baseline were in a major cytogenetic response and 95% of patients who had achieved 2–3-log reductions were in complete cytogenetic response. Also, 82% of patients who had not achieved a 1-log reduction had also not achieved major cytogenetic response.

With availability of RQ-PCR assays and limited sensitivity of cytogenetic analysis, one could make a case for stopping routine cytogenetic analysis after therapy commences. However, only cytogenetic analysis can identify emergence of additional chromosome abnormalities in the leukemic clone (clonal evolution, CE), and other chromosomal abnormalities (OCA) in Ph-negative metaphases. CE is considered one manifestation of the multistep progression of CML. It was originally described in patients with blastic phase CML, occurring in 50–80% of cases[31,32] and subsequently reported in 5–10% of patients presenting with chronic phase CML and in 30% of patients developing accelerated phase features. CE has been associated with poor prognostic features.[17,33,34] In patients treated with imatinib, CE prior to imatinib is associated with a lower probability of complete cytogenetic response[35] and shorter overall survival.[36] Chromosome 9q+ deletions were

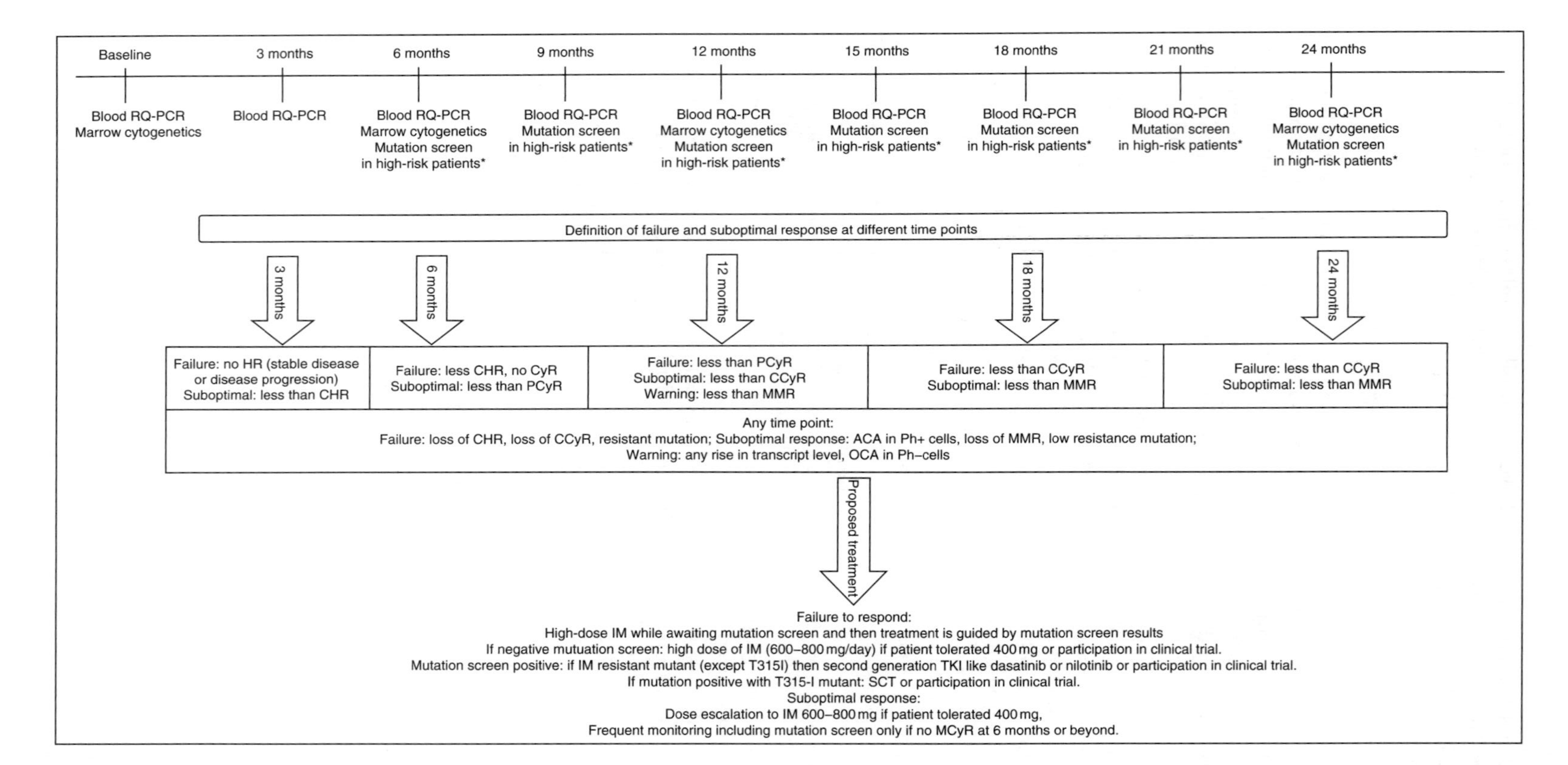

Figure 8.1 Current recommendation and guidelines for monitoring patients on kinase inhibitors. *Mutation screen in high-risk patients: <1-log reduction in BCR-ABL at 6 months or >2-fold rise in BCR-ABL and loss of MMR or >4-fold rise in BCR-ABL if MMR maintained. RQ-PCR, real-time quantitative polymerase chain reaction; HR, hematological response; CHR, complete hematological response (see text for criteria); CyR, cytogenetic response (65–95% Ph+ cells); PCyR, partial cytogenetic response (1–35% Ph+ cells); CCyR, complete cytogenetic response (no Ph+ cells); MCyR, major cytogenetic response; MMR, major molecular response; OCA, other chromosomal abnormality in Ph− cells (see text for details); IM, imatinib; TKI, tyrosine kinase inhibitors.

reported to be associated with less complete hematological response, less complete cytogenetic response, and shorter progression-free survival in one study,[37] but not in another study.[38]

OCA have been reported in the Ph-negative cells of about 5% of patients who achieved complete cytogenetic response with imatinib.[39–45] The most common abnormality is trisomy 8 (50%), but deletion of chromosome 7 alone or with other abnormalities is observed in about 15% of cases. In some cases OCA have been associated with the development of a myelodysplastic syndrome or acute myeloid leukemia, mainly in patients with a deletion of chromosome 7 and/or other complex abnormalities, but also in some patients with isolated trisomy 8. However, some patients remain in complete cytogenetic response and hematological remission after detection of OCA[43,45–48] and in some cases OCA may be transient. The presence of OCA without dysplastic features in the blood is probably not an indication for a change in therapy, based on our current understanding.

The next issue to consider is how frequently should marrow sampling be performed for cytogenetic analysis? Cytogenetic response at 3 and 6 months predicts complete cytogenetic response and progression-free survival at 24 months. However, cytogenetic response at 6 months is a better predictor than a cytogenetic response at 3 months.[49] Hence a reasonable approach would be to conduct bone marrow cytogenetic analysis at baseline, at 6 months, and then 6 monthly until a patient achieves MMR.[30] Patients with a significant rise in BCR-ABL level and loss of MMR should probably recommence marrow cytogenetic studies.[30] This approach would mean that some patients with OCA would not be identified. However, if signs of myelodysplasia, progressive anemia, or macrocytosis are identified, marrow studies would then be justified. If a clinician would change therapy in the setting of OCA with a normal blood picture, then regular marrow studies even for patients in MMR may be justified.

Real-time quantitative polymerase chain reaction

Competitive RT-PCR was used to follow patients on IFNα and following allogeneic stem cell transplantation. The introduction of real-time quantitative PCR (RQ-PCR) techniques (TaqMan (Applied Biosystem, Foster City, CA) and LightCycler system (Roche Applied Science, Indianapolis, IN)) not only simplified quantification of residual disease, but also contributed to increased precision and accuracy of the PCR measurements, making RQ-PCR the current standard for BCR-ABL quantification. The TaqMan assay is based on the use of the 5′ nuclease activity of *Taq* polymerase to cleave a non-extendable dual-labeled hybridization probe during the extension phase of the PCR assay. One fluorescent dye serves as a reporter and its emission spectra is quenched by the second fluorescent dye. The nuclease degradation of the probe releases the quenching dye resulting in an increase of fluorescence monitored by a detector in real time. Cycle threshold (Ct) values are calculated by determining the point at which the fluorescence crosses a threshold limit. An alternative RQ-PCR approach for detection and quantification of BCR-ABL fusion transcripts has been established using the LightCycler technology. Fluorescence monitoring of PCR amplification is based on the concept of fluorescence resonance energy transfer (FRET) between two adjacent hybridization probes carrying donor and acceptor fluorophores. Excitation of a donor fluorophore (fluorescein) with an emission spectrum that overlaps the excitation spectrum of an acceptor fluorophore results in non-radioactive energy transfer to the acceptor. Once conditions are established, the amount of fluorescence resulting from the two probes is proportional to the amount of PCR product.[50,51]

In RQ-PCR, the kinetics of PCR are followed during the linear amplification phase rather than at or near the end point where amplification plateaus. This eliminates the need for co-amplification of a competitor. The fluorescence-based technology enhances reproducibility since quantitation is determined during the exponential phase of the PCR. The real-time detection of accumulating product eliminates the need for post-PCR manipulation and, thus, the possibility of post-PCR contamination is reduced. The real-time technique is performed on an analyzer that incorporates a thermal cycler, fluorescence detection, and result calculation, which has greatly simplified quantitative PCR.

The IRIS trial provided evidence for the first time that a reduction of BCR-ABL transcripts was predictive of progression-free survival.[52] In the molecular analysis of the IRIS study a major molecular response was defined as ≥3-log reduction in BCR-ABL : BCR level when compared with the standardized median pretreatment level. This was established by calculating the median BCR-ABL level of 30 pretherapy samples. In this study 53% and 80% of patients who were in complete cytogenetic response achieved major molecular response at 12 and 48 months, respectively.[19] In a landmark analysis of the IRIS trial, achievement of MMR by 12 months was associated with 100% probability of transformation-free survival at 60 months.[19] Molecular response at 3 months is also a good indicator of subsequent response. Those patients who do not achieve a 1-log reduction by 3 months have a very low probability of achieving MMR (only 13% at 30 months). Patients who achieved >2-log and 1–2-log reductions at 3 months have 100% and 69% probability of achieving MMR.[53] Recently, a consensus group within the European LeukemiaNet proposed a definition of failure and suboptimal response at different time points.[25] 'Failure' means that continuing imatinib treatment at the current dose is no longer appropriate for these patients, who would likely benefit more from other treatments. 'Suboptimal response' means that the patient may still have substantial benefit from continuing imatinib, but that the long-term outcome of the treatment would not likely be as favorable. A 'Warning' means that standard-dose imatinib treatment may not be the best choice, and the patient requires more careful monitoring. Patients who fail to achieve optimal response are most likely to have some form of imatinib resistance, although poor compliance should be considered.

IMATINIB RESISTANCE

Imatinib resistance can be categorized as primary or acquired. Primary resistance is the failure to achieve specified levels of response. This has been defined as failure to achieve complete hematological response by 3 months (2–3% of patients) or major cytogenetic response by 6 months (approximately 15% of patients) despite a therapeutic dose of imatinib (at least 300 mg daily). Overall, 10–16% of newly diagnosed CML patients appear to have primary resistance to imatinib at 400 mg/day.[19,54] Primary resistance is more frequent in chronic phase patients who were treated with imatinib following IFNα failure or intolerance, 5% did not achieve complete hematological response and 40% did not achieve major cytogenetic response by 18 months.[55] Imatinib failure is also more common in advanced stage disease patients, 76% of patients in accelerated phase and 84% of patients in blast crisis failed to achieve major cytogenetic response.[56,57]

Currently mechanisms of primary resistance are not clear but it does not appear to be due to kinase domain mutations.[53] Recently, White *et al.* suggested OCT1-mediated imatinib influx may be a key determinant of molecular response to imatinib and patients with lower OCT1-mediated intracellular drug uptake and retention may have lower rates of MMR at 3 and 12 months.[21]

Acquired resistance can be defined as onset of advanced phase disease in a patient who previously had sustained complete hematological remission or loss of sustained complete hematological response without progression to advanced phase or loss of major cytogenetic response or loss of a complete cytogenetic response with a corresponding significant increase in BCR-ABL transcript numbers.[58]

In the IRIS trial the rate of all progression events was 18% after a median follow-up of 5 years, most of which occurred within the first 3 years of treatment.[19] The incidence of secondary resistance or progressive disease was higher (26%) in chronic phase patients who were previously treated with IFNα and substantially higher in accelerated (73%) and blast phases (95%) of CML.[54]

The most common mechanism of acquired resistance to imatinib is the reactivation of BCR-ABL kinase activity within leukemic cells despite the presence of imatinib. Point mutation in the BCR-ABL kinase domain is the most common cause (50–90% of cases) of acquired imatinib resistance;[59–64] other proposed mechanisms of acquired imatinib resistance are overexpression and amplification of the *BCR-ABL* gene,[59,60] activation of BCR-ABL independent pathways such as members of the SRC kinase family,[65] binding of imatinib to serum α1 acid glycoprotein, and increased drug efflux through the multidrug resistance protein.[66] The other concept which is evolving is 'leukemic stem cell resistance'. Leukemic stem cells may be in a quiescent state (G_0) which renders them resistant to imatinib and may be responsible for resistance and progression.[67]

More than 70 mutations have been identified in the kinase domain and an update of the reported mutations is represented in Figure 8.2. The mutations are located throughout the kinase domain including the ATP binding loop (P-loop), imatinib binding site, activation loop (A-loop), catalytic domain, and the carboxy terminal.

(1) P-loop mutations. The P-loop normally accommodates the phosphate group of ATP. It is a glycine-rich structure and encompasses amino acids 248–257. Upon binding of imatinib, the P-loop undergoes major downward displacement and forms a hydrophobic cage surrounding imatinib, which is stabilized by water-mediated hydrogen bonds between Y253 and N322. Mutations in the P-loop (L248V, G250E, Q252H/R,

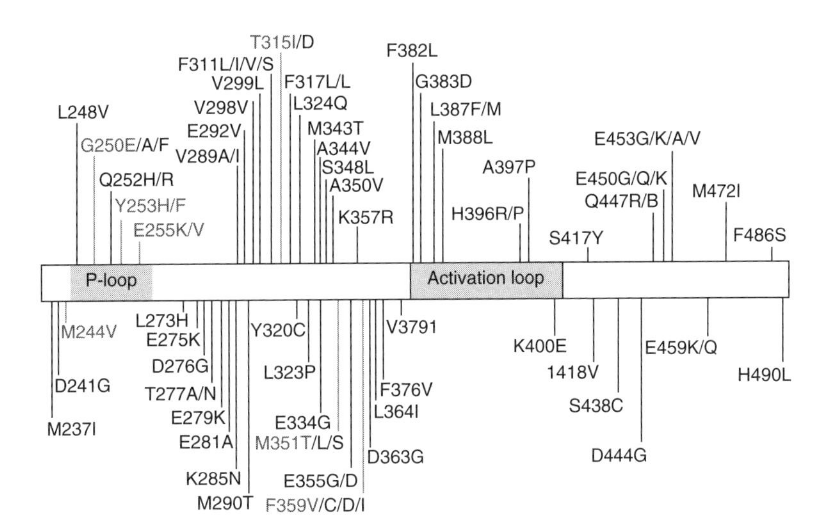

Figure 8.2 Linear representation of ABL kinase domain and relative position of mutations. There are more than 70 mutations reported; however, amino acid substitution at seven residues (M244V, G250E, Y253 H/F, E255K/V, T315I, M351T, and F359V) account for 85% of all resistance associated mutations.[86]

Y253F/H, and E255K) may lead to destabilization of the distorted shape and shift the equilibrium toward the active state, thus hindering the conformation of the P-loop required for imatinib binding. P-loop mutations comprise 45–50% of all mutations and have been associated with a poor prognosis compared with other mutations. We reported mortality of 92% in patients with P-loop mutations (median survival of 4.5 months after detection of the mutation), while only 21% of patients with mutations outside the P-loop died.[62] Two other groups also reported that P-loop mutation were associated with poorer prognosis and shorter survival compared with patients with other mutations.[68,69] *In vitro* analysis revealed that E255K, E255V, Y253H, Y253F, and G250E were highly resistant to imatinib with IC_{50} values greater than 10-fold higher than wild-type BCR-ABL.[64] However, Jabbour *et al.* did not find that P-loop mutations were associated with poorer prognosis.[70] A recent report has determined that some mutations in the P-loop may alter the transformation potency of BCR-ABL by altering substrate specificity and signal transduction pathway activation.[71] The two P-loop mutations that were tested, E255K and Y253F, displayed increased transformation potency compared with wild-type and the other mutants. While another common mutant M351T, displayed the least transforming potency.

(2) Mutations at the imatinib binding sites. Amino acids T315 ('gatekeeper position'), V289, F317, and F359 interact directly with imatinib via hydrogen bond (T315) or van der Waals interactions (V289, F317). T315I is largely insensitive not only to imatinib but also to second generation tyrosine kinase inhibitors including nilotinib and dasatinib. Substitution of threonine with the bulky isoleucine not only disrupts the hydrogen bond with imatinib but also allosterically interferes with drug binding. *In vitro* kinase analysis shows that T315I is highly resistant to imatinib with IC_{50} >10 μM. While F317L is less resistant with imatinib IC_{50} of 0.9 μM (3 times higher than wild-type BCR-ABL).[64]

(3) Mutations involving the activation loop (A-loop mutation). The activation loop comprises amino acids 381–402 and regulates the kinase activity. Mutations in the A-loop prevent the kinase from adopting its inactive conformation, which is required for imatinib binding.[72] A-loop mutations comprise 5% of all mutations and exhibit moderate imatinib resistance in cellular and *in vitro* kinase assays.

(4) Mutations of catalytic domain. Mutations of the catalytic domain comprise approximately 20% of all mutations with M351T being the most common. M351 contacts the ABL SH2 domain and helps to stabilize the autoinhibited conformation of ABL. The M351T mutation disrupts the interaction between the SH2 and the kinase domain and impairs autoinihibition, shifting the equilibrium toward the active conformation to which imatinib cannot bind.[72] M351T confers moderate imatinib resistance in *in vitro* kinase assay.[64]

(5) Mutations in the carboxy terminal. Mutations in the carboxy terminal have been detected in about 16% of all patients with mutations tested at our institution. The IC_{50} values for most of these mutations are unknown. An *in vitro* mutagenesis screen identified many additional mutations within and outside the kinase domain, which have not yet been recovered from patients. However, most of the studies sequenced the kinase domain and hence information regarding mutation outside the kinase domain is limited.

Although kinase domain mutations are common cause of acquired imatinib resistance, all mutations may not be associated with imatinib resistance.[73] By using sensitive assays, kinase domain mutations have been detected within 3 months of imatinib treatment exposure[74] or prior to imatinib therapy[68] and even at diagnosis.[75] However, these mutations were not always detected in patients who developed subsequent imatinib resistance. There are several technologies available for mutation detection and they vary in sensitivity. Direct sequencing can usually detect mutant clones representing >15–20% of total BCR-ABL,[60,61] while subcloning and sequencing has a sensitivity of 5–10% depending on the number of clones examined.[64] Denaturing high-performance liquid chromatography (D-HPLC) is a more sensitive method that is able to detect >0.1% mutant clone.[76,77]

As mutation analysis is costly and not readily available, it is imperative to select patients for detailed analysis, who are likely to have mutations. Mutations are most common in blast crisis. Our group have reported that accelerated phase patients have a 61% probability of developing mutations by 24 months of imatinib. Late chronic phase patients treated with prior IFNα had a 26% probability of mutations emerging by 2 years, whereas newly diagnosed patients had a 7% probability of a mutation.[78] Hence regular mutation screening would be appropriate for patients in the advanced phase of CML. However, monitoring newly diagnosed patients with regular mutation screens is probably not cost effective.[78] Selected chronic phase patients who have suboptimal cytogenetic and molecular response or have significant increases in BCR/ABL should be targeted.[78,79] We reported that 61% of patients who had more than a 2-fold rise in BCR-ABL transcripts had a mutation detectable by direct sequencing. Only 0.6% of patients with stable or decreasing BCR-ABL levels had a detectable mutation.[80] Another group reported that a serial rise in BCR-ABL transcripts may be more reliable than a single 2-fold rise in BCR-ABL transcripts.[81] This is highly dependent on the measurement reliability of the assay. The depth of BCR-ABL reduction from which change is detected is also relevant, and loss of threshold levels of response, such as loss of MMR may define patients in need of change in therapy, particularly if linked to a molecular cause such as kinase mutation.[82]

ADDITIONAL VALUE OF REAL-TIME QUANTITATIVE POLYMERASE CHAIN REACTION TO MONITOR COMPLIANCE

A greater than 2-fold rise in BCR-ABL transcripts and/or a persistent rise in consecutive RQ-PCR assays for BCR-ABL indicates the need for kinase domain mutation screening. However, not all patients with a rise in BCR-ABL transcripts have detectable mutations. Some of these patients will have acquired resistance without kinase domain mutations. Furthermore, in some cases poor compliance may lead to a pattern mimicking acquired resistance. An illustrative case from our center is a 37-year-old man diagnosed with CML-CP (Figure 8.3). After starting imatinib, BCR-ABL transcripts decreased for the first 9 months. However, because of an intercurrent psychiatric illness he ceased taking imatinib without informing his treating physician. Within 2 months of stopping imatinib BCR-ABL transcripts increased to baseline level. The kinase domain mutation screen was negative. After restarting imatinib BCR-ABL transcripts decreased steadily over the next 12 months. However, he again ceased imatinib. Within a short time of stopping imatinib BCR-ABL transcripts once again rapidly increased and again kinase domain mutation screen was negative. Imatinib was restarted under supervision and his BCR-ABL transcripts fell once again.

This case highlights that poor compliance should be considered if BCR-ABL transcripts rise and also highlights the additional role for regular RQ-PCR for BCR-ABL to monitor patient compliance.

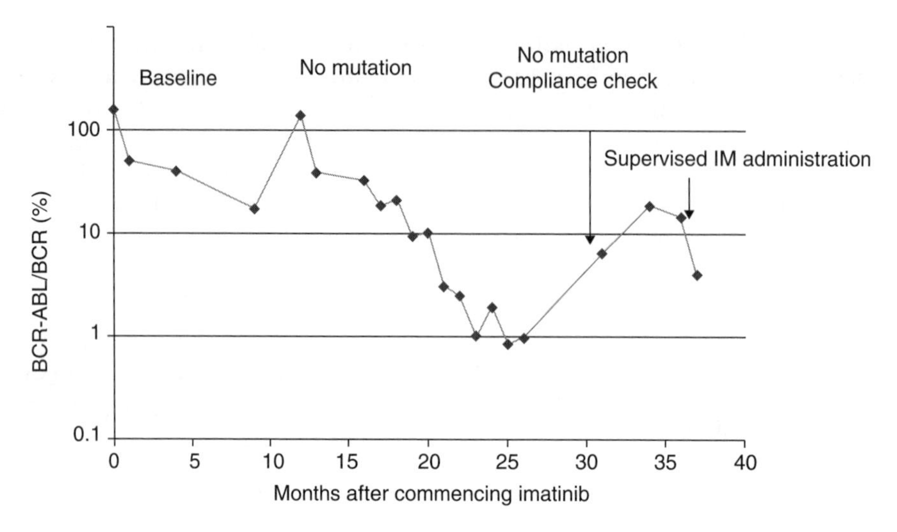

Figure 8.3 Role of real-time quantitative polymerase chain reaction (RQ-PCR) for BCR-ABL in monitoring patient compliance to imatinib (IM). Following initial response, BCR-ABL transcripts increased twice first at 12 months and then at 31 months after starting imatinib. On both occasions kinase domain mutation studies were negative. Both increases in BCR-ABL transcripts were owing to poor compliance to imatinib.

LIMITATIONS OF CURRENT MONITORING METHODOLOGY AND STRATEGIES FOR IMPROVEMENT

Sensitivity of PCR assay

RQ-PCR for BCR-ABL mRNA is by far the most sensitive assay in the context of residual disease analysis and can detect a single leukemia cell in a background of 10^5 to 10^6 normal cells. Therefore, PCR is up to 2–3 logs more sensitive than conventional methods. However, patients who have no residual disease detectable by RQ-PCR may still have up to a million leukemic cells that could contribute to subsequent relapse. Currently, MMR confers protection from progression-free survival (PFS).[19] Patients who achieved MMR by 12 months had 100% PFS at 5 years.[83] Current assays are not usually sensitive enough to detect BCR-ABL transcript levels below 4.5-log reduction from standardized baseline. Rousselot *et al.*[84] stopped imatinib in patients who had persistently negative RQ-PCR assays for more than 2 years on imatinib therapy. Half of their patients relapsed within 6 months of stopping imatinib. This indicates that many patients who are PCR negative still have residual disease capable of early relapse when imatinib is stopped. It would clearly be advantageous to increase the sensitivity of MRD monitoring to enable patient response to be monitored for longer and allow a more substantial response to be determined.

Standardization of RQ-PCR assay

Although RQ-PCR is currently the most sensitive test to monitor patients who achieve complete cytogenetic response, there is still considerable diversity in the way in which RQ-PCR for BCR-ABL is carried out and how the results are reported in different laboratories. Methods have not been standardized across all laboratories and guidelines for acceptable levels of reproducibility and sensitivity are still being established. In addition certified international reference and control methods are not available.

To address these issues there was an investigator meeting at the National Institutes of Health (NIH) in Bethesda in October 2005 and key recommendations made at this meeting were published in 2006.[85] It is beyond the scope of this chapter to include detailed guidelines. Here we discuss some of the key issues and recommendations.

International scale for reporting results

There are currently various different methods in use for reporting results of RQ-PCR data on individual patients. It is highly desirable that an international scale of measurement for BCR-ABL transcript levels is established. This would enable molecular response to be compared in trials assessing different drug regimens where RQ-PCR assays have been performed in different laboratories using various techniques.

A panel of experts proposed an international scale that could be applied at individual centers. The international scale would be anchored to the major molecular response as established in the IRIS trial and is fixed at 0.10%. To convert laboratory BCR-ABL values to the international scale a conversion factor for each laboratory must be determined. The conversion factor is derived from the value that is equivalent to the MMR value as established in the IRIS trial. The conversion factor should be formally tested with a series of quality control samples, with values established in reference laboratories.[86]

The proposed formula for individual conversion of laboratory BCR-ABL/control percentage values to the international scale is

$$\text{BCR-ABL(local value)} \times \text{conversion factor} = \text{BCR-ABL (international scale)}$$

SUMMARY

All newly diagnosed CML-CP patients should have blood counts, RQ-PCR for BCR-ABL on peripheral blood, and bone marrow cytogenetic tests at baseline (Figure 8.1). After starting imatinib patients should be followed by complete blood counts every 2 weeks until complete hematological response and then 6 weekly unless indicated otherwise. RQ-PCR for BCR-ABL should be conducted every 3 months. Bone marrow cytogenetics analysis should be undertaken at diagnosis, at 6 months, and then at 12 months, or if there is a significant rise in BCR-ABL. Mutation screening should take place in patients who have suboptimal response or have a significant rise in BCR-ABL.

ACKNOWLEDGMENT

We thank Susan Branford for help in the preparation of the manuscript.

REFERENCES

1. Talpaz M, Kantarjian HM, McCredie KB et al. Clinical investigation of human alpha interferon in chronic myelogenous leukemia. Blood 1987; 69: 1280–8.
2. Chase A, Grand F, Zhang JG et al. Factors influencing the false positive and negative rates of BCR-ABL fluorescence in situ hybridization. Genes Chromosomes Cancer 1997; 18: 246–53.
3. Tkachuk DC, Westbrook CA, Andreeff M et al. Detection of bcr-abl fusion in chronic myelogeneous leukemia by in situ hybridization. Science 1990; 250: 559–62.
4. Schoch C, Schnittger S, Bursch S et al. Comparison of chromosome banding analysis, interphase- and hypermetaphase-FISH, qualitative and quantitative PCR for diagnosis and for follow-up in chronic myeloid leukemia: a study on 350 cases. Leukemia 2002; 16: 53–9.
5. Morley A. Quantifying leukemia. N Engl J Med 1998; 339: 627–9.
6. Morgan GJ, Hughes T, Janssen JW et al. Polymerase chain reaction for detection of residual leukaemia. Lancet 1989; 1: 928–9.
7. Hughes TP, Morgan GJ, Martiat P, Goldman JM. Detection of residual leukemia after bone marrow transplant for chronic myeloid leukemia: role of polymerase chain reaction in predicting relapse. Blood 1991; 77: 874–8.
8. Kawasaki ES, Clark SS, Coyne MY et al. Diagnosis of chronic myeloid and acute lymphocytic leukemias by detection of leukemia-specific mRNA sequences amplified in vitro. Proc Natl Acad Sci USA 1988; 85: 5698–702.
9. Hochhaus A, Weisser A, La Rosee P et al. Detection and quantification of residual disease in chronic myelogenous leukemia. Leukemia 2000; 14: 998–1005.
10. Potter MN, Cross NC, van Dongen JJ et al. Molecular evidence of minimal residual disease after treatment for leukaemia and lymphoma: an updated meeting report and review. Leukemia 1993; 7: 1302–14.
11. Cross NC, Feng L, Chase A et al. Competitive polymerase chain reaction to estimate the number of BCR-ABL transcripts in chronic myeloid leukemia patients after bone marrow transplantation. Blood 1993; 82: 1929–36.
12. Delage R, Soiffer RJ, Dear K, Ritz J. Clinical significance of bcr-abl gene rearrangement detected by polymerase chain reaction after allogeneic bone

marrow transplantation in chronic myelogenous leukemia. Blood 1991; 78: 2759–67.
13. Lin F, Kirkland MA, van Rhee FV et al. Molecular analysis of transient cytogenetic relapse after allogeneic bone marrow transplantation for chronic myeloid leukaemia. Bone Marrow Transplant 1996; 18: 1147–52.
14. Lin F, van Rhee F, Goldman JM, Cross NC. Kinetics of increasing BCR-ABL transcript numbers in chronic myeloid leukemia patients who relapse after bone marrow transplantation. Blood 1996; 87: 4473–8.
15. Branford S, Hughes TP, Rudzki Z. Monitoring chronic myeloid leukaemia therapy by real-time quantitative PCR in blood is a reliable alternative to bone marrow cytogenetics. Br J Haematol 1999; 107: 587–99.
16. Hochhaus A, Lin F, Reiter A et al. Quantification of residual disease in chronic myelogenous leukemia patients on interferon-alpha therapy by competitive polymerase chain reaction. Blood 1996; 87: 1549–55.
17. Sokal JE, Gomez GA, Baccarani M et al. Prognostic significance of additional cytogenetic abnormalities at diagnosis of Philadelphia chromosome-positive chronic granulocytic leukemia. Blood 1988; 72: 294–8.
18. O'Brien SG, Guilhot F, Larson RA et al. Imatinib compared with interferon and low-dose cytarabine for newly diagnosed chronic-phase chronic myeloid leukemia. N Engl J Med 2003; 348: 994–1004.
19. Druker BJ, Guilhot F, O'Brien SG et al. Five-year follow-up of patients receiving imatinib for chronic myeloid leukemia. N Engl J Med 2006; 355: 2408–17.
20. White D, Saunders V, Lyons AB et al. In vitro sensitivity to imatinib-induced inhibition of ABL kinase activity is predictive of molecular response in patients with de novo CML. Blood 2005; 106: 2520–6.
21. White DL, Saunders VA, Dang P et al. OCT-1-mediated influx is a key determinant of the intracellular uptake of imatinib but not nilotinib (AMN107): reduced OCT-1 activity is the cause of low in vitro sensitivity to imatinib. Blood 2006; 108: 697–704.
22. Cilloni D, Messa F, Gottardi E et al. Sensitivity to imatinib therapy may be predicted by testing Wilms tumor gene expression and colony growth after a short in vitro incubation. Cancer 2004; 101: 979–88.
23. Crossman L, Loriaux M, Vartanian K et al. Gene expression profiling of CML CD34+ cells prior to imatinib therapy reveals differences between patients with and without subsequent complete cytogenetic response. ASH annual Meeting Abstracts 2005; 106: 1222a.
24. McLean LA, Gathmann I, Capdeville R et al. Pharmacogenomic analysis of cytogenetic response in chronic myeloid leukemia patients treated with imatinib. Clin Cancer Res 2004; 10: 155–65.
25. Baccarani M, Saglio G, Goldman J et al. Evolving concepts in the management of chronic myeloid leukemia: recommendations from an expert panel on behalf of the European LeukemiaNet. Blood 2006; 108: 1809–20.
26. Hughes TP, Branford S, Reynolds J et al. Maintenance of imatinib dose intensity in the first six months of therapy for newly diagnosed patients with CML is predictive of molecular response, independent of the ability to increase dose at a later point. ASH Annual Meeting Abstracts 2005; 106: 164a.
27. Hughes T, Branford S. Molecular monitoring of chronic myeloid leukemia. Semin Hematol 2003; 40: 62–8.
28. Kantarjian HM, Talpaz M, Cortes J et al. Quantitative polymerase chain reaction monitoring of BCR-ABL during therapy with imatinib mesylate (STI571; gleevec) in chronic-phase chronic myelogenous leukemia. Clin Cancer Res 2003; 9: 160–6.
29. Merx K, Muller MC, Kreil S et al. Early reduction of BCR-ABL mRNA transcript levels predicts cytogenetic response in chronic phase CML patients treated with imatinib after failure of interferon alpha. Leukemia 2002; 16: 1579–83.
30. Ross DM, Branford S, Moore S, Hughes TP. Limited clinical value of regular bone marrow cytogenetic analysis in imatinib-treated chronic phase CML patients monitored by RQ-PCR for BCR-ABL. Leukemia 2006; 20: 664–70.
31. Anastasi J, Feng J, Le Beau MM et al. The relationship between secondary chromosomal abnormalities and blast transformation in chronic myelogenous leukemia. Leukemia 1995; 9: 628–33.
32. Sessarego M, Panarello C, Coviello DA et al. Karyotype evolution in CML: high frequency of translocations other than the Ph. Cancer Genet Cytogenet 1987; 25: 73–80.
33. Kantarjian HM, Smith TL, McCredie KB et al. Chronic myelogenous leukemia: a multivariate analysis of the associations of patient characteristics and therapy with survival. Blood 1985; 66: 1326–35.
34. Swolin B, Weinfeld A, Westin J et al. Karyotypic evolution in Ph-positive chronic myeloid leukemia in relation to management and disease progression. Cancer Genet Cytogenet 1985; 18: 65–79.
35. Schoch C, Haferlach T, Kern W et al. Occurrence of additional chromosome aberrations in chronic myeloid leukemia patients treated with imatinib mesylate. Leukemia 2003; 17: 461–3.
36. Cortes JE, Talpaz M, Giles F et al. Prognostic significance of cytogenetic clonal evolution in patients with chronic myelogenous leukemia on imatinib mesylate therapy. Blood 2003; 101: 3794–800.
37. Huntly BJ, Guilhot F, Reid AG et al. Imatinib improves but may not fully reverse the poor prognosis

of patients with CML with derivative chromosome 9 deletions. Blood 2003; 102: 2205–12.

38. Quintas-Cardama A, Kantarjian H, Talpaz M et al. Imatinib mesylate therapy may overcome the poor prognostic significance of deletions of derivative chromosome 9 in patients with chronic myelogenous leukemia. Blood 2005; 105: 2281–6.
39. Abruzzese E, Gozzetti A, Zaccaria A. Ph-abnormal clones emerged during imatinib therapy: clinical report and clonal analyses on 23 patients from GIMEMA working party in CML registry. Blood 2004; 104: 803a, abstract 2936.
40. Bacher U, Hochhaus A, Berger U et al. Clonal aberrations in Philadelphia chromosome negative hematopoiesis in patients with chronic myeloid leukemia treated with imatinib or interferon alpha. Leukemia 2005; 19: 460–3.
41. Bumm T, Muller C, Al-Ali HK et al. Emergence of clonal cytogenetic abnormalities in Ph- cells in some CML patients in cytogenetic remission to imatinib but restoration of polyclonal hematopoiesis in the majority. Blood 2003; 101: 1941–9.
42. Jabbour E, Kantarjian H, O'Brien S et al. Chromosomal abnormalities in Philadelphia chromosome-negative metaphases appearing during Imatinib Mesylate therapy in patients with newly diagnosed chronic myeloid leukemia in chronic phase. Blood 2005; 106: 317a, abstract 1090.
43. Medina J, Kantarjian H, Talpaz M et al. Chromosomal abnormalities in Philadelphia chromosome-negative metaphases appearing during imatinib mesylate therapy in patients with Philadelphia chromosome-positive chronic myelogenous leukemia in chronic phase. Cancer 2003; 98: 1905–11.
44. O'Dwyer ME, Gatter KM, Loriaux M et al. Demonstration of Philadelphia chromosome negative abnormal clones in patients with chronic myelogenous leukemia during major cytogenetic responses induced by imatinib mesylate. Leukemia 2003; 17: 481–7.
45. Terre C, Eclache V, Rousselot P et al. Report of 34 patients with clonal chromosomal abnormalities in Philadelphia-negative cells during imatinib treatment of Philadelphia-positive chronic myeloid leukemia. Leukemia 2004; 18: 1340–6.
46. Abruzzese E, Gozzetti A, Zaccaria A. Ph-abnormal clones emerged during imatinib therapy: clinical report and clonal analyses on 23 patients from GIMEMA working party in CML registry. Blood 2004; 104: 803a, abstract 2936.
47. Deininger M, Kantarjian H, Hochhaus A et al. Good prognosis of CML patients with clonal cytogenetic abnormalities in Ph-negative cells. Blood 2005; 106: 315a, abstract 1082.
48. Jabbour E, Kantarjian H, O'Brien S et al. Chromosomal abnormalities in Philadelphia chromosome-negative metaphases appearing during Imatinib Mesylate therapy in patients with newly diagnosed chronic myeloid leukemia in chronic phase. Blood 2005; 106: 317a, abstract 1090.
49. Druker B, Gathmann I, Bolton AE, Larson RA. Probability and impact of obtaining a cytogenetic response to imatinib as intial therapy for chronic myeloid leukemia (CML) in chronic phase. Blood 2003; 102: 182a.
50. Wittwer CT, Herrmann MG, Moss AA, Rasmussen RP. Continuous fluorescence monitoring of rapid cycle DNA amplification. Biotechniques 1997; 22: 130–1, 134–8.
51. Wittwer CT, Ririe KM, Andrew RV et al. The LightCycler: a microvolume multisample fluorimeter with rapid temperature control. Biotechniques 1997; 22: 176–81.
52. Hughes TP, Kaeda J, Branford S et al. Frequency of major molecular responses to imatinib or interferon alfa plus cytarabine in newly diagnosed chronic myeloid leukemia. N Engl J Med 2003; 349: 1423–32.
53. Hughes T, Branford S. Molecular monitoring of BCR-ABL as a guide to clinical management in chronic myeloid leukaemia. Blood Rev 2006; 20: 29–41.
54. Shah NP. Loss of response to imatinib: mechanisms and management. Hematology Am Soc Hematol Educ Program 2005; 183–7.
55. Kantarjian H, Sawyers C, Hochhaus A et al. Hematologic and cytogenetic responses to imatinib mesylate in chronic myelogenous leukemia. N Engl J Med 2002; 346: 645–52.
56. Sawyers CL, Hochhaus A, Feldman E et al. Imatinib induces hematologic and cytogenetic responses in patients with chronic myelogenous leukemia in myeloid blast crisis: results of a phase II study. Blood 2002; 99: 3530–9.
57. Talpaz M, Silver RT, Druker BJ et al. Imatinib induces durable hematologic and cytogenetic responses in patients with accelerated phase chronic myeloid leukemia: results of a phase 2 study. Blood 2002; 99: 1928–37.
58. Goldman JM. Chronic myeloid leukemia – still a few questions. Exp Hematol 2004; 32: 2–10.
59. Gorre ME, Mohammed M, Ellwood K et al. Clinical resistance to STI-571 cancer therapy caused by BCR-ABL gene mutation or amplification. Science 2001; 293: 876–80.
60. Hochhaus A, Kreil S, Corbin AS et al. Molecular and chromosomal mechanisms of resistance to imatinib (STI571) therapy. Leukemia 2002; 16: 2190–6.
61. Branford S, Rudzki Z, Walsh S et al. High frequency of point mutations clustered within the adenosine triphosphate-binding region of BCR/ABL in patients with chronic myeloid leukemia or Ph-positive acute lymphoblastic leukemia who develop imatinib (STI571) resistance. Blood 2002; 99: 3472–5.

62. Branford S, Rudzki Z, Walsh S et al. Detection of BCR-ABL mutations in patients with CML treated with imatinib is virtually always accompanied by clinical resistance, and mutations in the ATP phosphate-binding loop (P-loop) are associated with a poor prognosis. Blood 2003; 102: 276–83.
63. Cowan-Jacob SW, Guez V, Fendrich G et al. Imatinib (STI571) resistance in chronic myelogenous leukemia: molecular basis of the underlying mechanisms and potential strategies for treatment. Mini Rev Med Chem 2004; 4: 285–99.
64. Shah NP, Nicoll JM, Nagar B et al. Multiple BCR-ABL kinase domain mutations confer polyclonal resistance to the tyrosine kinase inhibitor imatinib (STI571) in chronic phase and blast crisis chronic myeloid leukemia. Cancer Cell 2002; 2: 117–25.
65. Donato NJ, Wu JY, Stapley J et al. BCR-ABL independence and LYN kinase overexpression in chronic myelogenous leukemia cells selected for resistance to STI571. Blood 2003; 101: 690–8.
66. Gambacorti-Passerini C, Barni R, le Coutre P et al. Role of alpha1 acid glycoprotein in the in vivo resistance of human BCR-ABL(+) leukemic cells to the abl inhibitor STI571. J Natl Cancer Inst 2000; 92: 1641–50.
67. Graham SM, Jorgensen HG, Allan E et al. Primitive, quiescent, Philadelphia-positive stem cells from patients with chronic myeloid leukemia are insensitive to STI571 in vitro. Blood 2002; 99: 319–25.
68. Soverini S, Martinelli G, Rosti G et al. ABL mutations in late chronic phase chronic myeloid leukemia patients with up-front cytogenetic resistance to imatinib are associated with a greater likelihood of progression to blast crisis and shorter survival: a study by the GIMEMA Working Party on Chronic Myeloid Leukemia. J Clin Oncol 2005; 23: 4100–9.
69. Nicolini FE, Corm S, Le QH et al. Mutation status and clinical outcome of 89 imatinib mesylate-resistant chronic myelogenous leukemia patients: a retrospective analysis from the French intergroup of CML (Fi(phi)-LMC GROUP). Leukemia 2006; 20: 1061–6.
70. Jabbour E, Kantarjian H, Jones D et al. Frequency and clinical significance of BCR-ABL mutations in patients with chronic myeloid leukemia treated with imatinib mesylate. Leukemia 2006; 20: 1767–73.
71. Griswold IJ, MacPartlin M, Bumm T et al. Kinase domain mutants of Bcr-Abl exhibit altered transformation potency, kinase activity, and substrate utilization, irrespective of sensitivity to imatinib. Mol Cell Biol 2006; 26: 6082–93.
72. Deininger M, Buchdunger E, Druker BJ. The development of imatinib as a therapeutic agent for chronic myeloid leukemia. Blood 2005; 105: 2640–53.
73. Corbin AS, La Rosee P, Stoffregen EP et al. Several Bcr-Abl kinase domain mutants associated with imatinib mesylate resistance remain sensitive to imatinib. Blood 2003; 101: 4611–14.
74. Willis SG, Lange T, Demehri S et al. High-sensitivity detection of BCR-ABL kinase domain mutations in imatinib-naive patients: correlation with clonal cytogenetic evolution but not response to therapy. Blood 2005; 106: 2128–37.
75. Roche-Lestienne C, Lai JL, Darre S et al. A mutation conferring resistance to imatinib at the time of diagnosis of chronic myelogenous leukemia. N Engl J Med 2003; 348: 2265–6.
76. Irving JA, O'Brien S, Lennard AL et al. Use of denaturing HPLC for detection of mutations in the BCR-ABL kinase domain in patients resistant to Imatinib. Clin Chem 2004; 50: 1233–7.
77. Deininger MW, McGreevey L, Willis S et al. Detection of ABL kinase domain mutations with denaturing high-performance liquid chromatography. Leukemia 2004; 18: 864–71.
78. Hughes T. ABL kinase inhibitor therapy for CML: baseline assessments and response monitoring. Hematology Am Soc Hematol Educ Program 2006; 211–18.
79. Branford S, Rudzki Z, Parkinson I et al. Real-time quantitative PCR analysis can be used as a primary screen to identify patients with CML treated with imatinib who have BCR-ABL kinase domain mutations. Blood 2004; 104: 2926–32.
80. Branford S, Rudzki Z, Parkinson I et al. Real-time quantitative PCR analysis can be used as a primary screen to identify patients with CML treated with imatinib who have BCR-ABL kinase domain mutations. Blood 2004; 104: 2926–32.
81. Wang L, Knight K, Lucas C, Clark RE. The role of serial BCR-ABL transcript monitoring in predicting the emergence of BCR-ABL kinase mutations in imatinib-treated patients with chronic myeloid leukemia. Haematologica 2006; 91: 235–9.
82. Mauro MJ. Defining and managing imatinib resistance. Hematology Am Soc Hematol Educ Program 2006; 219–25.
83. Sherbenou DW, Wong MJ, Humayun A et al. Mutations of the BCR-ABL-kinase domain occur in a minority of patients with stable complete cytogenetic response to imatinib. Leukemia 2007; 21: 489–93.
84. Rousselot P, Huguet F, Rea D et al. Imatinib mesylate discontinuation in patients with chronic

myelogenous leukemia in complete molecular remission for more than 2 years. Blood 2007; 109: 58–60.

85. Hughes T, Deininger M, Hochhaus A et al. Monitoring CML patients responding to treatment with tyrosine kinase inhibitors: review and recommendations for harmonizing current methodology for detecting BCR-ABL transcripts and kinase domain mutations and for expressing results. Blood 2006; 108: 28–37.

86. Soverini S, Colarossi S, Gnani A et al. Contribution of ABL kinase domain mutations to imatinib resistance in different subsets of Philadelphia-positive patients: by the GIMEMA Working Party on Chronic Myeloid Leukemia. Clin Cancer Res 2006; 12: 7374–9.

Immunotherapy in chronic myeloid leukemia

9

Richard E Clark

It is clear that the immune system is particularly important in achieving the cure associated with allogeneic stem cell transplantation (SCT). This is especially true for chronic myeloid leukemia (CML), as supported by a number of clinical observations. In patients who remain leukemia free for many years after SCT, BCR-ABL transcripts often remain detectable in the first few weeks after transplantation, though they disappear by around 6 months after SCT, suggesting that an ongoing immune response may be important in conferring cure. T-cell depletion of the graft has been widely used to mitigate the effects of graft versus host disease, but is associated with an increased relapse rate. Post-SCT relapse of CML responds to infusions of donor T lymphocytes, and such responses may be curative.

Considerable laboratory work has been carried out in the past decade on the immune response to CML, and this has helped our understanding of how the host immune system may respond to malignancy. This information is now leading to clinical trials of immunotherapy in CML. Since BCR-ABL is not only central to the pathogenesis of CML, but also completely leukemia specific, the majority of clinical strategies have been directed against this antigen. Additional strategies have targeted other leukemia-associated antigens that are overexpressed in CML cells.

MOLECULAR FEATURES

The molecular biological features of CML are reviewed elsewhere in Chapter 2. The t(9;22)(q34;q11) translocation juxtaposes the distal part of the long arm of chromosome 9 to chromosome 22, creating the Philadelphia chromosome (Ph).[1] The chromosome 22 breakpoints are typically concentrated in the major breakpoint cluster region (M-bcr) of the *BCR* gene. In almost all CML patients, the *BCR* breakpoint occurs in or between exons e13 (formerly b2) and e14 (formerly b3) or exons e14 and e15 (formerly b4), and all *BCR* exons distal to the breakpoint are removed to chromosome 9. The chromosome 9 breakpoints occur over a large 200-kb region within the *ABL* gene. Because of splicing events during transcription, the 5′ part of the *BCR* gene becomes fused with the a2 exon of *ABL*. Almost all CML patients therefore express either e13a2 or e14a2 transcripts, which are translated to an e13a2 or e14a2 210-KDa BCR-ABL fusion protein. About 30% of Ph-positive acute lymphoblastic leukemia cases have the same molecular features. In the remaining 70%, there is juxtaposition of exon e1 of *BCR* to a2 of *ABL*, resulting in an e1a2 fusion transcript and a 190-kDa product.

BCR-ABL FUSION PEPTIDES

The amino acid sequences that span the BCR-ABL fusion junction are novel to the immune system, and are specific to leukemic cells. In the e14a2 transcript, a triplet codon is altered, and this creates a novel amino acid (lysine) at the actual BCR and ABL junction in the protein product. In the e13a2 transcript, a similar codon disruption also occurs, but this does not change the resultant amino acid.

The function of class I and II molecules of the major histocompatibility complex (MHC) is to present peptides on cell surfaces for scrutiny by T lymphocytes. Foreign protein antigens are ingested by antigen processing cells, which then degrade them to oligopeptides that are loaded onto class II MHC molecules. Endogenous antigens are degraded to smaller oligopeptides of 8–11 amino acids in length, which are assembled in the endoplasmic reticulum lumen into a stable complex with class I HLAα chain and β2 microglobulin. This complex is then exported to the cell surface, for recognition by cytotoxic T lymphocytes (CTL).

Several class I HLA molecules bind strongly to peptides spanning the BCR-ABL fusion junction. In a screen of 21 e13a2 and e14a2 junctional peptides for their binding to purified HLA molecules, the e14a2 junctional sequences KQSSKALQR, ATGFKQSSK, and HSATGFKQSSK showed affinity for HLA-A3.2 and -A11, and GFKQSSKAL showed affinity with HLA-B8.[2] This screen did not identify any peptides from the e13a2 junction that bound well to HLA class I. Mutations at or close to the anchor residue may improve the binding of e14a2 junctional peptides to HLA-A3[3] and HLA-A2.1,[4] and may improve the immunogenicity of BCR-ABL junctional peptides, including e13a2.[4]

We have shown that the HLA-A3/A11 associated e14a2 junctional peptide KQSSKALQR can be eluted from HLA molecules on the surface of HLA-A3 positive/e14a2 positive CML cells.[5] This demonstrates that BCR-ABL junctional peptides are present on CML cells in the context of HLA molecules, and therefore have the potential to be immunogenic. However, there are no additional data confirming that BCR-ABL junctional peptides are present in other HLA types, and to date we have been unable to demonstrate BCR-ABL junctional peptides in eluates from HLA-A201 positive patients.[6] This is in line with the *in vitro* observation that KQSSKALQR but not GFKQSSKAL may be generated by proteasomal cleavage of BCR-ABL.[7]

Fewer data are available concerning the HLA class II affinities of BCR-ABL peptides.[8,9] The 17-mer sequence ATGFKQSSKALQRPVAS, which evenly spans the e14a2 breakpoint, will elicit a CD4+ proliferative response especially in samples from DR*0401 and DR*0901 positive healthy subjects, which can be modified by mutations at various sites in the sequence.

IMMUNOGENICITY OF BCR-ABL JUNCTIONAL PEPTIDES

There is a broad correlation between the HLA binding affinity and the immunogenicity of BCR-ABL junctional peptides. Peptides from the e14a2 fusion junction that bind well to HLA-A3, -A11, and -B8 will generate specific class I HLA-restricted CTL responses in normal donors.[8,9] In all HLA-A3 positive donors tested, the A3/A11 binding peptide KQSSKALQR induced CTL that killed allogeneic HLA-A3 matched peptide-pulsed leukemia cell lines, CML cells from a HLA identical sibling, and unpulsed HLA matched but not mismatched e14a2 positive CML cells. CTL specific for e14a2 can also be generated from CML patients.[8,9] Using tetramer technology, we have shown that most HLA-A3 and/or HLA-B8 positive patients with e14a2 positive CML have circulating BCR-ABL specific CD8+ T-cells, especially if their leukemia is well controlled.[10]

These *in vitro* data suggest that CML patients have the capacity to respond to their own leukemic cells, and provide indirect evidence that CML cells are able to process and present endogenous e14a2 junctional peptides in the context of HLA, that can then serve as targets for class I HLA-restricted CTL. However, it is again important to note that these studies have only been carried out on a limited number of HLA types, principally HLA-A3, and almost exclusively on the e14a2 fusion junction.

These studies of *in vitro* CD8+ T-cell responses have typically used exogenous cytokines to replace any requirement for

CD4+ T cells. Several groups have demonstrated specific CD4+ T-cell responses to e14a2 fusion peptides in samples from healthy subjects,[8,9] and CD4+ T-cells specific for the e13a2 junction have been expanded from a healthy subject under conditions suitable for clinical use.[11] However, the limited available data suggest that CD4+ responses to BCR-ABL junctional peptides may be impaired in CML patients in comparison to healthy subjects.[12–14] This may be important, since if CD4+ responses are deficient *in vivo*, a net anergic response may arise.

OTHER LEUKEMIA-ASSOCIATED ANTIGENS

Because of concern that BCR-ABL may be a weak antigen, or may not bind well to some HLA types, several workers have focused on alternative antigens that are known to be overexpressed in CML cells. A 9-mer peptide from myeloperoxidase, the main component of neutrophil primary granules, binds well to HLA-A*0201, and will elicit CTL in normal donors which will kill HLA matched CML target cells.[15] CTL directed against PR1, a HLA-A*0201 restricted peptide from proteinase-3, another neutrophil granule protein overexpressed in CML, may circulate in CML patients,[16] and CTL with high avidity for their target are found in responding but not newly diagnosed patients.[17] The Wilms tumor gene product WT1 is overexpressed in most myeloid leukemias, and WT1-directed CTL circulate in CML patients.[16] CML progenitor cells may express sufficiently high levels of WT1 to elicit CTL, which leads to selective elimination of leukemic CD34+ progenitors,[18] and WT1 peptides may also elicit class II-restricted T-cell responses.[19] CD8+ T cells with specificity for PR1 and WT1 peptides have been reported in HLA-A2 positive healthy individuals.[16] T cells directed against the neutrophil granule protein elastase are reactive against CML cells.[20] This may be of relevance since in poorly controlled CML, circulating elastase levels may be high, and may contribute to pathogenesis.

Following allogeneic SCT, T cells of donor origin may be targeted to host hemopoiesis-specific antigens that are not necessarily leukemia specific, such as minor histocompatibility antigens (mHA).[21] Examples are HA-1 and HA-2, the expression of which is HLA-A2 restricted and limited to hemopoietic cells.[21] The Leiden group have extensively studied the role of immune responses to mHA after allogeneic SCT.[21] Infused donor CTL directed against mHA may confer remission in relapse after allogeneic SCT.[22]

DENDRITIC CELLS IN CHRONIC MYELOID LEUKEMIA

Dendritic cells can present BCR-ABL, since BCR-ABL specific CD4+ T-cell clones will produce γ-interferon on incubation with e14a2 positive monocyte-derived dendritic cells.[23] Dendritic cells from patients with e13a2 CML had no stimulatory activity, suggesting that dendritic cells presentation of e13a2 BCR-ABL might be inferior to e14a2 BCR-ABL. In untreated CML, many dendritic cells are BCR-ABL positive, and might therefore induce T-cell tolerance to BCR-ABL by endogenous expression on thymic dendritic cells. However, antigen processing and function by Ph-positive dendritic cells is abnormal,[24] though imatinib may change the dendritic cells population from predominant BCR-ABL positivity towards polyclonality as patients enter complete cytogenetic remission,[25] thus removing an important source of BCR-ABL peptide presentation.

Co-stimulatory molecule expression may be deficient in CML. In nude mice, immunization with leukemic cells with modified B7.1 expression is protective against later challenge with lethal doses of unmodified leukemic cells.[26] Furthermore, CD80 and CD86 expression may be low or absent on CML cells, but granulocyte-macrophage colony-stimulating factor (GM-CSF) and interleukin (IL)-4 may increase their apparent expression in cultured adherent cells, presumably by selection for Ph-positive dendritic cells. Cells primed in this way will elicit proliferative T-cell responses that are effective against unprimed CML cell targets.[27]

EFFECTS OF TYROSINE KINASE INHIBITORS ON THE IMMUNE SYSTEM

The tyrosine kinase inhibitor imatinib has revolutionized the outlook for CML over the past 5 years. However, there has been concern that it may have unwanted effects on the various cellular components of the immune system. Imatinib may restore the clonality of dendritic cells from Ph-positive to polyclonality,[25] and this is associated with return of dendritic cells function to normal.[28] However, it may interfere with the differentiation of monocytes and CD34+ progenitors into functional dendritic cells, impairing their ability to stimulate a primary T-cell response.[29] In addition, several studies have reported impaired T-cell proliferation,[30] and this effect may be as a result of inhibition of the kinase LCK. In contrast, an increase in interferon-γ producing T cells has been observed after 3 months of treatment, and imatinib may restore Th1 cell function toward normal, even in the absence of cytogenetic remission.[31] Overall, the effects may be of minor clinical importance, since there is no clinical evidence that imatinib treated patients have an increased susceptibility to infection. A possible explanation for these conflicting data is that many of these studies have used far higher imatinib concentrations that those achieved *in vivo*, even at high dosages.

At present there are no data on the immunological effects of either of the second generation tyrosine kinase inhibitors, dasatinib or nilotinib.

CLINICAL STRATEGIES

The effect of infusing expanded CTL directed against leukemic antigens has been examined in CML. Leukemia-reactive CTL from a HLA matched donor expanded *ex vivo* can induce remission in refractory advanced CML.[32] WT1 specific CTL will selectively kill leukemic precursors,[19] and high avidity CTL may be isolated that are useful in treatment.[33] Several other preclinical studies of cellular immunotherapy strategies have been carried out. In a mouse model of BCR-ABL positive leukemia, immunization of dendritic cells pulsed with the e14a2 BCR-ABL junctional peptide GFKQSSKAL may confer a BCR-ABL specific CTL response, and this was greater than in mice immunized with peptide alone.[34] Similar results have been reported after re-infusion of presumed Ph-positive dendritic cells in a CML patient.[35] Healthy donor dendritic cells transfected with an adeno-associated virus vector expressing the e14a2 BCR-ABL fusion region have been shown to prime HLA-restricted BCR-ABL specific CD4+ and CD8+ T cells *in vitro*, to levels comparable to those achieved using BCR-ABL peptides alone.[36] This strategy may have the advantage that multiple epitopes are generated, which may transcend the problem of HLA restriction for individual peptides. However, these studies of cellular immunotherapy require considerable resources, and their main value is of proof of principle rather than as clinical strategies for future widespread use. A recent trial has avoided choosing any particular antigen, by vaccinating imatinib treated patients with irradiated K562 cells engineered to produce GM-CSF, and several clinical responses have been described, with some molecular remissions.[37]

Vaccination of autologous multivalent heat shock protein (HSP) extracts is under investigation in a number of tumors. The rationale is that HSP chaperone intracellular peptides around the cell, and HSP–peptide complexes should therefore contain potentially immunogenic tumor associated peptides. A phase I study of this approach reported cytogenetic and/or molecular responses in 13 of 20 CML patients with minimal toxicity, though it was given concurrently with imatinib.[38] However, a phase II study in patients failing imatinib showed less impressive effects,[39] and at present it is uncertain whether HSP vaccination will find a place in CML therapy, especially because of the effort involved in preparing individual patient vaccines.

In contrast, peptide vaccination against specific antigens may be more generally applicable. WT1 peptide vaccination generates specific CTL,[40] and may induce remission in acute leukemia.[41] Clinical trials of WT1 peptide vaccination are now in progress in CML. A future extension of this may be the engineering of WT1 specific T cells by transducing WT1 specific T-cell receptor genes.[42,43] Vaccination studies are under way using the PR1 peptide.[44]

Three groups have immunized CML patients with BCR-ABL junctional peptides, aiming to induce a leukemia specific CTL and CD4+ response *in vivo*. Three of six CML patients treated at the highest dose levels generated BCR-ABL specific proliferative immune responses.[45] In a follow-up study, the same group showed that patients receiving imatinib can also mount CD4+ and in some cases CD8+ responses,[46] and some patients demonstrated cytogenetic and molecular responses. In a separate study using a very similar BCR-ABL peptide vaccination strategy, cytogenetic responses were observed in ten imatinib treated cases, and BCR-ABL transcripts became undetectable in three of the five cases of complete cytogenetic responders.[47]

We have recently reported a phase I study of BCR-ABL peptide vaccination in 19 e14a2 patients in first chronic phase, and on a stable dose of imatinib.[48] Either KQSSKALQR or GFKQSSKAL were used, dependent on the HLA class I type, and each peptide was also linked to PADRE (pan DR epitope) to augment CD4+ T-cell help. PADRE is a 15-mer which includes four non-natural amino acids, which binds with high or intermediate affinity to 15 of the 16 most common HLA-DR types. *In vitro*, PADRE induces CD4+ T-cell responses in virtually all individuals, and it has been used in several vaccination studies. Six vaccinations were given over 9 weeks, together with sargramostim. T-cell responses to PADRE were seen in all patients, confirming that the vaccine is visible to the immune system. Fourteen of 19 patients developed T-cell responses to BCR-ABL peptides, which were CD45RO+ indicating a memory cell phenotype. Thirteen of 14 patients in major cytogenetic response (MCR) at trial entry had at least a 1-log fall in BCR-ABL transcripts, in contrast to no benefit in any of five patients not in MCR at entry, underlining the view that immunotherapy is most likely to be effective in patients with well-controlled disease. The molecular responses typically occurred several months after completing vaccination, consistent with an effect at a primitive CML stem cell level. Vaccination improved the fall in BCR-ABL transcripts in patients who had previously received imatinib for more than 12 months,[48] suggesting that immunotherapy may be most effective if delayed until after disease reduction with conventional treatment.

In all these peptide vaccination studies, the toxicity profile is excellent, though some local delayed type hypersensitivity reactions have occurred. Overall, these observations suggest that BCR-ABL peptide vaccination may improve control of CML, especially in patients responding well to imatinib, but we do not currently know whether these cytogenetic and molecular responses are durable, and whether they were entirely owing to the vaccinations (or to other concurrent therapy especially imatinib). Randomized trials are therefore urgently required to address this further.

An interesting variation of BCR-ABL peptide vaccination is currently in phase I trial,[49] based on observations that amino acid substitutions at or near the anchor residues may increase the immunogenicity of both e13a2 and e14a2 junctional peptides.[4] These heteroclitic peptides induce CD8+ T-cell responses that cross-react with native junctional peptides, and might constitute a way to overcome the poor immunogenicity of e13a2 sequences.

CONCLUSIONS

A considerable body of *in vitro* data clearly indicate that the immune system is capable of responding against CML cells. However, the data do not cover all HLA and transcript types, and these studies have limited relevance to *in vivo* conditions, where the Ph-positive clone gradually expands over a long period of time.

Clearly, the immune system cannot operate optimally *in vivo*, since otherwise CML would never exist as a clinical phenotype. It is tempting to speculate that the emergence of CML depends not only on the Ph translocation and BCR-ABL, but also on the failure of the immune system to eradicate the Ph-positive clone, and this is supported by the demonstration of low levels of BCR-ABL transcripts in otherwise normal subjects.[50,51] Based on the premise that the immune system may have become tolerant to CML associated antigens, several clinical immunotherapy strategies have been tried. The majority of available data have examined BCR-ABL specific responses, because of their leukemia specificity. However, BCR-ABL specific responses may not be the only important immune mechanism in CML, especially following allografting. Recent data suggest that BCR-ABL may be a weaker immunogen than proteinase-3 or other CML related antigens, and it is possible that effects against multiple CML-related antigens may be additive.[52]

Immunotherapy in CML may therefore be approaching an awkward dilemma. On the one hand, it is tempting to now advocate large randomized studies of, for example, peptide vaccination, to determine whether this adds anything to the responses now achievable with tyrosine kinase inhibitors. A more cautious alternative approach will be to continue to adapt and refine protocol details in multiple smaller focused studies, in the hope that a more effective strategy can then be explored in larger randomized studies. As in other areas of its biology and clinical behavior, CML will continue to point the way for better understanding and treatment of more common tumors.

REFERENCES

1. Deininger MWN, Goldman JM, Melo JV. The molecular biology of chronic myeloid leukemia. Blood 2000; 96: 3343–56.
2. Bocchia M, Wentworth PA, Southwood S et al. Specific binding of leukemia oncogene fusion protein peptides to HLA Class I molecules. Blood 1995; 85: 2680–4.
3. Greco G, Fruci D, Accapezzato D et al. Two bcr-abl junction peptides bind HLA-A3 molecules and allow specific induction of human cytotoxic T lymphocytes. Leukemia 1996; 10: 693–9.
4. Pinilla-Ibarz J, Korontsvit T, Zakhaleva V, Roberts W, Scheinberg DA. Synthetic peptide analogs derived from bcr/abl fusion proteins and the induction of heteroclitic human T-cell responses. Haematologica 2005; 90: 1324–32.
5. Clark RE, Dodi IA, Hill SC et al. Direct evidence that leukaemic cells present HLA-associated immunogenic peptides derived from the BCR-ABL b3a2 fusion protein. Blood 2001; 98: 2887–93.
6. Clayton JE, Rusakiewicz S, McArdle S et al. Unpublished observations.
7. Posthuma EF, van Bergen CA, Kester MG et al. Proteosomal degradation of BCR/ABL protein can generate an HLA-A*0301-restricted peptide, but high-avidity T cells recognizing this leukemia-specific antigen were not demonstrated. Haematologica 2004; 89: 1062–71.
8. Clark RE, Christmas SE. BCR-ABL fusion peptides and cytotoxic T cells in chronic myeloid leukaemia. Leuk Lymphoma 2001; 42: 871–80.
9. Clark RE. The immune response to chronic myeloid leukaemia. In: Romero RF, ed. Focus on Leukemia Research. New York: Nova Science Publishers, 2005: 27–60.
10. Butt NM, Rojas JM, Wang L et al. Circulating BCR-ABL specific CD8+ cells are detectable in chronic myeloid leukaemia patients and healthy subjects. Haematologica 2005; 90: 1315–23.
11. Crough T, Nieda M, Morton J et al. Donor-derived b2a2-specific T cells for immunotherapy of patients with chronic myeloid leukemia. J Immunother 2002; 25: 469–75.
12. Pawelec G, Max H, Halder T et al. BCR/ABL leukaemia oncogene fusion peptides selectively bind to certain HLA-DR alleles and can be recognised by T cells found at low frequency in the repertoire of normal donors. Blood 1996; 88: 2118–24.
13. Bertazzoli C, Marchesi E, Passoni L et al. Differential recognition of a BCR/ABL peptide by lymphocytes from normal donors and chronic myeloid leukemia patients. Clin Cancer Res 2000; 6: 1931–5.
14. Abu-Eisha HM, Butt NM, Clark RE, Christmas SE. Evidence that a BCR-ABL fusion peptide does not induce lymphocyte proliferation or cytokine production in vitro. Leuk Res 2007; 31: 1675–81.
15. Braunschweig I, Wang C, Molldrem JJ. Cytotoxic T lymphocytes (CTL) specific for myeloperoxidase-derived HLA-A2-restricted peptides specifically lyse AML and CML cells. Blood 2000; 96: 761a, abstract.
16. Rezvani K, Grube M, Brenchley JM et al. Functional leukemia-associated antigen-specific memory CD8+ T cells exist in healthy individuals and in patients with chronic myelogenous leukemia before and

after stem cell transplantation. Blood 2003; 102: 2892–900.
17. Molldrem JJ, Lee PP, Kant S et al. Chronic myelogenous leukemia shapes host immunity by selective deletion of high-avidity leukemia-specific T cells. J Clin Invest 2003; 111: 639–47.
18. Gao L, Bellantuono I, Elsässer A et al. Selective elimination of leukemic CD34+ progenitor cells by cytotoxic T lymphocytes specific for WT1. Blood 2000; 95: 2198–203.
19. Müller L, Knights A, Pawelec G. Synthetic peptides derived from the Wilms' tumor 1 protein sensitize human T lymphocytes to recognize chronic myelogenous leukemia cells. Hematol J 2003; 4: 57–66.
20. Fujiwara H, El Ouriaghli F, Grube M et al. Identification and in vitro expansion of CD4+ and CD8+ T cells specific for human neutrophil elastase. Blood 2004; 103: 3076–83.
21. Falkenburg JHF, van de Corput L, Marijt EWA, Willemze R. Minor histocompatibility antigens in human stem cell transplantation. Exp Hematol 2003; 31: 743–51.
22. Marijt WA, Heemskerk MH, Kloosterboer FM et al. Hematopoiesis-restricted minor histocompatibility antigens HA-1- or HA-2-specific T cells can induce complete remissions of relapsed leukemia. Proc Natl Acad Sci U S A 2003; 100: 2742–7.
23. Yasukawa M, Ohminami H, Kojima K et al. HLA class II-restricted antigen presentation of endogenous bcr-abl fusion protein by chronic myelogenous leukemia-derived dendritic cells to CD4(+) T lymphocytes. Blood 2001; 98: 1498–505.
24. Dong R, Cwynarski K, Entwistle A et al. Dendritic cells from CML patients have altered actin organization, reduced antigen processing, and impaired migration. Blood 2003; 101: 3560–7.
25. Wang L, Butt NM, Atherton MG, Clark RE. Dendritic cells become BCR-ABL negative in chronic myeloid leukaemia successfully treated with imatinib. Leukemia 2004; 18: 1025–7.
26. Matulonis UA, Dosiou C, Lamont C et al. Role of B7-1 in mediating an immune response to myeloid leukemia cells. Blood 1995; 85: 2507–515.
27. Coleman S, Fisher J, Hoy T, Burnett AK, Lim SH. Autologous MHC-dependent leukaemia-reactive T lymphocytes in a patient with chronic myeloid leukaemia. Leukemia 1996; 10: 483–7.
28. Sato N, Narita M, Takahashi M et al. The effects of STI571 on antigen presentation of dendritic cells generated from patients with chronic myelogenous leukemia. Hematol Oncol 2003; 21: 67–75.
29. Appel S, Boehmler AM, Grunebach F et al. Imatinib mesylate affects the development and function of dendritic cells generated from CD34+ peripheral blood progenitor cells. Blood 2004; 103: 538–44.
30. Boissel N, Rousselot P, Raffoux E et al. Imatinib mesylate minimally affects bcr-abl+ and normal monocyte-derived dendritic cells but strongly inhibits T cell expansion despite reciprocal dendritic cell-T cell activation. J Leukoc Biol 2006; 79: 747–56.
31. Aswald JM, Lipton JH, Aswald S, Messner HA. Increased IFN-gamma synthesis by T cells from patients on imatinib therapy for chronic myeloid leukemia. Cytokines Cell Mol Ther 2002; 7: 143–9.
32. Falkenburg JHF, Wafelman AR, Joosten P et al. Complete remission of accelerated phase chronic myeloid leukemia by treatment with leukemia-reactive cytotoxic T lymphocytes. Blood 1999; 94: 1201–8.
33. Savage P, Gao L, Vento K et al. Use of B cell-bound HLA-A2 class I monomers to generate high-avidity, allo-restricted CTLs against the leukemia-associated protein Wilms tumor antigen. Blood 2004; 103: 4613–15.
34. He L, Feng H, Raymond A et al. Dendritic-cell-peptide immunization provides immunoprotection against bcr-abl-positive leukemia in mice. Cancer Immunol Immunother 2001; 50: 31–40.
35. Lim SH, Coleman S, Bailey-Wood R. In vitro cytokine-primed leukaemia cells induce in vivo T cell responsiveness in chronic myeloid leukaemia. Bone Marrow Transplant 1998; 22: 1185–90.
36. Sun J-Y, Krouse RS, Forman SJ et al. Immunogenicity of a p210 BCR-ABL fusion domain candidate DNA vaccine targeted to dendritic cells by a recombinant adeno-associated virus vector in vitro. Cancer Res 2002; 62: 3175–83.
37. Smith B, Kasamon YL, Miller CB et al. K562/GM-CSF vaccination reduces tumor burden, including achieving molecular remissions, in chronic myeloid leukemia (CML) patients (PTS) with residual disease on imatinib mesylate (IM). J Clin Oncol 2006; 24: 6509, abstract.
38. Li Z, Qiao Y, Liu B et al. Combination of imatinib mesylate with autologous leukocyte-derived heat shock protein and chronic myelogenous leukemia. Clin Cancer Res 2005; 11: 4460–8.
39. Marin D, Mauro M, Goldman J et al. Preliminary results from a phase II trial of AG-858, an autologous heat shock protein-peptide vaccine, in combination with imatinib in patients with chronic phase chronic myeloid leukemia (CML) resistant to prior imatinib monotherapy. Blood 2005; 106: 318a, abstract.
40. Oka Y, Tsuboi A, Kawakami M et al. Development of WT1 peptide cancer vaccine against hematopoietic malignancies and solid cancers. Curr Med Chem 2006; 13: 2345–52.
41. Mailander V, Scheibenbogen C, Thiel E et al. Complete remission in a patient with recurrent acute myeloid leukemia induced by vaccination with WT1 peptide in the absence of hematological or renal toxicity. Leukemia 2004; 18: 165–6.
42. Tsuji T, Yasukawa M, Matsuzaki J et al. Generation of tumor-specific, HLA class I-restricted human Th1 and Tc1 cells by cell engineering with tumor

peptide-specific T-cell receptor genes. Blood 2005; 106: 470–6.

43. Xue SA, Gao L, Hart D et al. Elimination of human leukemia cells in NOD/SCID mice by WT1-TCR gene-transduced human T cells. Blood 2005; 106: 3062–7.
44. Rusakiewicz S, Molldrem JJ. Immunotherapeutic peptide vaccination with leukemia-associated antigens. Curr Opin Immunol 2006; 18: 599–604.
45. Pinilla-Ibarz J, Cathcart K, Korontsvit T et al. Vaccination of patients with chronic myelogenous leukaemia with bcr-abl oncogene breakpoint fusion peptides generates specific immune responses. Blood 2000; 95: 1781–7.
46. Cathcart K, Pinilla-Ibarz J, Korontsvit T et al. A multivalent bcr-abl fusion peptide vaccination trial in patients with chronic myeloid leukemia. Blood 2004; 103: 1037–42.
47. Bocchia M, Gentili S, Abruzzese E et al. Effect of a p210 multipeptide vaccine associated with imatinib or interferon in patients with chronic myeloid leukaemia and persistent residual disease: a multicentre observational trial. Lancet 2005; 365: 657–62.
48. Rojas JM, Knight K, Wang L et al. The immune response to BCR-ABL peptide immunisation is variable and transient in chronic myeloid leukaemia: results from the EPIC study. Haematologica 2006; (Suppl s1). 177, abstract.
49. Maslak PG, Dao T, Gupta S et al. Pilot trial of a synthetic breakpoint peptide vaccine in patients with chronic myeloid leukemia (CML) and minimal disease. J Clin Oncol 2006; 24: 6514, abstract.
50. Bose S, Deininger M, Gora-Tybor J et al. The presence of typical and atypical BCR-ABL fusion genes in leukocytes of normal individuals: biologic significance and implications for the assessment of minimal residual disease. Blood 1998; 92: 3362–7.
51. Biernaux C, Loos M, Sels A et al. Detection of major bcr-abl gene expression at a very low level in blood cells of some healthy individuals. Blood 1995; 86: 3118–22.
52. Elmaagacli AH, Koldehoff M, Peceny R et al. WT1 and BCR-ABL specific small interfering RNA have additive effects in the induction of apoptosis in leukemic cells. Haematologica 2005; 90: 326–34.

Potential treatment algorithms and future directions for patients with chronic myeloid leukemia

10

Tariq I Mughal, John M Goldman

INTRODUCTION

Since the introduction of imatinib mesylate, the 'first generation' tyrosine kinase inhibitor (TKI), into the clinic in 1998, the drug has become the preferred treatment for the majority, if not all, newly diagnosed patients with chronic myeloid leukemia (CML) in chronic phase (CP), except perhaps for children.[1,2] Imatinib reduces substantially the number of CML cells in a patient's body, resulting in a complete cytogenetic remission in a significant proportion of patients but complete molecular responses only in a minority and then only after some years of treatment and probably in less than 50% of patients.[3] The next (second) generation TKIs, dasatinib and nilotinib, appear to be more potent than imatinib and are now in the clinic, for the treatment of imatinib-resistant/refractory CML and Philadelphia chromosome (Ph)-positive acute lymphoblastic leukemia (ALL).[4,5] Other candidate drugs include bosutinib (SKI-606), INNO-406 (NS-187), and an aurora kinase inhibitor, MK-0457 (VX680). Allogeneic stem cell transplantation (alloSCT), however, remains the only therapeutic modality that can clearly produce long-term complete molecular remission associated, presumably, with eradication of all residual leukemia stem cells.[6,7] In this chapter we address the current treatment algorithms for patients with CML, with an emphasis on the non-transplant therapies, and speculate on some of the challenges for the future. AlloSCT is discussed in Chapter 7.

A POTENTIAL TREATMENT ALGORITHM FOR A NEWLY DIAGNOSED PATIENT WITH CHRONIC MYELOID LEUKEMIA IN CHRONIC PHASE

Until the end of the 20th century it was standard practice to recommend alloSCT to all patients less than 50 years of age with newly diagnosed CML in CP provided they had suitable HLA-identical sibling or 'HLA-matched' unrelated donors.[8] Patients presenting in the advanced phases of CML usually received combination chemotherapy, often followed by an alloSCT if a 'second' CP could be achieved. The treatment algorithm for the newly diagnosed patients changed dramatically once the impressive success of imatinib in inducing complete hematological response and complete cytogenetic responses in the majority of newly diagnosed patients with CML in CP was recognized. Thereafter, imatinib became the preferred first-line therapy worldwide (Chapter 5).

Imatinib inhibits the enzymatic action of the activated BCR-ABL tyrosine kinase by occupying the ATP-binding pocket of the ABL-kinase component of the BCR-ABL oncoprotein, thereby blocking the capacity of the enzyme to phosphorylate downstream effector molecules. It also binds to an adjacent part of the kinase domain (KD) in a manner that holds the activation loop of the BCR-ABL oncoprotein in its inactive conformation (Figure 10.1).[10]

For patients who started imatinib in untreated ('early') chronic phase in the IRIS

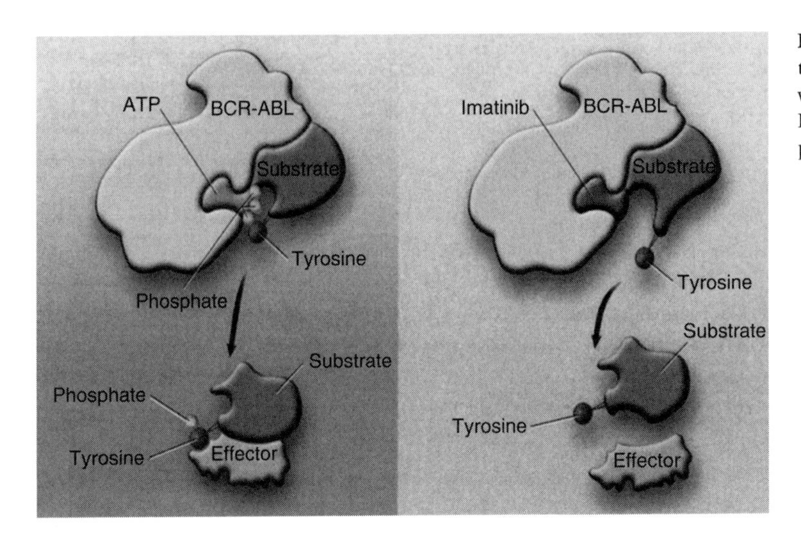

Figure 10.1 How imatinib therapy might work in patients with chronic myeloid leukemia. From reference 9, with permission.

study (a phase III randomized trial of interferon alfa (IFNα) and cytarabine compared to imatinib mesylate) imatinib induced cumulative best complete hematological remissions in 98% and cumulative best complete complete cytogenetic response in about 83% at 6 years; the corresponding figures following a 5-year follow-up were 98% and 83%, respectively.[3,11] The actual proportion of patients who remain in complete cytogenetic response whilst on imatinib at 6 years is about 60% (Figure 10.2).[1] About 2% of all patients in CP progress to advanced phase disease each year, which contrasts with estimated annual progression rates of >15% for patients treated with hydroxyurea and about 10% for patients receiving IFNα, either with or without cytarabine. Indeed, preliminary evidence suggests that this annual rate of progression, about 2%, actually diminishes as the years pass and for patients who have been on therapy beyond the 4th and 5th years is zero (Figure 10.3).[11] Complete molecular responses are, however, less common and imatinib will probably not eradicate all residual CML in the vast majority of patients.

Nevertheless, the drug prolongs overall survival very substantially compared with historical data for patients receiving IFNα or hydroxyurea.[12] Furthermore, of patients who achieve a ≥3-log reduction in BCR-ABL transcripts, the majority remain alive in continuing complete cytogenetic response at 5 years after initiation of imatinib.[13] Therefore, a topical issue is whether total eradication of all residual leukemia stem cells is actually necessary, since the survival of small numbers of residual leukemia stem cells might well be compatible with an individual patient's long-term survival. Conversely, if such a population of cells was a possible source of subsequent relapse, the notion of two contrasting therapeutic algorithms for patients based on prognostic factors, both disease-related such as the Sokal or Hasford risk score, and treatment-related, such as the European Group for Blood and Marrow Transplantation (EBMT) transplant risk score, can be considered.[15,16] The Sokal risk score, though derived in the pre-imatinib era, has recently been validated for use in imatinib-treated patients. It is likely that other candidate disease-related prognostic factors, such as gene expression profiling, will be found useful in the near future.[17,18] Clearly the most robust prognostic indicators to imatinib treatment, so far, are the cytogenetic and molecular responses. It is of considerable interest that the latest analysis of the IRIS cohort suggests that the actual time to achieve a complete cytogenetic response does not appear to affect the long-term outcome.[19] This is at variance with the current definitions of response, such as those proposed by the European LeukemiaNet, which consider anything less than a complete cytogenetic response at 12 months to be suboptimal (Table 10.1).[20] The relationship between the level of residual disease and risk of disease progression is, however, well recognized. Patients who consistently attain a 3-log reduction in the concentration of BCR-ABL transcripts, compared to the baseline, appear to have a lower risk of disease progression compared to those who attain lesser degrees of molecular responses.

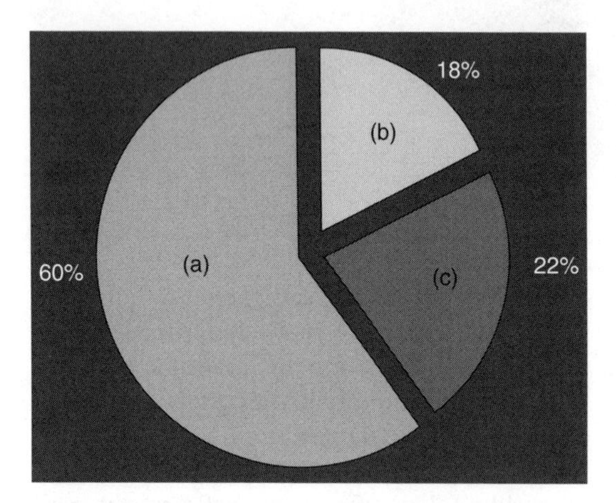

Figure 10.2 Responses on imatinib at 6 years for the IRIS cohort. CCyR, complete cytogenetic response. Adapted from reference 11, with permission. (a) In CCyR on Imatinib. (b) No CCyR. (c) Discontinued.

For the vast majority of patients, imatinib is the first-line treatment of choice. The standard starting dose of initial imatinib is 400 mg/day, though several studies suggest that higher doses, up to 800 mg daily, might give better results with a greater proportion of patients achieving a complete molecular response.[21,22] Such studies also suggest better progression-free and transformation-free survival, but with potentially more side-effects, particularly myelosuppression. The higher dose imatinib studies are still on-going and until the longer-term results are available, it is reasonable to start newly diagnosed patients in CP on 400 mg/day.

The alternative treatment option should involve an early allogeneic SCT for the small minority of patients who would benefit from an immediate alloSCT compared with continuing imatinib irrespective of the outcome from imatinib. A retrospective analysis from the Center for International Blood and Marrow Transplant Research (CIBMTR) and the EBMT suggests that for adult patients,

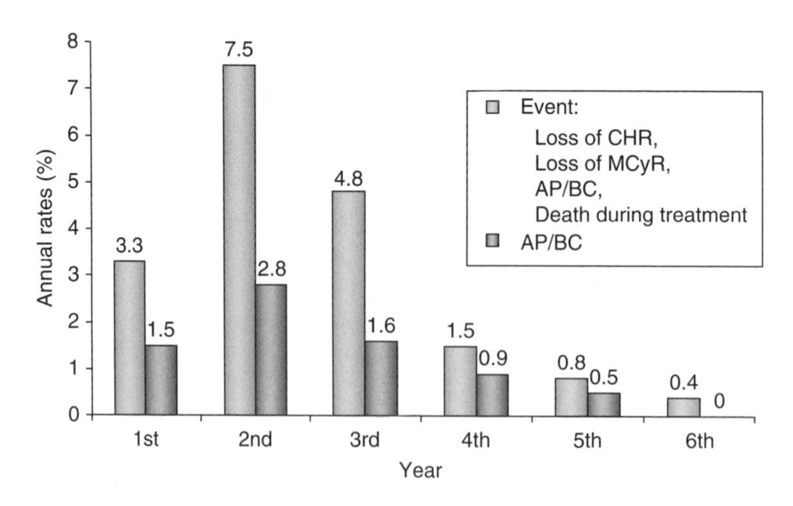

Figure 10.3 IRIS study following a 6-year follow-up: annual events in all patients. CHR, complete hematological response; MCyR, major cytogenetic response; AP/BC accelerated phase/blast crisis. Adapted from reference 11, with permission.

Table 10.1 Definitions of failure and suboptimal response in patients with early chronic phase chronic myeloid leukemia treated with 400 mg/day imatinib

Time	*Failure*	*Suboptimal response*	*Warnings*
Diagnosis	–	–	High risk Del9q+ AOA in Ph+ cells
3 months	No HR	< CHR	
6 months	< CHR No CyR	< PCyR	
12 months	< PCyR	< CCyR	< MMolR
18 months	< CCyR	< MMolR	
Anytime	Loss of CHR Loss of CCyR Mutation	ACA in Ph+ cells Loss of MMolR Mutation	Any ↑ BCR-ABL transcript level OCA in Ph– cells

From reference 20, with permission.
*Low level of insensitivity to imatinib.
ACA, additional chromosomal abnormalities; HR, hematological response; CHR, complete HR; CyR, cytogenetic response; PCyR, partial CyR; CCyR, complete CyR; MMolR, major molecular response; OCA, other chromosomal abnormalities.

including those with low risk for transplant related mortality by EBMT criteria, it is not possible to identify a cohort who would clearly benefit from an immediate SCT versus continuing imatinib irrespective of the outcome from imatinib.[23] The outcome for children, those with a potential syngeneic donor and possibly those with high-risk disease by Sokal or Hasford criteria, is uncertain. The current EBMT recommendations, however, suggest that patients with high-risk disease and a low transplant risk should probably still be considered for an early alloSCT. Such a cohort, if treated with imatinib in the first instance should probably not receive a second TKI on relapse (see below) and rather proceed to SCT. With regard to children, many pediatric hematologists still recommend initial treatment by alloSCT for patients under the age of 16 who have HLA-identical siblings, largely because of a lack of adequate data pertaining to the use of imatinib as first-line therapy in children.

The current safety analysis of imatinib is quite impressive, with very few potentially serious long-term effects. There was initially concern about the potential for myocardial toxicity, but the recent IRIS analysis has confirmed that the risk is no higher than that of the normal population.[24,25] There remains, however, a concern for the older patients who are anemic and may have pre-existing cardiac disease. It is therefore appropriate to exercise caution under these circumstances. There has also been some concern about the potential to induce secondary malignancies, in particular acute myeloid leukemia, and a small excess of urothelial tumors were reported in one small series.[26,27] Other rare, but potentially serious adverse effects have included cerebral edema.[28,29] Myelotoxicity appears to be dose related and reversible. When higher doses of imatinib are used, many patients require adjunctive therapy with myeloid growth factors, which can be given quite safely.

A POTENTIAL TREATMENT ALGORITHM FOR A PATIENT WITH CHRONIC MYELOID LEUKEMIA IN CHRONIC PHASE WHO IS RESISTANT OR INTOLERANT TO IMATINIB

About 20% of patients with CML in early CP eventually become resistant to imatinib.[30] Resistance is more common in patients who start imatinib in late CP. It occurs in about 70% of patients treated in myeloid blast crisis and in all of the patients in lymphoid blast crisis. Resistance, both primary and secondary, is now being increasingly recognized in a significant minority of patients in chronic phase. Primary resistance is actually very rare and can be associated with low levels of the human organic cation transporter 1 (hOCT1), which are associated with poor intracellular uptake of imatinib, or with a poorly compliant patient.[31,32] The mechanism for secondary or acquired resistance whereby patients respond well initially and then lose their response, appear quite different.[33] The principal mechanism underlying this form of resistance appears to involve expansion of a Ph-positive clone bearing a BCR-ABL kinase domain (KD) mutation. It can also arise from a variety of other mechanisms, including amplification of the *BCR-ABL* fusion gene, relative overexpression of BCR-ABL oncoprotein and overexpression of P-glycoprotein that enhances the cellular removal of imatinib. Structural studies suggest that not all mutations are equivalent; T315I, E255K, and some (but not all) P-loop mutations are associated with resistance to imatinib, probably because they interfere with imatinib binding to the BCR-ABL KD.[34]

Currently there is debate about the significance of these mutations in CML, particularly since some mutations have been identified at very low levels in newly diagnosed patients and probably reflect the natural evolution of the CML stem cells. Therefore, the emergence of a mutation, particularly in patients who appear to be responding to imatinib, should not by itself be considered as a failure of treatment.[35,36] Currently over 70 different mutations have been characterized and the precise significance of each appears to be different, with only a minority being associated directly with resistance to imatinib. It is of interest that one of the very first mutations described in 2001, the so-called 'gate-keeper' or T315I mutation, remains a principal cause for resistance not only to the original ABL tyrosine kinase inhibitor, imatinib, but also to the second generation drugs such as dasatinib and nilotinib.[37,38] This mutation arises as a consequence of threonine being replaced by isoleucine at ABL position 315. The isoleucine is a much larger amino acid compared with threonine and impairs the actual binding of the various inhibitors by steric hindrance.

There is also debate at present about the optimal treatment strategy for patients who remain in complete cytogenetic response (on imatinib treatment), but develop a molecular relapse.[39] It is likely that such a cohort may fare best either by increasing the dose of imatinib, or, as appears more likely, by switching to an alternative TKI, such as dasatinib or nilotinib.[40] Studies in progress should help define this particular enigma in the near future.

For patients who develop *de facto* resistance to imatinib, there are a number of clinical trials in progress, assessing the benefits of adding other treatments to imatinib, based on *in vitro* studies suggesting potential synergism between imatinib and a number of conventional as well as investigational agents.[39,41] Preliminary results from trials assessing the combination of imatinib with IFNα are encouraging, but only relatively small doses of IFNα can be tolerated in combination with full dose imatinib. More recent efforts are being directed towards use of the long-acting form of IFNα, pegylated IFNα, which was introduced a decade ago in the hope of reducing many of the IFNα-related toxic effects. An Italian study confirmed complete cytogenetic response in 63% of the cohort, but 58% of the patients experienced toxicity, both hematological (50%) and non-hematological (50%).[42]

Small series of patients subjected to combinations of imatinib and low-dose cytarabine showed a complete cytogenetic response in 57% of patients, but an excessive number of side-effects, both hematological and non-hematological, were noted. Over 50% of all patients discontinued therapy at 9 months because of toxicity. Recently, there has been considerable interest in combining imatinib with hypomethylating agents, such as 5-azacitidine and 5-aza-2′-deoxycitidine

Table 10.2 Collated responses in patients with imatinib-resistant or imatinib-intolerant chronic myeloid leukemia in various phases receiving dasatinib 70 mg twice daily. Minimum follow-up of >12 months for all studies

	Chronic phase (n = 387)	*Advanced phase (n = 174)*	*Myeloid blast crisis (n = 109)*	*Lymphoid blast crisis (n = 48)*	*Ph+ ALL (n = 46)*
Complete hematological response	91%	64%	34%	35%	41%
Major cytogenetic response	59%	39%	33%	52%	56%
Complete cytogenetic response	49%	32%	26%	46%	54%

Ph+ ALL, Philadelphia chromosome-positive acute lymphoblastic leukemia.

(decitabine), both of which disrupt the chromatin by inhibiting DNA methylation and thus lead to gene silencing.[43] Both agents are active when used independently in small pilot studies, and preclinical studies show synergy when imatinib is added, particularly with decitabine. Other investigational approaches include combining imatinib with a farnesyl transferase inhibitor (FTI), such as lonafarnib (SCH66336) or tipifarnib (R115777).[44,45] Homoharringtonine, a semi-synthetic plant alkaloid that enhances apoptosis of CML cells, is active in combination with imatinib in imatinib-resistant/refractory patients.[46] Pilot studies using other agents such as arsenic trioxide and bortezomib in combination with imatinib are also in progress.

The majority of patients who are resistant/intolerant to imatinib should receive dasatinib or nilotinib, both of which are currently approved for this indication in many parts of the world. Dasatinib, in contrast to imatinib, is a thiazole-carboxamide structurally unrelated to imatinib. Furthermore, it binds to the ABL KD regardless of the conformation of the activation loop, be it open or closed. It also inhibits some of the SRC family kinases.[47,48] Preclinical studies showed that dasatinib was 300-fold more potent than imatinib and is active against 18 of 19 tested imatinib-resistant KD mutant subclones, with the notable exception of the T315I mutant.[49]

Current experience with dasatinib in patients with CP CML resistant/refractory to imatinib suggest that about 90% of patients have a complete hematological response and 52% of patients have a complete cytogenetic response.[50] About 25% of patients with the more advanced phases of CML and Ph-positive ALL also have reasonable responses (Table 10.2). Responses are seen in patients with most of the currently known ABL KD mutations, except the T315I mutation. Hematological toxicity is common, particularly in those with the advanced phases of CML and Ph-positive ALL. These include neutropenia (49%), thrombocytopenia (48%), and anemia (20%). Non-hematological toxicity includes diarrhea, headaches, superficial edema, pleural effusions, and occasional pericardial effusions. Grade 3/4 side-effects are rare and grade 3/4 pleural effusions occurred in 6% of patients. The recently completed 'dose and schedule' study confirmed the notion that a lower dose of dasatinib (100 mg/day) was as effective as the previously approved higher dose (70 mg bid) in terms of the hematological, and major and complete cytogenetic responses, including the time to achieve these responses, but the toxicity profile confirmed a much lower incidence of pleural and pericardial effusions.[51]

Dasatinib is also being assessed as a potential first-line treatment and studies involving patients in CP, following at least 3 months of dasatinib therapy, show 89% complete hematological response and 79% complete cytogenetic response.[52] These data compare well with first-line responses to imatinib. The toxicity profile appears to be similar to that seen in the imatinib-resistant studies, but the number of patients entered so far is quite small. The drug has also been tested in patients with CML in advanced phases whose disease was resistant to both imatinib and nilotinib; remarkably, 57% hematological responses, including 43% complete hematological response, were observed. Among those patients who had a hematological response, 32% had a cytogenetic response, including two patients who exhibited a complete cytogenetic response.

Nilotinib, like imatinib, works by binding to a closed (inactive) conformation of the ABL KD, with a much higher affinity than imatinib. Like imatinib, it inhibits the dysregulated tyrosine kinase activity by occupying the ATP-binding pocket of the ABL kinase component of the BCR-ABL oncoprotein and blocking the capacity of the enzyme to phosphorylate downstream effector molecules. *In vitro* studies suggest that nilotinib is about 30–50-fold more potent than imatinib. Nilotinib is also active in 32 of the currently 33 imatinib-resistant cell lines with mutant ABL kinases, but has no activity against the T315I mutation.

Current phase II studies in patients who are resistant or intolerant to imatinib are still in progress, and preliminary results suggest a complete hematological response in about 70% and a 40% complete cytogenetic response in these patients (Figure 10.4).[53,54] Patients in the advanced phases of CML also respond, but to a lesser degree. The most common treatment-related toxicity is myelosuppression, followed by headaches, pruritus, and rashes. Overall, 22% of the CP patients experienced thrombocytopenia, with 19% having either grade 3/4 severity; 16% had neutropenia and a further 16% had anemia. Most of the non-hematological side-effects were of a grade 1/2 severity. All, including the hematological effects were fully reversible. About 19% of all patients experience arthralgias and about 14% experience fluid retention, particularly pleural and pericardial effusions. Importantly, patients with the imatinib-acquired T315I mutation appear to be refractory to nilotinib. Nilotinib is also being tested as first-line therapy for newly diagnosed patients in chronic phase. Preliminary results confirm the drug to be more potent than imatinib and further patient accrual continues.[55]

As discussed earlier, based on current EBMT experience, it is reasonable to consider an early alloSCT for those patients who are resistant to imatinib and have high-risk disease, by Sokal and Hasford risk stratification, and a low transplant risk, by EBMT criteria, and wish to be transplanted, rather than subjecting them to the next generation TKI. An alternative would be to prescribe a second TKI for a defined period and then proceed with an

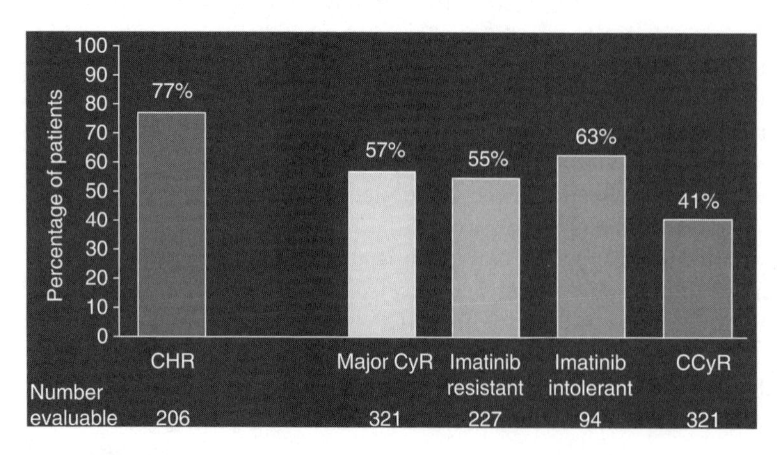

Figure 10.4 Summary of the phase II results of nilotinib in patients with chronic phase chronic myeloid leukemia resistant/refractory to imatinib after ≥6 months of treatment. Median time to complete hematological response (CHR) was 1 month and to major cytogenetic response (CG) was 2.8 months. CCyR, complete cytogenetic response. Adapted from reference 54, with permission.

alloSCT if the response is suboptimal. In practice, however, many patients will opt to receive a trial of a next generation TKI.

A POTENTIAL TREATMENT ALGORITHM FOR A PATIENT WITH CHRONIC MYELOID LEUKEMIA IN CHRONIC PHASE WHO IS RESISTANT TO ALL CURRENTLY AVAILABLE TYROSINE KINASE INHIBITORS

For patients who are resistant/refractory to the current generation of TKIs, and are under the age of 50 years, it is probably best to consider an alloSCT, provided that a suitable donor is identified and the patient remains in CP. For those with advanced phase disease, one could offer combination chemotherapy or if appropriate a clinical trial assessing one of the new agents active against the T315I mutation, and then consider alloSCT if a second CP is achieved.[56] Clearly, this is an area which is evolving rapidly; it is difficult to make firm recommendations at present.

Patients who proceed to an alloSCT after prior treatment with imatinib appear to have a higher relapse incidence than those who have not previously received imatinib.[14] This most likely represents a selection bias for relatively resistant disease. Preliminary data based on small patient series do not, however, suggest that prior treatment with imatinib increases the probability of transplant-related mortality (Figure 10.5).[57,58] Moreover, patients with KD mutations appear to fare as well post-transplant as those lacking such mutations. The experience with alloSCT after initial treatment of advanced phase disease with imatinib is still limited.

FUTURE APPROACHES

Following the realization that a molecular remission and 'cure' might not be possible with imatinib alone, and the notion that the graft-versus-leukemia effect is the principal reason for success in patients with CML subjected to an allograft, many efforts are being directed to exploring the potential of developing an active specific immunotherapy strategy for patients with CML by inducing an immune response to a tumor-specific antigen.[59] At the same time, better understanding of the resistance mechanisms to imatinib, and indeed dasatinib and nilotinib, has paved the way towards the development of more potent drugs, both TKI and others.

The principle involves generating an immune response to the unique amino acid sequence of p210 at the fusion point.

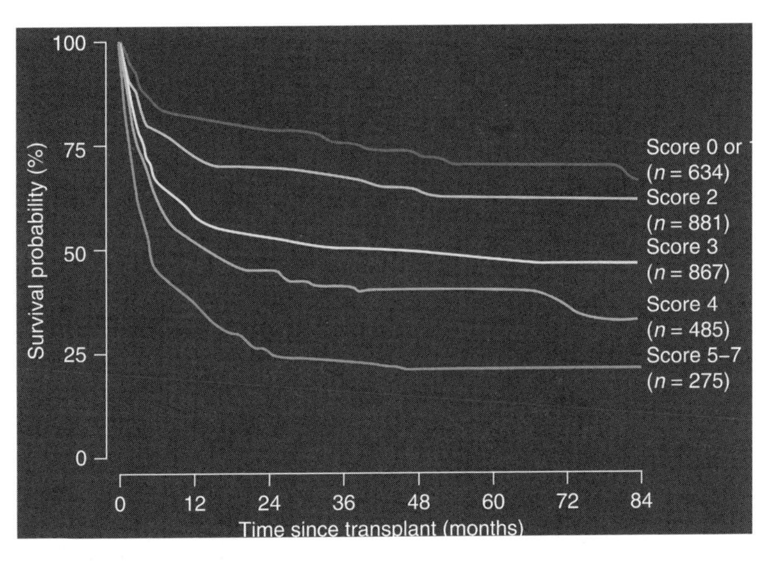

Figure 10.5 Overall survival probability after allogeneic bone marrow transplantation for chronic myeloid leukemia after imatinib treatment according to pretransplant risk score (Gratwohl score).

Clinical responses to the BCR-ABL peptide vaccination, including complete cytogenetic responses, have been reported in a small series. In contrast to previous earlier unsuccessful attempts, the current series included administration of granulocyte-macrophage colony-stimulating factor as an immune adjuvant, and patients were only enrolled if they had measurable residual disease and human leukocyte alleles known to which the selected fusion peptides were predicted to bind avidly.[60,61] If these results can be confirmed, vaccine development against BCR-ABL and other CML-specific antigens could become an attractive treatment for patients who have a minimal residual disease status with imatinib. Other targets for vaccine therapy now being studied include peptides derived from the Wilms tumor-1 protein, proteinase-3, elastase, and PRAME, all of which are overexpressed in CML cells.[62–64]

From the next generation TKI perspective, the largest current experience is with bosutinib (SKI-606). Bosutinib is an oral dual ABL/SRC kinase inhibitor, like dasatinib. It appears to be about 200 times more potent than imatinib, and unlike imatinib and dasatinib, does not inhibit other targets such as KIT or platelet-derived growth factor receptor.[65] The preliminary results of treating patients with CML in CP and advanced phase, as well as Ph-positive ALL, appear encouraging, and the toxicity profile appears reasonable, with gastrointestinal and cutaneous toxicities being the major grade 3/4 adverse effects. Another drug of interest, currently in phase I studies, is INNO-406 (previously called NS-187).[66] This drug inhibits the ABL and LYN kinases, and preclinical studies have confirmed its candidacy for the treatment of imatinib-resistant CML.

Other specific inhibitors of signal transduction pathways downstream of BCR-ABL have been tested alone and in combination with imatinib. Some of these agents, such as 17-allylaminogeldanamycin (17-AAG), are just entering formal clinical trials or might do so in the near future. 17-AAG, a drug which degrades the BCR-ABL oncoprotein by inhibiting the heat shock protein 90, a molecular chaperone required for stabilization of BCR-ABL, has just entered phase I studies.[67] 17-AAG appears to have activity in patients with the E255K and T315I mutations. It also downregulates *BCR-ABL* mRNA, though the precise mechanism remains unclear. Another novel TKI, PD166326, also appears to have significant activity in patients with the H396P and M351T mutations.[68] This agent also appears to be superior to imatinib in murine models. Other potential agents include rapamycin, an mTOR inhibitor, and wortmannin, which is a PI3K inhibitor not currently available in a formulation suitable for clinical use. Rapamycin synergizes with imatinib in inhibiting BCR-ABL-transformed cells, including those that are imatinib resistant.

Strategies being developed to overcome the T315I mutants include the aurora kinase inhibitor MK-0457 (previously known as VX-680).[56] Preliminary clinical studies confirm hematological and cytogenetic responses in patients with the T315I mutant imatinib-refractory CML, but the trials have been suspended at present pending investigation of potential myocardial toxicity. Efforts are also being directed to downregulating survivin, a key member of the inhibitor of apoptosis family of proteins, in both imatinib-sensitive and imatinib-resistant CML patients.[69]

CONCLUSIONS

The substantial understanding of the molecular features and pathogenesis of CML has provided important insights into targeting treatment to specific molecular defects. The successful introduction of imatinib as targeted therapy for CML has made the approach to management of the newly diagnosed patient fairly complex. The second generation of TKI, dasatinib and nilotinib, have shown to have significant activity in selected patients in both CP and the more advanced phases of the disease, who are resistant to imatinib. Efforts are also in progress assessing the potential first-line role of both these drugs.[70] The notion that the graft-versus-leukemia effect is the principal reason for success in patients with CML subjected to an allograft has renewed interest in immunotherapy. The use of kinase inhibitors in conjunction with various immunotherapeutic strategies is now being studied.

For the moment, the various treatment options should be assessed carefully in terms of the relative risk–benefit ratios and a management strategy developed accordingly. For the minority of patients, who are either children or in whom the risk of transplant-related mortality is relatively low but with high Sokal risk stratification, it appears reasonable to recommend an early alloSCT. It would also be reasonable to contemplate an early SCT for patients who have an identical twin donor. For all other patients (who constitute the vast majority), it is best to commence imatinib at 400 mg/day, increasing to a maximum of 800 mg/day in patients with a suboptimal response.

Patients who are resistant/refractory to imatinib should receive dasatinib, or nilotinib when the latter drug is approved. For those who are resistant/refractory to these drugs, it is best to consider an alloSCT, provided that a suitable donor is identified or after an appropriate clinical trial assessing emerging drugs for those with a T315I mutation. Clearly, this is an area which is evolving rapidly; it is difficult to make firm recommendations at present.

Finally, *pari passu* with all the non-transplant treatment efforts, efforts in improving the technology of alloSCT, such as the ability to prevent GVHD without abrogation of graft-versus-leukemia, are also in progress. If successful, they might restore alloSCT as an alternative treatment option for some newly diagnosed patients, who might otherwise have to continue lifelong to take a TKI at not inconsiderable expense.

REFERENCES

1. Goldman JM. How I treat chronic myeloid leukemia in the imatinib era. Blood 2007; 110: 2828–37.
2. Mughal TI, Goldman JM. Targeting cancers with tyrosine kinase inhibitors: lessons learned from chronic myeloid leukaemia. Clin Med 2006; 6: 526–8.
3. Druker BJ, Guilhot F, O'Brien SG et al. Five-year follow-up of patients receiving imatinib for chronic myeloid leukemia. N Engl J Med 2006; 355: 2408–17.
4. Talpaz M, Shah NP, Kantarjian H et al. Dasatinib in imatinib-resistant Philadelphia chromosome positive leukemias. N Engl J Med 2006; 354: 2531–41.
5. Kantarjian H, Giles F, Wunderle L et al. Nilotinib in imatinib-resistant Philadelphia chromosome-positive leukemias. N Engl J Med 2006; 354: 2542–51.
6. Maziarz RT, Mauro MJ. Transplantation for chronic myelogenous leukemia: yes, no, maybe so. An Oregan perspective. Bone Marrow Transplant 2003; 32: 459–69.
7. Mughal TI, Yong A, Szydlo R et al. The probability of long-term leukaemia free survival for patients in molecular remission 5 years after allogeneic stem cell transplantation for chronic myeloid leukaemia in chronic phase. Br J Haematol 2001; 115: 569–74.
8. Mughal TI, Goldman JM. Molecularly targeted treatment of chronic myeloid leukemia: beyond the imatinib era. Front Biosci 2006; 1: 209–20.
9. Goldman JM, Mughal TI. Chronic myeloid leukemia. In: Postgraduate Haematology, 5th edition. Hoffbrand AV, Catovsky D, Tuddenham EGD, eds. Oxford: Wiley Blackwell, 2005; 603–18.
10. Druker BJ, Tamura S, Buchdunger E et al. Effects of a selective inhibitor of the Abl tyrosine kinase on the growth of the BCR-ABL positive cells. Nat Med 2000; 2: 561.
11. Hochhaus A, on behalf of the IRIS investigators. Outcomes post imatinib for patients on the IRIS trial: a 6 year follow-up. Blood 2007; 110: abstract 25.
12. Kantarjian HM, Talpaz M, O'Brien S et al. Survival benefit with imatinib mesylate versus interferon-α based regimens in newly diagnosed chronic-phase chronic myelogenous leukemia. Blood 2006; 108: 1835–40.
13. Hughes T, Branford S. Molecular monitoring of BCR-ABL as a guide to clinical management in chronic myeloid leukaemia. Blood Rev 2006; 20: 29–41.
14. Deininger M, Schleuning M, Greinix H et al. The effect of prior exposure to imatinib on transplant-related mortality. Haematologica 2006; 91: 452–9.
15. Gratwohl A, Hermans J, Goldman JM et al. Risk assessment for patients with chronic myeloid leukaemia before allogeneic bone marrow transplantation. Lancet 1998; 352: 1087–92.
16. NCCN guidelines for the management of CML 2.2007 [Accessed March 2008 at http://www.nccn.org/professionals/physicians_gls/PDF/cml.pdf].
17. Yong AS, Szydlo RM, Goldman JM et al. Molecular profiling of CD34+ cells identifies low expression of CD7 along with high expression of proteinase 3 and elastase as predictors of longer survival in patients with CML. Blood 2006; 107: 205–12.
18. Brazma D, Grace C, Howard J et al. Genomic profile of chronic myelogenous leukemia: imbalances

associate with disease progression. Genes Chromosomes Cancer 2007; 46: 1039–50.
19. Guilhot H, on behalf of the IRIS investigators. Time to complete cytogenetic response does not affect long term outcomes for patients with CML-CP on imatinib therapy. Blood 2007; 110: 16a, abstract 27.
20. Baccarani M, Saglio G, Goldman JM et al. Evolving concepts in the management of chronic myeloid leukemia: recommendations from an expert panel on behalf of the European LeukemiaNet. Blood 2006; 108: 1809–20.
21. Aoki E, Kantarjian H, O'Brien S et al. High-dose imatinib mesylate treatment in patients (pts) with untreated early chronic phase (CP) chronic myeloid leukemia (CML): 2.5 year follow-up. J Clin Oncol 2006; 24: 18s, abstract 6535.
22. Kantarjian HM, Hochaus A, Cortes J et al. Nilotinib for the treatment of patients with CML-CP resistant/refractory to imatinib: Responses in patients > 6 months of treatment. Blood 2007; 110: 226a, abstract 725.
23. Giralt S. Allogeneic hematopoietic progenitor cell transplantation for the treatment of CML in the era of tyrosine kinase inhibitors: lessons learned to date. Clin Lymph Myeloma 2007; 7: S102–4.
24. Schiffer CA. BCR-ABL tyrosine kinase inhibitors for chronic myelogenous leukemia. N Engl J Med 2007; 357: 258–65.
25. Kerkela R, Grazette L, Yacobi R et al. Cardiotoxicity of the cancer therapeutic agent imatinib mesylate. Nat Med 2006; 12: 908–16.
26. Atallah E, Kantarjian H, Cortes J. In reply to 'Cardiotoxicity of the cancer therapeutic agent imatinib mesylate'. Nat Med 2007; 13: 14.
27. Kovitz C, Kantarjian HM, Garcia-Manero G, Abbruzzo LV, Cortes J. Myelodysplastic syndromes and acute leukemia developing after imatinib mesylate therapy for chronic myeloid leukemia. Blood 2006; 108: 2811–13.
28. Roy L, Guilhot J, Martineau G, Larchée R, Guilhot F. Unexpected occurrence of second malignancies in patients treated with interferon followed by imatinib mesylate for chronic myelogenous leukemia. Leukemia 2005; 19: 1689–92.
29. Ebonether M, Stentoft J, Ford J et al. Cerebral edema as a possible complication of treatment with imatinib. Lancet 2002; 359: 1751–2.
30. Strebhardt K, Ullrich A. Another look at imatinib mesylate. N Engl J Med 2006; 355: 2481–2.
31. Apperley J. Part I: Mechanisms of resistance to imatinib in chronic myeloid leukaemia. Lancet Oncol 2007; 8: 1018–29.
32. Druker BJ. Circumventing resistance to kinase-inhibitor therapy. N Engl J Med 2006; 354: 2594–6.
33. Shah NP, Tran C, Lee FY et al. Overriding imatinib resistance with a novel ABL kinase inhibitor. Science 2004; 305: 399–401.
34. White DL, Saunders VA, Dang P et al. OCT-1 mediated influx is a key determinant of the intracellular uptake of imatinib but not nilotinib (AMN107): reduced OCT-1 activity is the cause of low in vitro sensitivity to imatinib. Blood 2006; 108: 697–704.
35. Branford S, Rudzki Z, Walsh S et al. Detection of BCR-ABL mutations in patients with CML treated with imatinib is virtually always accompanied by clinical resistance, and mutations in the ATP phosphate-binding loop (P-loop) are associated with a poor prognosis. Blood 2003; 102: 276–83.
36. Guilhot F. Mutation detection in CML: is it a useful tool? Blood 2005; 106: 1897–8.
37. Deininger M, Buchdunger E, Druker BJ. The development of imatinib as a therapeutic agent for chronic myeloid leukemia. Blood 2005; 105: 2640–53.
38. Mughal TI, Goldman JM. Emerging strategies for the treatment of mutant Bcr-Abl T315I myeloid leukemias. Clin Lymph Myeloma 2007; (Suppl 2): S81–4.
39. Apperley J. Part II: Management of resistance to imatinib in chronic myeloid leukaemia. Lancet Oncol 2007; 8: 1116–28.
40. Kantarjian HM, Pasquini R, Hamerschlak N et al. Dasatinib or high-dose imatinib for chronic-phase chronic myeloid leukemia after failure of first-line imatinib: a randomized phase 2 trial. Blood 2007; 109: 5143–50.
41. Cortes J, Kantarjian H. New targeted approaches in chronic myeloid leukemia. J Clin Oncol 2005; 23: 6316–24
42. Baccarani M, Martinelli G, Rosti G et al. Imatinib and pegylated human recombinant interferon-alpha2b in early chronic-phase chronic myeloid leukemia. Blood 2004; 104: 4245–51.
43. Issa J-P, Gharibyan V, Cortes J et al. Phase II study of low-dose decitabine in patients with chronic myelogenous leukemia resistant to imatinib mesylate. J Clin Oncol 2005; 23: 3948–56.
44. Cortes J, Albitar M, Thomas D et al. Efficacy of the farnesyl transferase inhibitor R115777 in chronic myeloid leukemia and other hematologic malignancies. Blood 2003; 101: 1692–7.
45. Cortes J, O'Brien S, Verstovsek S et al. Phase I study of lonafarnib (SCH66336) in combination with imatinib for patients (pts) with chronic myeloid leukemia (CML) after failure to imatinib. Blood 2004; 104: 288a, abstract 1009.
46. O'Brien S, Kantarjian H, Keating M et al. Homoharringtonine therapy induces responses in patients with chronic myelogenous leukemia in late chronic phase. Blood 1995; 86: 3322–6.
47. Mughal TI. Dasatinib, a novel Abl-Src kinase inhibitor, in the management of patients with Philadelphia chromosome-positive leukemias. Clin Leuk 2006; 1: 15–18.

48. Quintas-Cardama A, Kantarjian HM, Jones D et al. Dasatinib (BMS-354825) is active in Philadelphia chromosome-positive chronic myelogenous leukaemia after imatinib and nilotinib(AMN107) therapy failure. Blood 2007; 109: 497–9.
49. Muller MC, Erben P, Schenk T et al. Response to dasatinib after imatinib failure according to type of pre-existing BCR-ABL mutations. Blood 2006; 108: abstract 225.
50. Hochhaus A, Kantarjian HM, Baccarani M et al. Dasatinib induces notable hematologic and cytogenetic responses in chronic-phase chronic myelogenous leukaemia after failure of imatinib therapy. Blood 2007; 109: 2303–9.
51. Hochhaus A, Kim DW, Rousselot P et al. Dasatinib (SPRYCEL) 50mg or 70mg BID versus 100mg or 140mg QD in patients with chronic myeloid leukaemia in chronic-phase (CML-CP) or myeloid blast (CML-MB) phase who are imatinib-resistant (Im-r) or -intolerant (Im-i). Blood 2006; 108: 224A, abstract 745.
52. Cortes J, O'Brien S, Jones D et al. Dasatinib in patients with previously untreated chronic myelogenous leukaemia in chronic phase. Blood 2007; 110, abstract 30.
53. Mughal TI. Nilotinib in the post-imatinib era for the treatment of Philadelphia chromosome positive leukemias. Clin Leuk 2006; 1: 84–6.
54. Kantarjian HM, Giles F, Gatterman N et al. Nilotinib formerly AMN107, a highly selective BCR-ABL tyrosine kinase inhibitor is effective in patients with Philadelphia chromosome-positive chronic myelogenous leukemia in chronic phase following imatinib resistance or intolerance. Blood 2007; 110: 3540–6.
55. Cortes J et al. Nilotinib in newly diagnosed patients with chronic myelogenous leukemia in chronic phase. Blood 2007; 110: 17a.
56. Giles F, Cortes J, Jones D et al. MK-0457, a novel tyrosine inhibitor, is active in patients with chronic myeloid leukemia or acute lymphoblastic leukemia with T315I BCR-ABL mutation. Blood 2007; 2: 500–2.
57. Oehler, Gooley T, Synder DS et al. The effects of imatinib mesylate treatment before allogeneic transplantation for chronic myeloid leukemia. Blood 2007; 109: 1782–9.
58. Srivastava PK. Immunotherapy of human cancer: lessons from mice. Nat Immunol 2000; 1: 363–6.
59. Rojas JM, Knight K, Wang L, Clark FE. Clinical evaluation of BCR-ABL peptide immunisation in chronic myeloid leukaemia: results of the EPIC study. Leukemia 2007; 21: 2287–95.
60. Molldrem JJ, Lee PP, Wang C et al. Evidence that specific T lymphocytes may participate in the elimination of chronic myelogenous leukemia. Nat Med 2000; 6: 1018–23.
61. Bocchia M, Gentili S, Abruzzese E et al. Effect of a p210 multipeptide vaccine associated with imatinib or interferon in patients with chronic myeloid leukaemia and persistent residual disease: a multicentre observational trial. Lancet 2005; 365: 657–9.
62. Zeng Y, Graner MW, Thompson S et al. Induction of BCR-ABL-specific immunity following vaccination with chaperone rich lysates from BCR-ABL+ tumor cells. Blood 2005; 105: 2016–22.
63. Oka Y, Tsuboi A, Taguchi T et al. Induction of WTI (Wilms tumor gene)-specific cytotoxic T lymphocytes by WTI peptide vaccine and the resultant cancer regression. Proc Natl Acad Sci U S A 2004; 101: 13885–90.
64. Cortes J, Kantarjian H, Baccarani M et al. A phase1/2 study of SKI-606, a dual inhibitor of Src and Abl kinases, in adult patients with Philadelphia chromosome positive (Ph+) chronic myelogenous leukemia (CML) or acute lymphoblastic leukemia (ALL) relapsed, refractory or intolerant of imatinib. Blood 2006; 108: 54a, abstract 168.
65. Tao W, Sun T, Craig A et al. The ATP competitor INNO-406 (NS-187) inhibits proliferation and survival of mouse cells expressing several imatinib mesylate resistant Bcr/Abl mutants and cells from CML patients. Blood 2006; 108: 618a, abstract 2179.
66. Rao R, Fiskus W, Herger B et al. Inhibition of histone deactylase (HDAC) 6 and/or heat shock protein (HSP) 90: a strategy to abrogate multi-level protective responses to misfolded proteins induced by proteasome inhibitors in human leukemia cells. Blood 2006; 108: 80a, abstract 257.
67. Wolff NC, Veach DR, Tong WP et al. PD166326, a novel tyrosine kinase inhibitor, has greater antileukemic activity than imatinib mesylate in a murine model of chronic myelogenous leukemia. Blood 2005; 105: 3995–4003.
68. Carter BZ, Mak DH, Schober WD et al. Regulation of surviving expression through Bcr-Abl/MAPK cascade: targeting surviving overcomes imatinib resistance and increases imatinib sensitivity in imatinib-responsive CML cells. Blood 2006; 107: 1555–63.
69. Jabbour E, Cortes J, Ghanem H, O'Brien S, Kantarjian HM. Targeted therapy in chronic myeloid leukemia. Expert Rev Anticancer Ther 2008; 8: 99–110.
70. Mughal TI, Cross NC, Cortes J et al. Chronic myeloid leukemia: some topical challenges. Leukemia 2007; 21: 1347–52.

History of *BCR-ABL*-negative chronic myeloproliferative disorders

11

Tiziano Barbui

Current classification of the myeloproliferative disorders (MPD) by the World Health Organization (WHO) includes Philadelphia chromosome (Ph)-positive chronic myeloid leukemia (CML) and Ph-negative clonal hematological diseases. The most frequent of this latter group are polycythemia vera (PV), essential thrombocythemia (ET), and idiopathic myelofibrosis (IMF). Less common conditions encompass systemic mastocytosis, chronic eosinophilic leukemia, chronic myelomonocytic leukemia, and chronic neutrophilic leukemia.

The focus of this chapter is to summarize the history of the main biological and clinical developments achieved in the three most common Ph-negative MPD.

The history of PV began in 1892 with the initial description by Vaquez of a single patient who showed a particular form of cyanosis associated with persistent, autonomous, and extreme erythrocytosis.[1] A decade after this description, Osler delineated PV as a new clinical entity characterized by 'cyanosis with polycythemia and enlarged spleen with symptoms somewhat indefinite and with pathology quite obscure'.[2] These clinicians thought PV was marked only by the increase of red cell count not secondary to congenital heart disease and failed to recognize that the process resulted from a global bone marrow proliferation, as evidenced by concomitant hyperplasia of granulocytic and megakaryocytic cell lines. As a consequence, erythrocytosis was considered the most prominent cause of clinical manifestations and, accordingly, much of the research regarding the pathogenesis of PV focused on erythropoiesis.

At about the time efforts were made to distinguish PV from secondary diseases associated with erythrocytosis, true polycythemia was differentiated from chronic relative polycythemia occurring in patients with intravascular fluid depletion and without splenomegaly. The concept of secondary polycythemia was further elucidated by Gaisbock in 1905 who described the association of polycythemia with hypertension and regarded this picture as a separate entity distinct from PV.[3] Subsequently, many other authors reported cases of polycythemia associated with obesity, anxiety, and smoking. Noteworthy was the observation by Russell and Conley that, in contrast to patients with PV, individuals with secondary polycythemia had little improvement in symptoms after phlebotomy, suggesting that in these secondary erythrocytoses there was no cause–effect relationship between the increased hematocrit and vascular disturbances.[4] These early publications set the stage for more reliable and accurate classification of the polycythemic states.

The measurement of red cell mass (RCM) by the *in vitro* labeling of autologous erythrocytes with [^{51}Cr] sodium chromate, as described by the International Committee for Standardization in Hematology in 1973, was considered an essential element in establishing the diagnosis of absolute erythrocytosis.[5] Further advances in the differential diagnosis of polycythemic states came from the work done in France by Najean and co-workers.[6] These investigators demonstrated that the simultaneous measurement of red cell and plasma volume was more reliable than either the hematocrit evaluation or the measurement of a single volume to differentiate PV from primary thrombocythemia, pure erythrocytosis, and spurious and secondary polycythemia.

The first to describe the natural history of PV were Rosenthal and Bassen in 1938.[7] By reviewing the reported cases, they divided the clinical course of PV into the asymptomatic phase, the subsequent polycythemic and symptomatic phase and the terminal phase, called by the authors 'anemic and spent phase'. These investigators pointed out the chronicity of the disease and recognized that acute leukemia and myelofibrosis were part of its natural evolution. In 1954, Wasserman advanced a hypothetical concept for the course of PV and distinguished subsequent stages of this disorder.[8] The first stage is featured by pure erythrocytosis with increase of hematocrit but with normal platelet and leukocyte counts and no splenomegaly. This description may correspond to an initial phase of PV or to the so called 'idiopathic erythrocytosis' that was the object of subsequent clinical studies in Europe.[9] The second stage, according to Wasserman,[8] included the overt picture of PV and the subsequent phases represented the evolution to myelofibrosis that can be suspected when an apparent spontaneous remission of PV is occurring. The incidence, type of complications and causes of death were reported some years later in 1962. European investigators followed up a cohort of PV patients left untreated and calculated a median survival varying from 6 to 18 months from diagnosis.[10] With modern therapy, the life expectancy of PV patients in the first decade after diagnosis is not different from that of a matched population whereas a slight difference is seen after 10 years, owing to increase of malignancy.[11]

In contrast to PV, the history of ET and IMF is less rich. The first description of ET was reported by Epstein and Goedel in 1934,[12] but it should be mentioned that there was considerable controversy as to whether this condition truly represented a distinct entity. McCabe *et al.* claimed that if patients were followed for a sufficient length of time, some other underlying hematological diseases would eventually emerge.[13] It was not until the classic papers of Gunz[14] and Ozer *et al.*[15] in 1960, both of whom critically reviewed their experience and other reported cases of hemorrhagic thrombocythemia, that ET became widely accepted as a separate myeloproliferative disorder. However, despite its recognition, the lack of uniform diagnostic criteria made ET the least well-defined of the chronic MPD.

IMF was recognized in 1879 when Heuck described two cases that differed from classical CML on the finding of extramedullary erythropoiesis and bone marrow fibrosis.[16] It became apparent that IMF was a unique pathological entity after the work of Ward and Block in 1971, who presented evidence that this myeloid disorder had to be distinct from the others.[17]

The term 'myeloproliferative disorders' was coined by Dameshek in 1951 and this concept survives to the present day.[18] Dameshek was the first to recognize that PV, ET, and IMF, together with CML, were related diseases with common clinical and laboratory features. His initial schema also included megakaryocytic leukemia and erythroleukemia. The different clinical course, the laboratory features and the subsequent discovery of the Philadelphia (Ph^1) in 1960, led to the separation of CML from PV, ET, and IMF. These latter were classified as Ph-negative MPD. To elucidate his unifying theory, Dameshek postulated two different pathogenetic mechanisms: the first was that, in response to unrecognized stimulus, the myeloid, erythroid, megakaryocytic, and fibroblastic elements of the bone marrow proliferated *en masse*. The second possibility he advanced, was that the entire process of excessive myeloproliferation could be the result of a lack or diminution of inhibitory factors controlling the hematopoiesis. He also suggested that dormant embryonal hematopoietic cells in extramedullary sites could become activated.

It was 20 years later, in 1974, that hematopoietic stem cells derived from bone marrow or peripheral blood of PV patients were found to proliferate in serum containing cultures in the absence of exogenous erythropoietin.[19] Initially, some concerns were raised regarding these experiments since these 'endogenous erythroid colonies' or 'EECs', could be driven by minimal traces of erythropoietin (EPO) contamination in the serum but, subsequently, any doubts were dispelled by using an improved serum and EPO-free medium. EECs are one of the current WHO criterion for the diagnosis of PV.

At a similar time, studies based on X-chromosome inactivation in women with PV found that these disorders were derived from a clone of a single multipotent hematopoietic stem cell.[20] Thus, the question of whether PV was a benign condition, as interpreted by Osgood[21] and by Ward and Block,[17] or a neoplastic process, as claimed by Wasserman[8] years before, was answered. In 1960, CML became the first cancer associated with a specific cytogenetic marker (the Ph chromosome) which subsequently was shown to harbor a reciprocal chromosomal translocation t(9;22)(q34;q11). From the 1980s onwards, new insights into the molecular pathogenesis of the Ph-negative MPD were discovered. It was demonstrated that, in analogy with what had been discovered about CML, MPD have altered common components in the signal transduction pathways activated by growth factors. In the 1980s, German pathologists Burkhardt *et al.* described typical histopathological features from bone marrow biopsy material for the diagnosis and classification of each of the three Ph-negative MPD ET, PV, and IMF.[22] These pathological findings, currently confirmed by the majority of pathologists, inspired the WHO to include bone marrow morphology in the diagnostic criteria of MPD.[23] The recent discovery of a single acquired point mutation in the Janus kinase 2 *(JAK2)* gene in the majority of PV patients and in about half of ET and IMF cases, has provided an unique pathogenetic explanation for many clinical and biological features of MPDs and has permitted revision of the classification of these disorders.[24]

As far as the history of therapy is concerned, the application of venesection as a form of treatment was introduced in the years between 1903 and 1908.[25] In the late 1930s, Lawrence introduced radiophosphorus as treatment for PV[26] and the first recorded case of acute leukemia associated with the use of radiophosphorus was reported some years later.[27] In a panel discussion organized in 1955 by Dameshek the two modalities of treatment, venesection and radiophosphorus, were discussed and a consensus was reached to recommend radiophosphorus as the first-line therapy of PV.[28] However, Dameshek dissented and claimed that venesection had to be the first preferable therapy. At a similar time, new chemotherapeutic agents became available, so that thiotepa, busulfan, chlorambucil, cyclophosphamide, and melphalan were considered as alternatives to venesection or radiotherapy. These drugs were thought to have advantages over phlebotomy since they were able to control not only the excessive erythrocytosis but also the thrombocytosis, leukocytosis, and splenomegaly.

A great impetus to solve the uncertainties in the management of these disorders was given by Wasserman who established in 1967 the Polycythemia Vera Study Group (PVSG). This consortium included hematologists from the US and Europe with particular interest in PV and other MPD. The goals of this group were to define very stringent diagnostic criteria for future clinical trials, to delineate the epidemiology, natural history and pathophysiology, and to determine the optimal treatment.

With respect to PVSG diagnostic criteria, it should be underlined that, to enroll patients in clinical trials, the demonstration of elevation of red cell mass and plasma was required.[29] Since its creation, the group has conducted a total of 14 separate studies addressing questions on PV, ET, and IMF. Under the auspices of the National Cancer Institute, a randomized, controlled trial that compared the efficacy of phlebotomy alone with that of radiophosphorus and chlorambucil was designed (protocol 01). The results of this trial and those of studies 05 (aspirin plus persantin) and 08 (hydroxyurea) significantly influenced the worldwide clinical practice regarding PV.

From these studies, the recommended treatment for PV was phlebotomy for low-risk patients and hydroxyurea for high-risk cases. The leukemogenicity played by hydroxyurea, currently recommended as first-line therapy when cytoreductive therapy is indicated, is still a matter of concern and the dilemma of whether acute leukemia may be owing to the drug or represents an evolution of the underlying MPD remains unanswered. The conclusion of the PVSG 05 randomized clinical trial was that aspirin plus persantin, at the doses employed in the study, should not be used prophylactically. The hypothesis that low-dose aspirin could be helpful in PV was reconsidered in Europe and the multicenter, multinational European study called ECLAP (European Collaborative Low dose Aspirin in Polycythemia), supported by a grant from the Biomed 2 Program of the European Union and by unrestricted grants from Bayer and Bayer Italia, showed that aspirin was able to reduce the combined end-points of major thrombotic events without increasing the risk of hemorrhage.[30]

The clinical course and therapy of ET were also among the goals of the PVSG and an *ad hoc* subcommittee initiated, during the latter half of the 1970s, a series of studies showing that hydroxyurea and not melphalan had to be the drug of choice when indicated.[29] In the following years, however, some long-term follow-up studies revealed that a proportion of ET patients given hydroxyurea developed acute leukemia and myelodysplasia. This problem became a big issue and cast doubt on the use of hydroxyurea. Moreover, while it was clear that this drug was able to normalize platelet count in ET, no formal demonstration was available that this was associated with a decrease thrombotic rate.

The history of treatment in IMF is quite poor. Large and controlled clinical trials are lacking and, still today, therapy is symptomatic and does not influence overall survival. Curative approaches by using hematopoietic stem cell transplantation are being currently explored but further studies are required to confirm in larger series of patients the recently reported optimistic results registered in small size retrospective and phase II studies.

In the past decade, large randomized clinical trials have been carried out by European Investigators in PV and ET and some important questions on the natural history, risk factors, and therapy have been addressed.[31] In addition, the European collaborative experience shows that large, long-term networks of centers treating these rare diseases are mandatory to ensure even epidemiological representation, using a sufficient number of patients to allow statistical power. The recent description of the *JAK2* mutation has opened new horizons for therapy. Whether JAK2-targeted molecules will alter the natural history of these disorders, as imatinib for CML, remains to be demonstrated.

In conclusion, from the observation of Vaquez in 1892 to the recent discovery of *JAK2* mutation, the history of these relatively rare diseases serves as an ideal model to evaluate the incremental progress of our understanding, first measured over centuries and now in months.

REFERENCES

1. Vaquez HM. Sur une forme speciale de cyanose s'accompagnant d'hyperglobulie excessive et persistente. C R Soc Biol (Paris) 1892; 44: 384–8.
2. Osler W. Chronic cyanosis with polycythemia and enlarged spleen. Am J Med Sci 1903; 126: 187–201.
3. Gaisbock F. Die bedentung der blutdruckmessung fur die arztliche praxis. Deutch. Arch Klin Med 1905; 83: 363–409.
4. Russell RP, Conley CL. Benign polycythemia: Gaisbock's syndrome. Arch Intern Med 1964; 114: 734–40.
5. International Committee for Standardization in Hematology (ICSH). Standard techniques for the measurement of red cell and plasma volume. Br J Haematol 1973; 25: 795–814.
6. Najean Y, Cacchione R, Dresch C, Rain JD. Interet pratique de la mesure du volume globulaire dans le poliglobulies. Nouv Presse Med 1975; 4: 1633–6.
7. Rosenthal N, Bassen FA. Course of polycythemia. Arch Intern Med 1938; 62: 903–17.
8. Wasserman LR. Polycythemia vera – its course and treatment: relation to myeloid metaplasia and leukaemia. Bull N Y Acad Med 1954; 30: 343–75.

9. Pearson TC, Wetherly-Mein G. The course and complications of idiopathic erythrocytosis. Clin Lab Haematol 1979; 1: 189–96.
10. Chievitz E, Thiede T. Complication and causes of death in polycythemia vera. Acta Med Scand 1962; 172: 513–23.
11. Finazzi G, Barbui T. How we treat patients with polycythemia vera. Blood 2007; 109: 5104–11.
12. Epstein E, Goedel A. Haemorrhagische thrombocythemie bei vascularer schrumpfmilz. Virchow's Archiv Abteilung 1934; 293: 233–47.
13. McCabe WR, Bird RM, Mc Laughlin RA. Is primary hemorrhagic thrombocythemia a clinical myth? Ann Intern Med 1955; 43: 182–90.
14. Gunz FW. Hemorrhagic thrombocythemia: a critical review. Blood 1960; 15: 706–23.
15. Ozer FL, Truax WE, Miesch DC. Primary hemorrhagic thrombocythemia. Am J Med 1960; 28: 807–23.
16. Heuck G. Zwei falle von leukamie mit eigenthumlichen blut-resp. Knochenmarksbefund. Arch Patol Anat Physiol Virchows 1879; 78: 475–96.
17. Ward HP, Block MH. The natural history of agnogenic myeloid metaplasia and a critical evaluation with the myeloid proliferative disorders. Medicine 1971; 50: 357–420.
18. Dameshek W. Some speculations on the myeloproliferative syndromes. Blood 1951; 6: 372–5.
19. Prchal JF, Axelrad AA. Bone-marrow responses in polycythemia vera. N Engl J Med 1974; 290: 1382.
20. Adamson JW, Fialkow PJ, Murphy S, Steinmann L. Polycythemia vera: stem cell and probable clonal origin of the disease. N Engl J Med 1976; 295: 913–16.
21. Osgood EE. Polycythemia vera: age relationships and survival. Blood 1965; 6: 243–56.
22. Burkhardt R, Bartl R, Jaeger K et al. Chronic myeloproliferative disorders. Pathol Res Pract 1984; 179: 131–86.
23. WHO classification of the chronic myeloproliferative diseases (CMPD) polycythemia vera, chronic idiopathic myelofibrosis, essential thrombocythemia and CMPD unclassifiable. In: Jaffe ES, Harris NL, Stein H, Vardiman JW, eds. WHO Classification of Tumours. Pathology and Genetics of Tumours of Hematopoiesis and Lymphoid Tissues. Lyon, France: IARC Press, 2001: 31–42.
24. Campbell PJ, Green AR. The myeloproliferative disorders. N Engl J Med 2006; 355: 2452–66.
25. Berlin NI. The closing of the Wasserman-Polycythemia Vera Study Group era. Semin Hematol 1997; 34: 1–5.
26. Lawrence JH. Polycythemia: physiology, diagnosis and treatment based on 303 cases. Modern Medical Monographs. New York: Grune and Stratton, 1955; 13–136.
27. Tinney WS, Hall BE, Giffin HZ. Hematologic complications of polycythemia vera. Proc Staff Meet Mayo Clin 1943; 18: 227–30.
28. Dameshek W, Lawrence JH, Rosenthal L et al. Panels in therapy: III The treatment of polycythemia vera. Blood 1955; 10: 655–61.
29. Berk PD, Wasserman LR, Fruchtman SM et al. Treatment of polycythemia vera: a summary of clinical trials conducted by the Polycythemia Vera Study Group. In: Wasserman LR, Berk PD, Berlin NI, eds. Polycythemia Vera and Myeloproliferative Disorders. Philadelphia, PA: WB Saunders, 1995.
30. Landolfi R, Marchioli R, Kutti J et al. Efficacy and safety of low-dose aspirin in polycythemia vera. N Engl J Med 2004; 350: 114–24.
31. Barbui T, Finazzi G. Therapy of polycythemia vera and essential thrombocythemia is driven by the cardiovascular risk. Semin Thromb Hemost 2007; 33: 321–9.

BCR-ABL-negative atypical chronic myeloproliferative disorders

12

Sonja Burgstaller, Andreas Reiter, Nicholas CP Cross

INTRODUCTION

Chronic myeloproliferative disorders (MPD) include a spectrum of diseases characterized by excess clonal proliferation of one or more myeloid lineages in the bone marrow with cell maturation being relatively normal. Excess proliferation results in increased numbers of leukocytes, red cells, and/or platelets in the peripheral blood, and is frequently associated with splenomegaly and hepatomegaly. The original classification proposed by Dameshek included four related chronic MPD, often referred to as 'classical' MPD and currently called chronic myeloid leukemia (CML), polycythemia vera (PV), essential thrombocythemia (ET), and primary myelofibrosis (PMF).[1] Although many people considered that CML was distinct from the other three disorders, Dameshek's suggestion that his classification 'may prove useful and even productive' was dramatically borne out by the finding that chronic MPD, at least as far as we know at present, have a common root cause: aberrant activation of tyrosine kinase signaling as a result of specific acquired mutations that results in clonal, stem cell-derived hyperproliferation. The importance of tyrosine kinases was of course highlighted by the finding and characterization of *BCR-ABL* in CML,[2–4] but a clear pointer towards the wider involvement of this class of signaling proteins in the pathogenesis of MPD came from the study of so-called 'atypical' MPD, a heterogeneous group of diseases that are the subject of this review.

BCR-ABL-NEGATIVE CHRONIC MYELOID LEUKEMIA AND RELATED ATYPICAL DISORDERS

Conventional cytogenetic evaluation detects the reciprocal translocation t(9;22)(q34;q11) in the majority of cases of CML. In about 10% of cases, variant translocations are seen that involve one or more chromosomes in addition to chromosomes 9 and 22.[5] The vast majority of these variant cases turn out to be positive for the *BCR-ABL* fusion gene when tested by molecular methods such as reverse transcriptase polymerase chain reaction (RT-PCR) to detect *BCR-ABL* mRNA or using fluorescent *in situ* hybridization (FISH) to detect the juxtaposition of the *BCR* and *ABL* genes. In addition to these variant cases, a further 5–10% of patients with a provisional or suspected diagnosis of CML do not have rearrangements of chromosomes 9 or 22. Approximately half of these turn out to be *BCR-ABL* positive on further investigation and half are *BCR-ABL* negative, the latter often being referred to as '*BCR-ABL*-negative CML'.

Although the entity '*BCR-ABL*-negative CML' is not recognized by the WHO classification system,[6] it remains a useful (if somewhat vague) umbrella term for a heterogeneous but clearly related spectrum of disorders that bear a resemblance to CML at presentation but are found to be negative for the Philadelphia chromosome and the *BCR-ABL* fusion. Patients may or may not have dysplastic features and thus span the WHO-defined category of chronic MPDs (CMPDs) and myelodysplastic/myeloproliferative diseases (MDS/MPD). In the WHO system, patients with *BCR-ABL*-negative CML may be correctly classified as atypical CML (aCML), chronic neutrophilic leukemia (CNL), chronic eosinophilic leukemia (CEL), chronic myelomonocytic leukemia (CMML), juvenile myelomonocytic leukemia (JMML), or, for cases that do not fit into any of these categories, CMPD-unclassified or MDS/MPD-unclassified. Collectively, these entities plus systemic mastocytosis (SM) are often referred to as 'atypical' or 'non-classic' MPD to distinguish them from the four 'classical' MPD.

From a clinical point of view, patients with *BCR-ABL*-negative CML have a more aggressive clinical course, poorer response to treatment, and shorter survival than those with typical CML. In a series of 76 cases from a single institution over a 32-year period, the median overall survival was only 2 years, with a median age at presentation of 66 years.[7] Of those who died, one-third had transformed to myeloid blast crisis; the remainder died from other causes. Multivariate analysis indicated that age greater than 65 years, hemoglobin <10 g/dl, and leukocyte count $>50 \times 10^9$/l were independent predictors of a poor prognosis and that these factors could be used to distinguish a high-risk group with a median survival of only 9 months from a lower-risk group with a median survival of 38 months.[7]

CHALLENGES AT THE BEGINNING OF THE CURRENT CENTURY

As described in detail below, it has become evident that constitutive activation of tyrosine kinase signaling plays a central role in the pathogenesis of MPD, including *BCR-ABL*-negative CML and related diseases. Collectively, however, abnormalities of tyrosine kinases or downstream signaling components are only seen in about one-third of cases. A major challenge, therefore, is the identification of causal molecular changes in the remaining cases.

Activated tyrosine kinases are excellent drug targets, as dramatically demonstrated by the effects of imatinib in CML.[8] Since imatinib is also active against some other kinases including platelet-derived growth factor receptor (PDGFR)α and PDGFRβ kinases, this paradigm has been widened to include some atypical MPD. However, effective compounds are not yet available to target all activated tyrosine kinases or related abnormalities.

An accurate diagnosis including morphology, karyotyping, and molecular genetics will become increasingly important to reach the aim of direct individualized treatment. In addition, new molecular findings need to be incorporated into disease classification systems.

THE MOLECULAR PATHOGENESIS OF *BCR-ABL*-NEGATIVE MYELOPROLIFERATIVE DISORDERS

Overview

The following sections describe the molecular abnormalities that have been identified to date in atypical MPD along with their clinical implications. The mechanism by which these abnormalities result in hyperproliferation of specific cell lineages is not considered in any detail.

The vast majority of patients with atypical *BCR-ABL*-negative MPD present with a normal or aneuploid karyotype – that is, gains or losses of whole chromosomes, most commonly +8.[7] Thus, for most cases there are no clues at this level of analysis to indicate what underlying abnormalities are driving aberrant proliferation of myeloid cells. However, a small subset of patients, perhaps 1%, harbor reciprocal chromosomal translocations that facilitate molecular investigation. Many of these translocations are recurrent, although all are very uncommon. The t(5;12)(p13;q31-33) was the first recurrent abnormality to be described and, to date, more than 50 cases with this translocation have been reported. Many other translocations have been described only in single individuals, but at least six recurrent breakpoint clusters have emerged at chromosome bands 4q11-12, 5q31-33, 8p11-12, 9p34, 9q34, and 13q12.

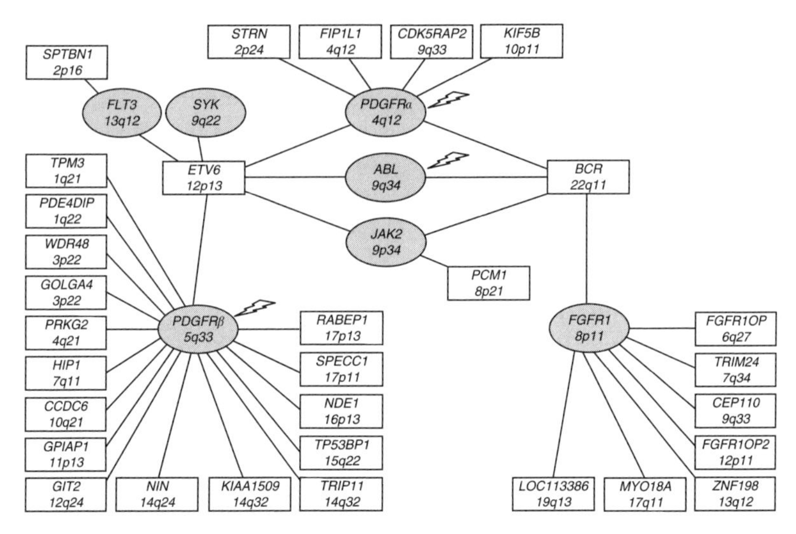

Figure 12.1 Network of 39 tyrosine kinase fusion genes in atypical myeloproliferative disorders and related conditions. Fusions involving *ABL*, *PDGFRα* and *PDGFRβ* have either been shown to be sensitive or are predicted to be sensitive to imatinib, dasatinib, nilotinib (and possibly other tyrosine kinase inhibitors) as indicated by the jagged arrowheads.

Cloning of these translocations has revealed that they frequently target and activate protein tyrosine kinases, with the breakpoint clusters above involving *PDGFRA*, *PDGFRB*, *FGFR1*, *JAK2*, *ABL*, and *FLT3*, respectively (Figure 12.1). Most of these fusions are not specific to any particular WHO-defined entity and so the following sections are therefore based on their molecular classification. Fusion genes are largely formed by cytogenetically visible chromosomal translocations and indeed the only fusion that is not usually associated with a visible karyotypic aberration is *FIP1L1-PDGFRA*. Consequently, conventional cytogenetic analysis remains an important part of the diagnostic work up for atypical MPD, along with histopathological and molecular analysis. Cytogenetics often serves as a critical pointer towards the presence of a particular fusion gene which can then be specifically tested for by RT-PCR and other techniques.

In all cases known to date, fusion genes encode proteins in which the N-terminal region of a partner gene is fused in-frame to the C-terminal region of the kinase, including the catalytic domain. The partner gene provides a promoter to drive transcription of the fusion in hemopoietic progenitor cells and, in nearly all cases, an oligomerization domain that is essential for kinase activation. In contrast to their normal counterparts, fusion tyrosine kinases are constitutively active and no longer dependent on upstream signals to transmit proliferative, anti-apoptotic, and other signals. In model systems, fusion tyrosine kinases transform growth factor-dependent cell lines to factor independence and give rise to CML-like diseases when expressed appropriately in mice. Some point mutations in tyrosine kinases and downstream signaling components have also been identified, all of which serve to activate signaling.

PDGFRA fusion genes

PDGFRα is a class III protein tyrosine kinase encoded by *PDGFRA* at 4q12. To date, six *PDGFRA* fusion genes have been described in association with atypical MPD, the first of which was a fusion of *BCR* and *PDGFRA* seen in two patients with *BCR-ABL*-negative CML, peripheral blood eosinophilia, and a t(4;22)(q12;q11).[9] Subsequently, other patients with *BCR-PDGFRA* were reported in the setting of acute pre-B-cell acute lymphoblastic leukemia (ALL) and secondary *BCR-ABL*-negative CML after treatment for diffuse large B-cell lymphoma.[10,11] *BCR-PDGFRA* shows molecular heterogeneity, with different *BCR* exons involved. Most gene fusions are spliced to give rise to clean exon to exon chimeric mRNAs but, unusually, the *PDGFRA* breakpoints cluster within an exon (exon 12). The consequences of this are described in more detail below. Other patients with *BCR-PDGFRA* aCML have been reported, and we have also identified a patient who progressed to B-cell ALL (B-ALL), one who presented with B-ALL, and another that had T-lymphoblastic extramedullary disease. These findings strongly suggest that *BCR-PDGFRA* disease, like CML, is a stem cell disorder.[9,10]

The second partner gene to be identified was *FIP1L1*. *FIP1L1-PDGFRA* is generated by a cytogenetically cryptic 800-kb interstitial deletion on chromosome 4q12[12,13] and is currently the second most common tyrosine kinase fusion in MPD after *BCR-ABL*. Although seen in very occasional cases of atypical CML, it is almost always associated with CEL, presenting as hypereosinophilic syndrome (HES) or SM with eosinophilia. In addition, these patients typically show splenomegaly, increased serum vitamin B_{12}, and mast cell tryptase levels. Noteworthy is the extreme male preponderance in this subtype of leukemia reported in many previous studies.[14–17] In a series of 376 UK patients with persistent unexplained hypereosinophilia the *FIP1L1–PDGFRA* fusion was detectable in 40 (11%) of patients, only one of whom was female.[18] The frequency with which *FIP1L1-PDGFRA* is seen in other series has varied widely between 3 and 56%[14,15,19–21] and the principal reason for this appears to be different patient selection criteria. The fusion has been recently described in two patients after receiving combination chemotherapy for non-Hodgkin lymphoma and Langerhans cell histiocytosis, respectively.[22,23] These two cases raise the possibility of a therapy-related genetic lesion.

The use of imatinib treatment for patients with HES started before the underlying molecular target had been identified, and the clear responses of some patients paved the way for the finding of the *FIP1L1-PDGFRA* fusion. Between 2001 and 2003 a total of 24 patients with HES received imatinib with more than half achieving a complete hematological remission.[24–29] Subsequently, Cools and colleagues showed that five patients harbored the *FIP1L1-PDGFRA* fusion, all of whom responded to imatinib. However, four patients with durable responses to imatinib did not reveal *FIP1L1-PDFGRA*, indicating that an unidentified target of imatinib may be the driving force behind these cases of HES.[12] However, subsequent studies have suggested that durable responses to imatinib in *FIP1L1-PDGFRA*-negative cases are uncommon[29] which in turn suggests that novel mutations in imatinib responsive genes in HES are also very uncommon.

Other *PDGFRA* fusion partners that have been recently identified in single patients are *KIF5B*, *CDK5RAP2*, *ETV6* and *STRN*.[30–32] *KIF5B* is located at 10p11 and encodes kinesin family member 5B, a microtubule-based motor protein involved in transport organelles. The *KIF5B-PDGRA* fusion was identified in a single patient with a complex karyotype involving chromosomes 3, 4, and 10.[30] *CDK5RAP2* is located at 9q33 and encodes a protein that is believed to be involved in centrosomal regulation; fusion to *PDGFRA* resulted from insertion of part of chromosome 9 into chromosome 4.[31] *STRN* encodes striatin, a scaffolding protein that targets proteins such as the estrogen receptor to the cell membrane, facilitating the assembly of other proteins required for rapid receptor activation. *STRN-PDGFRA* and *ETV6-PDGFRA* were seen in conjunction with a t(2;4)(p24;q12) and t(4;12)(q2?3;p1?2), respectively.[32]

For five of the six fusions, the breakpoints within *PDGFRA* are located within exon 12, which, after splicing, leads to an mRNA fusion in which the partner gene is joined to a truncated *PDGFRA*. Intron-derived sequences are often incorporated into the mature RNA and the region encoding the negative regulatory WW-like domain within the PDGFRα juxtamembrane region is disrupted. Stover and colleagues showed that FIP1L1 is highly unusual in that is does not appear to have a self-dimerization motif and, more surprisingly, FIP1L1 appears to be completely dispensable for activation of PDGFRα.[33] Truncation of the PDGFRα WW-like domain appears to be sufficient to activate the kinase in the absence of an oligomerization domain provided by the partner protein.[33] It remains unclear why the WW-like domain is truncated with other fusion partners that do provide an oligomerization domain (such as BCR), and also why truncation of this domain is not usually seen for fusions involving PDGFRβ.

PDGFRB fusion genes

To date, 16 *PDGFRB* fusions have been described in the context of MPD (Figure 12.1). All are associated with visible chromosomal translocations of 5q31-33 with published partners at 1q21 (*TPM3* and *PDE4PIP*), 3p22 (*WDR48* and *GOLGA4*), 4q21 (*PRKG2*), 7q11 (*HIP1*), 10q21 (*CCDC6/H4*), 11p13 (*GPIAP1*), 12p13 (*ETV6*), 12q24 (*GIT2*), 14q24 (*NIN*), 14q32 (*KIAA1509*), 15q22 (*TP53BP1*), 16p13 (*NDE1*), 17p13 (*RABEP1*), and 17p11 (*SPECC1/HCMOGT1*).[34–45] A 17th partner gene, *TRIP11* (also known as *CEV14*) has been identified in a patient with a t(5;14)(q33;q32) appearing during progression of underlying acute myeloid leukemia (AML) as a secondary abnormality.[46]

Of these fusions, *ETV6-PDGFRB* is the most frequently described, although it is still very uncommon. Patients usually present with peripheral-blood eosinophilia, monocytosis, and splenomegaly. The phenotype of *PDGFRB*-rearranged patients with other partners is somewhat more diverse and fusions have been described in patients with aCML, CMML, CEL, MDS, PMF, AML, and CMPD-unclassified. Eosinophilia is usually present, but lack of eosinophilia does not necessarily exclude involvement of *PDGFRB*. Similarly, the finding of a translocation that targets 5q31-33 does not definitely mean that *PDGFRB* is involved, even in cases with pronounced eosinophilia.[47–49] This is an important point since only those cases with a bona fide PDGFRβ fusion are likely to be responsive to imatinib treatment.

Patients with *PDGFRB* rearrangements have a very wide age range (2–84 years) with the median age at presentation being about 40 years. As for *PDGFRA* fusions, men are affected more often than women with an approximately 8 : 1 male : female ratio. The reasons for this are unknown. The clinical course of patients with *PDGFRB* fusions is highly variable, but since the number of patients reported with different translocations is very small an accurate definition of the disease is not possible. Some cases progress to acute leukemia and the overall impression is that the median time to transformation is several years and probably similar to CML. The 2-year survival rate of 18 evaluable patients with *PDGFRB* fusions was given as only 55%,[48] but this rate was based on published case reports with limited follow-up, so this estimate may be considerably biased towards more aggressive cases.

PDGFRB genomic breakpoints are usually intronic (intron 10) and consequently encode fusion proteins that retain the WW domain, which is almost identical to the corresponding domain in PDGFRα. However, variant breakpoints have been reported that involve exon 12 for *NIN-PDGFRB*[39] and *PRKG2-PDGFRB*,[44] exon 10 for *GIT2-PDGFRB*, and exon 11 with *GPIAP1-PDGFRB* fusion.[44] *PDGFRB* exon 12 breakpoints result in a loss of the WW domain,[39,44] indicating that it is not required for constitutive activation of the PDGFRβ kinase.

FGFR1 fusion genes

The involvement of 8p11 was first described in 1984 in a patient with a t(6;8)(q27;p11) who presented with a *BCR-ABL*-negative MPD in combination with a T-cell lymphoma. Subsequently other similar cases were reported with distinct translocations but a common breakpoint at 8p11-12, leading Macdonald to postulate that they constituted a new nosological entity which he termed the '8p11 myeloproliferative syndrome (EMS)'.[50] Others noted the similarity and unusual features associated with the t(8;13)(p11;q12)[51] and the name 'stem cell leukemia-lymphoma syndrome (SCLL) also emerged. Molecular proof that EMS/SCLL is indeed a distinct syndrome came with the finding that the translocations disrupt another receptor tyrosine kinase, *FGFR1*.

To date, eight different *FGFR1* fusion partners have been described in EMS at 6q27 (*FGFR1OP1/FOP*), 7q34 (*TRIM24/TIF1*), 9q33 (*CEP110*), 12p11 (*FGFR1OP2*), 13q12 (*ZNF198;* also known as *RAMP, FIM* or *ZMYM2*), 17q11 (*MYO18A*), 19q13 (*LOC113386/HERV-K*), and 22q11 (*BCR*).[52–61] No cytogenetically invisible fusion involving *FGFR1* has so far been reported and all mRNA fusions described to date involve *FGFR1* exon 9.

The vast majority of EMS patients present with typical features of an MPD, i.e. leukocytosis, hypercellular bone marrow, and splenomegaly. Eosinophilia in the peripheral blood and/or bone marrow is usually but not always present. EMS can resemble CMML and aCML, but the distinguishing feature of this condition is the strikingly high incidence of coexisting non-Hodgkin lymphoma, which immunohistochemical investigation usually reveals to be of T-cell phenotype. Lymphadenopathy can occur either at the time of diagnosis or during the course of the disease. Such lymphadenopathy is not unique to EMS and has been described in association with other tyrosine kinase fusions, notably *FIP1L1-PDGFRA*.[62]

Clinically, EMS typically exhibits a very aggressive pattern of behavior with transformation to AML or occasionally B-ALL. The median time to transformation is only 6–9 months according to published case reports but again it is unclear to what extent these are biased towards more aggressive cases. Certainly we are aware of anecdotal patients who have been maintained for 2 years or more in chronic phase on interferon alfa or even hydroxyurea but, nevertheless, it seems clear that EMS cases should be considered for early allogeneic bone marrow transplantation[50] and currently this is the only technique that can result in long-term molecular remission.[63]

Despite the small number of cases reported in the literature, some trends indicating a correlation between the identity of the partner gene and the clinical phenotype have emerged. Patients exhibiting a t(8;22) and *BCR-FGFR1* fusion seem to show a phenotype that is more similar to classic *BCR-ABL*-positive CML than to patients with other *FGFR1* fusions, although one case that was studied in detail also showed evidence of lymphoproliferation.[64–66]

Some *BCR-FGFR1* cases also showed basophilia, a feature that is uncommon in *BCR-ABL*-negative MPD. Biphenotypic presentation of an MPD in association with a T-cell non-Hodgkin lymphoma seems to be more common in patients with a t(8;13) compared with other translocations.[50] Patients with a t(8;9) present relatively frequently with thrombocytosis and monocytosis,[50] whereas some patients with a t(6;8) were diagnosed initially as having PV.[67] Detailed mouse modeling of the *BCR-FGFR1* and *ZNF198-FGFR1* fusions demonstrated that the GRB2 binding site (Y177) was primarily responsible for the CML-like phenotype, confirming the suggestion that the partner genes may play a direct role in specifying the precise clinical phenotype.[68]

Although different partner proteins are involved in a wide range of cellular processes, it is notable that several (e.g. NIN, FGFR1OP1/FOP, CEP110, PCM1, CDK5RAP2) are components of the centrosome. The FGFR1OP1-FGFR1 fusion protein has been shown to be located almost exclusively at centrosomes and actively signals from this position. Delavel *et al.* hypothesize that the centrosome, which is linked to the microtubules, is close to the nucleus, and is connected to the Golgi apparatus and the proteasome, could serve to integrate multiple signaling pathways controlling cell division, cell migration, and cell fate. Abnormal kinase activity at the centrosome may be an efficient way to pervert cell division in malignancy.[69]

FLT3 mutations and fusion genes

The FMS-like tyrosine kinase 3 (*FLT3*) gene is located at chromosome 13q12 and plays an important role in normal hematopoiesis. Although activating internal tandem duplications (ITD) or point mutations are more common in acute leukemias, they have been described in 5% of cases with aCML[70] and 13% of patients with CMPD or CMPD/MDS.[71] Recently, two patients with *FLT3* fusion genes have been identified. *ETV6-FLT3* was found in a patient with a *BCR-ABL*-negative MPD with hypereosinophilia and at (12;13)(p13;q12),[72] and *SPTBN1-FLT3* was found in a patient with aCML as a consequence of a t(2;13)(p16;q12).[70] Both the *FLT3* ITD and *ETV6-FLT3* induce a myeloproliferative phenotype in mouse models, indicating that constitutive activation of *FLT3* may be sufficient to induce an MPD-like disorder, but insufficient to recapitulate the AML phenotype.[73,74]

JAK2 mutations and fusion genes

The first reports of the involvement of *JAK2* in human MPD were published in 1997, when the fusion of *ETV6* to *JAK2* was described in two patients with a t(9;12)(p24;p13) and childhood ALL and in one patient with a t(9;15;12)(p24;q15;p13) and a *BCR-ABL*-negative CML.[75,76] Two further *JAK2* partner genes in patients with aCML have subsequently been identified: *PCM1* in association with a t(8;9)(p21-23;p23-24) and *BCR* in association with t(9;22)(p24;q11).[77,78] Several additional cases with *PCM1-JAK2* have now been identified in the context of a diverse range of hematological malignancies including myeloid and lymphoid disorders including T-cell lymphoma.[79–81] As seen for *PDGFR* fusions, *JAK2* fusions are predominantly seen in males.

More recently, *JAK2* has emerged as a critical factor in classical MPD with the finding of the V617F mutation in more than 95% of patients with PV and roughly 50% of patients with ET and PMF.[82] In addition, V617F has been detected in a range of atypical MPD: 17–19% of *BCR-ABL*-negative CML, 3–13% of CMML, roughly one-quarter of CNL, and occasional cases with HES or SM. V617F was not detectable in any case of MPD with rare tyrosine kinase fusion genes or in any individual case with *BCR-ABL*-positive CML.[83–85] In addition, V617F has been reported in cases of MDS with a myeloproliferative component.[86–89]

It is not clear why different individuals with V617F show different phenotypes with preferential expansion of erythroid, granulocyte, megakaryocyte, monocyte, or eosinophil lineages. Accumulating evidence suggests that this difference is unlikely to be owing to the identity of the cell in which the mutation arises but rather may be caused by the constitutional genetic background of the individual or by acquired changes that may precede or be subsequent to V617F. Thus far, there are no data regarding the prognostic significance of V617F in *BCR-ABL*-negative CML or other atypical MPD.

KIT mutations

KIT is required for the growth, differentiation, and functional activation of human mast cells and activating mutations of this receptor are seen in the great majority of cases of SM, a disease that is described in detail elsewhere in this book but is also included here briefly for completeness. Most SM cases are positive for the activating mutation D816V, although the incidence in different studies is highly variable owing to patient selection, sensitivity of the molecular method, and the source of the specimen that is analyzed. However, if sensitive methods are used, especially in combination with purification or enrichment of mast cells, then more that 80% of cases are D816V positive. Of the remaining cases, other mutations have been described that affect the same amino acid (D816Y, D816F, D816H) plus a range of other rare changes (D820G, V560G, F522C, E839K, V530I, K509I).[90] In addition to SM, KIT mutations play a pathogenetic role in a variety of other malignancies, including AML and gastrointestinal stromal tumors (GIST).[91] Whereas mutations located in the juxtamembrane or extracellular domains of KIT are sensitive to imatinib, the kinase loop mutation D816V is highly resistant. However, *in vitro* data with several compounds including PKC412, dasatinib, and nilotinib show some promising results.[92–95] and clinical trials with these compounds are underway.

RAS, *PTPN11*, and *NF1* mutations

In addition to activation of tyrosine kinases, mutations affecting downstream signaling components have been identified in some MPD. RAS proteins are small GTPases that play a critical role in transducing signals from upstream receptors, including tyrosine kinases. Activating *RAS* mutations are widespread in malignancy and within the MPD approximately 50% of aCML/CMML cases were found to harbor activating *NRAS* or *KRAS* mutations.[96,97] However, these studies used sensitive allele-specific hybridization methods and it is possible that many changes were only present in minor subclones. A more recent analysis using less sensitive methods found only 13% of patients with *BCR-ABL*-negative CML to have activating *RAS* mutations, all of which were in *NRAS*.[83] Activating kinase mutations, kinase fusion genes, and *NRAS* mutations are almost always mutually exclusive, presumably because they are functionally redundant. In one study, the presence of a *RAS* mutation was not found to be of prognostic value.[7]

Activation of the RAS pathway is particularly prominent in JMML. *NRAS* and *KRAS* mutations are seen in about 20% of cases[98] and some of these mutations appear to be associated with disease that improves spontaneously over time.[99] RAS may also be activated indirectly by gain of function mutations *PTPN11* or biallelic loss of function mutations of *NF1*, with these abnormalities being seen in roughly one-third and one-quarter of JMML cases, respectively.[100,101] *RAS*, *NF1*, and *PTPN11* mutations are almost always mutually exclusive, suggesting that mutations in these genes have the same functional consequences. Other abnormalities are seen in a small proportion of JMML cases, including V617F[102] plus some of the tyrosine kinase fusions detailed above.

The association between JMML and *NF1* was initially suspected because some children with neurofibromatosis type 1, a disease caused by inherited *NF1* mutations, also developed JMML. *NF1* is a large gene which has not been screened comprehensively in adult atypical MPD; however, the apparent lack of association between neurofibromatosis and adult MPD suggests that *NF1* mutations may not play an important role in these diseases. We have not detected *PTPN11* mutations in *BCR-ABL*-negative CML and also failed to find abnormalities in a number of other genes including *BRAF* and several tyrosine kinases[83] plus more recently *MPL515* or *JAK2* exon 12 (unpublished data).

CLINICAL IMPLICATIONS OF MOLECULAR ABNORMALITIES

For most patients with *BCR-ABL*-negative CML, hydroxyurea remains the basic treatment to control elevated leukocyte counts. The great majority of patients are too old to consider stem cell transplantation but some achieve durable complete hematological remission and occasionally cytogenetic remission with interferon alfa.[103] However, the finding of deregulated tyrosine kinases opened up the possibility of targeted signal transduction therapy following the paradigm of imatinib in CML.

Patients with rearrangements of *PDGRA* or *PDGFRB* show excellent responses to treatment with imatinib achieving a high rate of durable hematological and cytogenetic responses.[12,30,31,39,40,49] Recently published data indicate that the majority of patients exhibiting a *FIP1L1-PDGFRA* fusion gene reached a molecular remission under treatment with imatinib, including patients receiving low-dose imatinib (100 or 200 mg/day).[18,29] Treatment with imatinib as monotherapy or as maintenance after intensive chemotherapy was also highly effective in *FIP1L1-PDGFRA*-positive secondary AML with seven of seven patients disease-free and in complete hematological and complete molecular remission after a median time of 20 months on imatinib.[62] Overall, these striking results suggest that imatinib should be the treatment of choice for all patients with *PDGFRA* or *PDGFRB* fusion genes.

Similar to resistance occurring in patients treated with imatinib in chronic phase CML, an acquired point mutation of the FIP1L1-PDGFRA fusion protein has been described.[12,104] This T674I mutation is located in an analogous position to the T315I mutation that leads to resistance to imatinib in the setting of CML.[47] Sorafenib is a potent inhibitor of B-RAF and VEGFR, and was also shown to inhibit FLT3, KIT, and PDGFR. This compound, which was recently approved for the treatment of metastatic renal cell carcinoma, has been shown to be a potent inhibitor of *FIP1L1-PDGFRA* and its imatinib-resistant T674I mutation.[105] In addition, it has been shown that PKC412 and nilotinib are able to inhibit effectively the T674I mutant *in vivo* and *in vitro*, respectively.[106,107]

Imatinib is not active against JAK2 or FGFR1, and thus alternative compounds are needed to target diseases driven by abnormalities in these kinases. PKC412 inhibits *ZNF198-FGFR1* kinase activity *in vitro* and induced a partial response in a patient with this fusion and

Table 12.1 Conventional and molecular classification of atypical myeloproliferative disorders (MPD)

	Usually associated with	*Abnormalities*
Molecularly defined entities		
PDGFRA-rearranged MPD	CEL, SM-eo	>95% *FIP1L1-PDGFRA*; 5 other *PDGFRA* fusions
PDGFRB-rearranged MPD	CEL, aCML, CMML	50% *ETV6-PDGFRB*; 15 other *PDGFRB* fusions
8p11 myeloproliferative syndrome	aCML, CMML, CEL (+T-NHL)	8 *FGFR1* fusions
JAK2-rearranged MPD	aCML, CEL, AML, other	>90% *PCM1-JAK2*; 2 other *JAK2* fusions
SM		>80% *KIT* D816V; 5% other *KIT* mutations
Partially molecularly defined entities		
JMML, CNL, aCML, CMML, unclassified MPD		30% *PTPN11* mutations; 20% *RAS* mutations; 20% *NF1* mutations
		5–50% V617F *JAK2*; 5% *FLT3* ITD; 10% *RAS*
Molecularly undefined entities		
Includes the majority of cases of CEL, CNL, CMML, aCML, CNL, and unclassified MPD or MDS/MPD that are negative for the abnormalities above, plus a small proportion of cases of JMML and SM		

CEL, chronic eosinophilic leukemia; SM-eo, systemic mastocytosis associated with eosinophilia; aCML, atypical chronic myeloid leukemia; CMML, chronic myelomonocytic leukemia; NHL, non-Hodgkin lymphoma; AML, acute myeloid leukemia; JMML, juvenile myelomonocytic leukemia; CNL, chronic neutrophilic leukemia; MDS, myelodysplastic syndrome.

advanced phase disease;[108] however, thus far we are unaware of any patient who has achieved a good cytogenetic response to PKC412. Other small molecule inhibitors are in development that may ultimately prove to be more effective.[109]

The results of trials with second generation tyrosine kinase inhibitors, including dasatinib (BMS354825) and nilotinib (AMN107), show that these molecules are active against a number of different imatinib-resistant ABL kinase domain mutations seen in *BCR-ABL*-positive CML.[110,111] In addition, these compounds are active against fusions involving PDGFRα and PDGFRβ in cell lines and mice (but not JAK2 or FGFR1), but treatment of *PDGFR*-rearranged patients has not yet been described.[112]

Overall, constitutive activation of tyrosine kinase signaling is confirmed as the pathogenetic hallmark of *BCR-ABL*-negative CML. Currently, the molecular basis is understood, at least partially, for about one-third of cases and ongoing research is focused on elucidating the pathogenesis of the remaining cases. An increasing molecular knowledge of disease subsets and intimate association of particular abnormalities with specific therapies is a strong driver towards a new, molecular based classification of atypical MPD and an indication of how this might currently look is shown on Table 12.1. Currently, effective targeted therapy is possible for only a small proportion of cases; however, several candidate molecules are in development that are likely to be of wider benefit.

REFERENCES

1. Dameshek W. Some speculations on the myeloproliferative syndromes. Blood 1951; 6: 372–5.
2. Shtivelman E, Lifshitz B, Gale RP et al. Fused transcript of abl and bcr genes in chronic myelogenous leukaemia. Nature 1985; 315: 550–4.
3. Stam K, Heisterkamp N, Grosveld G et al. Evidence of a new chimeric bcr/c-abl mRNA in patients with chronic myelocytic leukemia and the Philadelphia chromosome. N Engl J Med 1985; 313: 1429–33.
4. Lugo TG, Pendergast AM, Muller AJ et al. Tyrosine kinase activity and transformation potency of bcr-abl oncogene products. Science 1990; 247: 1079–82.
5. Chase A, Huntly BJ, Cross NCP. Cytogenetics of chronic myeloid leukaemia. Best Pract Res Clin Haematol 2001; 14: 443–71.
6. Vardiman JW, Harris NL, Brunning RD. The World Health Organization (WHO) classification of the myeloid neoplasms. Blood 2002; 100: 2292–302.
7. Onida F, Ball G, Kantarjian HM et al. Characteristics and outcome of patients with Philadelphia chromosome negative, bcr/abl negative chronic myelogenous leukemia. Cancer 2002; 95: 1673–84.
8. Druker BJ, Guilhot F, O'Brien SG et al. Five-year follow-up of patients receiving imatinib for chronic myeloid leukemia. N Engl J Med 2006; 355: 2408–17.
9. Baxter EJ, Hochhaus A, Bolufer P et al. The t(4; 22) (q12; q11) in atypical chronic myeloid leukaemia fuses BCR to PDGFRA. Hum Mol Genet 2002; 11: 1391–7.
10. Trempat P, Villalva C, Laurent G et al. Chronic myeloproliferative disorders with rearrangement of the platelet-derived growth factor alpha receptor: a new clinical target for STI571/Glivec. Oncogene 2003; 22: 5702–6.
11. Safely AM, Sebastian S, Collins TS et al. Molecular and cytogenetic characterization of a novel translocation t(4; 22) involving the breakpoint cluster region and platelet-derived growth factor receptor-alpha genes in a patient with atypical chronic myeloid leukaemia. Genes Chromosomes Cancer 2004; 40: 44–50.
12. Cools J, DeAngelo DJ, Gotlib J et al. A tyrosine kinase created by fusion of the PDGFRA and FIP1L1 genes as a therapeutic target of imatinib in idiopathic hypereosinophilic hyndrome. N Engl J Med 2003; 348: 1201–14.
13. Griffin JH, Leung J, Bruner RJ et al. Discovery of a fusion kinase in EOL-1 cells and idiopathic hypereosinophilic syndrome. Proc Natl Acad Sci U S A 2003; 100: 7830–5.
14. Pardanani A, Ketterling RP, Li CY et al. FIP1L1-PDGFRA in eosinophilic disorders: prevalence in routine clinical practice, long-term experience with imatinib therapy, and a critical review of the literature. Leuk Res 2006; 30: 965–70.
15. Pardanani A, Brockman SR, Paternoster SF et al. FIP1L1-PDGFRA fusion: prevalence and clinicopathologic correlates in 89 consecutive patients with moderate to severe eosinophilia. Blood 2004; 104: 3038–45.
16. Klion AD, Noel P, Akin C et al. Elevated serum tryptase levels identify a subset of patients with a myeloproliferative variant of idiopathic hypereosinophilic syndrome associated with tissue fibrosis, poor prognosis, and imatinib responsiveness. Blood 2003; 101: 4660–6.
17. Klion AD, Robyn J, Akin C et al. Molecular remission and reversal of myelofibrosis in response to imatinib mesylate treatment in patients with the

myeloproliferative variant of hypereosinophilic syndrome. Blood 2004; 103: 473–8.

18. Jovanovic JV, Score J, Waghorn K et al. Low-dose imatinib mesylate leads to rapid induction of major molecular responses and achievement of complete molecular remission in FIP1L1-PDGFRA positive chronic eosinophilic leukaemia. Blood 2007; 109: 4635–40.
19. Vandenberghe P, Wlodarska I, Michaux L et al. Clinical and molecular features of FIP1L1-PDGFRA (+) chronic eosinophilic leukemias. Leukemia 2004; 18: 734–42.
20. Roche-Lestienne C, Lepers S, Soenen-Cornu V et al. Molecular characterization of the idiopathic hypereosinophilic syndrome (HES) in 35 French patients with normal conventional cytogenetics. Leukemia 2005; 19: 792–8.
21. Bacher U, Reiter A, Haferlach T et al. A combination of cytomorphology, cytogenetic analysis, fluorescence in situ hybridization and reverse transcriptase polymerase chain reaction for establishing clonality in cases of persisting hypereosinophilia. Haematologica 2006; 91: 817–20.
22. Tanaka Y, Kurata M, Togami K et al. Chronic eosinophilic leukemia with the FIP1L1-PDGFRalpha fusion gene in a patient with a history of combination chemotherapy. Int J Hematol 2006; 83: 152–5.
23. Ohnishi J, Kandabashi K, Maeda Y et al. Chronic eosinophilic leukaemia with FIP1L1-PDGFRA fusion and T674I mutation that evolved from Langerhans cell histiocytosis with eosinophilia after chemotherapy. Br J Haematol 2006; 134: 547–9.
24. Pardanani A, Reeder T, Porrata L et al. Imatinib therapy for hypereosinophilic syndrome and eosinophilic disorders. Blood 2003; 101: 3391–7.
25. Schaller JL, Burkland GA. Case report: rapid and complete control of idiopathic hypereosinophilia with imatinib mesylate. Med Gen Med 2001; 3: 9.
26. Gleich GJ, Leiferman KM, Pardanani A et al. Treatment of hypereosinophilic syndrome with imatinib mesylate. Lancet 2002; 359: 1577–8.
27. Ault P, Cortes J, Koller C et al. Response of idiopathic hypereosinophilic syndrome to treatment with imatinib mesylate. Leuk Res 2002; 26: 881–4.
28. Cortes J, Ault P, Koller C et al. Efficacy of imatinib mesylate in the treatment of idiopathic hypereosinophilic syndrome. Blood 2003; 101: 4714–16.
29. Baccarani M, Cilloni D, Rondoni M et al. Imatinib mesylate induces complete and durable responses in all patients with the FIP1L1-PDGFRα positive hypereosinophilic syndrome. Results of a multicenter study. Haematologica 2007; 92: 1173–9.
30. Score J, Curtis C, Waghorn K et al. Identification of a novel imatinib responsive KIF5B-PDGFRA fusion gene following screening for PDFGRA overexpression in patients with hypereosinophilia. Leukemia 2006; 20: 827–32.
31. Walz C, Curtis C, Schnittger S et al. Transient response to imatinib in a chronic eosinophilic leukemia associated with ins(9;4)(q33;q12q25) and a CDK5RAP-PDGFRA fusion gene. Genes Chromosomes Cancer 2006; 45: 950–6.
32. Curtis CE, Grand FH, Musto P et al. Two novel imatinib-responsive PDGFRA fusion genes in chronic eosinophilic leukaemia. Br J Haematol 2007; 138: 77–81.
33. Stover EH, Chen J, Folens C et al. Activation of FIP1L1-PDGFRα requires disruption of the juxtamembrane domain of PDGFRα and is FIP1L1-independent. Proc Natl Acad Sci U S A 2006; 103: 8078–83.
34. Rosati R, La Starza R, Bardi A et al. PDGFRB fuses to TPM3 in the t(1;5)(q23;q33) of chronic eosinophilic leukemia and to NDE1 in the t(5;16)(q33;p13) of chronic myelomonocytic leukemia. Haematologica 2006; 91(Suppl 1): 214.
35. Wilkinson K, Velloso ER, Lopes LF et al. Cloning of the t(1;5)(q23;q33) in a myeloproliferative disorder associated with eosinophilia: involvement of PDGFRB and response to imatinib. Blood 2003; 102: 4187–90.
36. Ross TS, Bernard OA, Berger R et al. Fusion of Huntingtin interacting protein 1 to platelet-derived growth factor beta receptor (PDGFbetaR) in chronic myelomonocytic leukemia with t(5;7)(q33;q11.2). Blood 1998; 91: 4419–26.
37. Kulkarni S, Heath C, Parker S et al. Fusion of H4/D10S170 to the platelet-derived growth factor receptor beta in BCR-ABL-negative myeloproliferative disorders with a t(5;10)(q33;q21). Cancer Res 2000; 60: 3592–8.
38. Golub TR, Barker GF, Lovett M et al. Fusion of PDGF receptor beta to a novel ets-like gene, tel, in chronic myelomonocytic leukemia with t(5;12) chromosomal translocation. Cell 1994; 77: 307–16.
39. Vizmanos JL, Novo FJ, Roman JP et al. NIN, a gene encoding a CEP110-like centrosomal protein, is fused to PDGFRB in a patient with a t(5;14)(q33;q24) and an imatinib-responsive myeloproliferative disorder. Cancer Res 2004; 64: 2673–6.
40. Levine RL, Wadleigh M, Sternberg DW et al. KIAA1509 is a novel PDGFRB fusion partner in imatinib-responsive myeloproliferative disease associated with a t(5;14)(q33;q32). Leukemia 2005; 19: 27–30.
41. Grand FH, Burgstaller S, Kuhr T et al. p53-Binding protein 1 is fused to the platelet-derived growth factor receptor beta in a patient with a t(5;15)(q33;q22) and an imatinib-responsive eosinophilic myeloproliferative disorder. Cancer Res 2004; 64: 7216–19.
42. Magnusson MK, Meade KE, Brown KE et al. Rabaptin-5 is a novel fusion partner to platelet-derived growth factor beta receptor in chronic myelomonocytic leukemia. Blood 2001; 98: 2518–25.

43. Morerio C, Acquila M, Rosanda C et al. HCMOGT-1 is a novel fusion partner to PDGFRB in juvenile myelomonocytic leukemia with t(5;17)(q33;p11.2). Cancer Res 2004; 64: 2649–51.
44. Walz C, Metzgeroth G, Haferlach C et al. Characterization of three new imatinib-responsive fusion genes in chronic myeloproliferative disorders generated by disruption of the platelet-derived growth factor receptor β gene. Haematologica 2007; 92: 163–9.
45. Curtis C, Apperley JF, Dang R et al. The platelet-derived growth factor receptor beta fuses to two distinct loci at 3p21 in imatinib responsive chronic eosinophilic leukemia. Blood 2005; 109: 61–4.
46. Abe A, Emi N, Tanimoto M et al. Fusion of the platelet-derived growth factor receptor beta to a novel gene CEV14 in acute myelogenous leukemia after clonal evolution. Blood 1997; 90: 4271–7.
47. Gotlib J. Molecular classification and pathogenesis of eosinophilic disorders: 2005 update. Acta Haematol 2005; 114: 7–25.
48. Steer EJ, Cross NCP. Myeloproliferative disorders with translocations of chromosome 5q31-33: role of the platelet-derived growth factor receptor β. Acta Haematol 2002; 107: 113–22.
49. David M, Cross NCP, Burgstaller S et al. Durable response to imatinib in patients with PDGFRB fusion gene-positive and BCR-ABL-negative chronic myeloproliferative disorders. Blood 2007; 109: 61–4.
50. Macdonald D, Reiter A, Cross NCP. The 8p11 myeloproliferative syndrome: a distinct clinical entity caused by constitutive activation of FGFR1 [review]. Acta Haematol 2002; 107: 101–7.
51. Inhorn RC, Aster JC, Roach SA et al. A syndrome of lymphoblastic lymphoma, eosinophilia, and myeloid hyperplasia/malignancy associated with t(8;13)(p11;q11): description of a distinctive clinicopathologic entity. Blood 1995; 85: 1881–7.
52. Belloni E, Trubia M, Gasparini P et al. 8p11 myeloproliferative syndrome with a novel t(7;8) translocation leading to fusion of the FGFR1 and TIF1 genes. Genes Chromosomes Cancer 2005; 42: 320–5.
53. Guasch G, Mack GJ, Popovici C et al. FGFR1 is fused to the centrosome-associated protein CEP110 in the 8p12 stem cell myeloproliferative disorder with t(8;9)(p12;q33). Blood 2000; 95: 1788–96.
54. Grand EK, Grand FH, Chase AJ et al. Identification of a novel gene, FGFR1OP2, fused to FGFR1 in the 8p11 myeloproliferative syndrome. Genes Chromosomes Cancer 2003; 40: 78–83.
55. Xiao S, Nalabolu SR, Aster JC et al. FGFR1 is fused with a novel zinc-finger gene, ZNF198, in the t(8;13) leukaemia/lymphoma syndrome. Nat Genet 1998; 18: 84–7.
56. Smedley D, Hamoudi R, Clark J et al. The t(8;13)(p11;q11-12) rearrangement associated with an atypical myeloproliferative disorder fuses the fibroblast growth factor receptor 1 gene to a novel gene RAMP. Hum Mol Genet 1998; 7: 637–42.
57. Popovici C, Adelaide J, Ollendorff V et al. Fibroblast growth factor receptor 1 is fused to FIM in stem-cell myeloproliferative disorder with t(8;13). Proc Natl Acad Sci U S A 1998; 95: 5712–17.
58. Reiter A, Sohal J, Kulkarni S et al. Consistent fusion of ZNF198 to the fibroblast growth factor receptor-1 in the t(8;13)(p11;q12) myeloproliferative syndrome. Blood 1998; 92: 1735–42.
59. Walz C, Chase A, Schoch C et al. The t(8;17)(p11;q23) in the 8p11 myeloproliferative syndrome fuses MYO18A to FGFR1. Leukemia 2005; 19: 1005–9.
60. Guasch G, Popovici C, Mugneret F et al. Endogenous retroviral sequence is fused to FGFR1 kinase in the 8p12 stem-cell myeloproliferative disorder with t(8;19)(p12;q13.3). Blood 2003; 101: 286–8.
61. Fioretos T, Panagopoulos I, Lassen C et al. Fusion of the BCR and the fibroblast growth factor receptor-1 (FGFR1) genes as a result of t(8; 22)(p11; q11) in a myeloproliferative disorder: the first fusion gene involving BCR but not ABL. Genes Chromosomes Cancer 2001; 32: 302–10.
62. Metzgeroth G, Walz C, Score J et al. Recurrent finding of the FIP1L1-PDGFRA fusion gene in eosinophilia-associated acute myeloid leukemia and lymphoblastic T-cell lymphoma. Leukemia 2007; 21: 1183–8.
63. Suzan F, Guasch G, Terre C et al. Long-term complete haematological and molecular remission after allogeneic bone marrow transplantation in a patient with a stem cell myeloproliferative disorder associated with t(8;13)(p12;q12). Br J Haematol 2003; 121: 312–14.
64. Demiroglu A, Steer EJ, Heath C et al. The t(8;22) in chronic myeloid leukemia fuses BCR to FGFR1: transforming activity and specific inhibition of FGFR1 fusion proteins. Blood 2001; 98: 3778–83.
65. Fioretos T, Panagopoulos I, Lassen C et al. Fusion of the BCR and the fibroblast growth factor receptor-1 (FGFR1) genes as a result of t(8; 22)(p11; q11) in a myeloproliferative disorder: the first fusion gene involving BCR but not ABL. Genes Chromosomes Cancer 2001; 32: 302–10.
66. Murati A, Arnoulet C, Lafage-Pochitaloff M et al. Dual lympho-myeloproliferative disorder in a patient with t(8;22) with BCR-FGFR1 gene fusion. Int J Oncol 2005; 26: 1485–92.
67. Vizmanos JL, Hernandez R, Vidal MJ et al. Clinical variability of patients with the t(6;8)(q27;p12) and FGFR1OP-FGFR1 fusion: two further cases. Hematol J 2004; 5: 534–7.
68. Roumiantsev S, Krause DS, Neumann CA et al. Distinct stem cell myeloproliferative/T-lymphoma syndromes induced by ZNF198-FGFR1 and BCR-FGFR1 fusion genes from 8p11 transolcations. Cancer Cell 2004; 5: 287–98.

69. Delaval B, Letard S, Lelievre H et al. Oncogenic tyrosine kinase of malignant hemopathy targets the centrosome. Cancer Res 2005; 65: 7231–40.
70. Grand FH, Iqbal S, Zhang L et al. A constitutively active SPTBNI-FLT3 fusion in atypical chronic myeloid leukemia is sensitive to tyrosine kinase inhibitors and immunotherapy. Exp Hematol 2007; 35: 1723–7.
71. Lin P, Jones D, Medeiros LJ et al. Activating FLT3 mutations are detectable in chronic and blast phase of chronic myeloproliferative disorders other than chronic myeloid leukaemia. Am J Clin Pathol 2006; 126: 530–3.
72. Vu HA, Xinh PT, Masuda M et al. FLT3 is fused to ETV6 in a myeloproliferative disorder with hypereosinophilia and a t(12;13)(p13;q12) translocation. Leukemia 2006; 20: 1414–21.
73. Kelly LM, Liu Q, Kutok JL et al. FLT3 internal tandem duplication mutations associated with human acute myeloid leukemias incuce myeloproliferative disease in a murine bone marrow transplant model. Blood 2002; 99: 310–18.
74. Baldwin BR, Li L, Tse KF et al. Transgenic mice expressing Tel-FLT3, a constitutively activated form of FLT3, develop myeloproliferative diasease. Leukemia 2007; 21: 764–71.
75. Lacronique V, Boureux A, Valle VD et al. A TEL-JAK2 fusion protein with constitutive kinase activity in human leukemia. Science 1997; 278: 1309–12.
76. Peeters P, Raynaud SD, Cools J et al. Fusion of TEL, the ETS-variant gene 6 (ETV6), to the receptor-associated kinase JAK2 as a result of t(9;12) in a lymphoid and t(9;15;12) in a myeloid leukemia. Blood 1997; 90: 2535–40.
77. Reiter A, Walz C, Watmore A et al. The t(8;9)(p22;p24) is a recurrent abnormality in chronic and acute leukemia that fuses PCM1 to JAK2. Cancer Res 2005; 65: 2662–7.
78. Griesinger F, Hennig H, Hillmer F et al. A BCR-JAK2 fusion gene as the result of a t(9;22)(p24;q11.2) translocation in a patient with a clinically typical chronic myeloid leukemia. Genes Chromosomes Cancer 2005; 44: 329–33.
79. Adelaide J, Perot C, Gelsi-Boyer V et al. A t(8;9) translocation with PCM1-JAK2 fusion in a patient with T-cell lymphoma. Leukemia 2006; 20: 536–7.
80. Bousquet M, Quelen C, De Mas V et al. The t(8;9)(p22;p24) translocation in atypical chronic myeloid leukemia yields a new PCM1-JAK2 fusion gene. Oncogene 2005; 24: 7248–52.
81. Murati A, Gelsi-Boyer V, Adelaide J et al. PCM1-JAK2 fusion in myeloproliferative disorders and acute erythroid leukemia with t(8;9) translocation. Leukemia 2005; 19: 1692–6.
82. Delhommeau F, Pisani DF, James C et al. Oncogenic mechanisms in myeloproliferative disorders. Cell Mol Life Sci 2006; 63: 2939–53.
83. Jones AV, Kreil S, Zoi K et al. Widespread occurrence of the JAK2 V617F mutation in chronic myeloproliferative disorders. Blood 2005; 106: 2162–8.
84. Jelinek J, Oki Y, Gharibyan V et al. JAK2 mutation 1849G > T is rare in acute leukemias but can be found in CMML, Philadelphia-chromosome negative CML and megakaryocytic leukemia. Blood 2005; 106: 3370–3.
85. Steensma DP, Dewald GW, Lasho TL et al. The JAK2 V617F activating tyrosine kinase mutation is an infrequent event in both "atypical" myeloproliferative disorders and the myelodysplastic syndrome. Blood 2005; 106: 1207–9.
86. Ohyashiki K, Aota Y, Akahane D et al. The JAK2 V617F tyrosine kinase mutation in myelodysplastic syndromes (MDS) developing myelofibrosis indicates the myeloproliferative nature in a subset of MDS patients. Leukemia 2005; 19: 2359–60.
87. Ingram W, Lea NC, Cervera J et al. The JAK2 V617F mutation identifies a subgroup of MDS patients with isolated deletion 5q and a proliferative bone marrow. Leukemia 2006; 20: 1319–21.
88. Szpurka H, Tiu R, Murugesan G et al. Refractory anemia with ringed sideroblasts associated with marked thrombocytosis (RARS-T), another myeloproliferative condition characterized by JAK2 V617F mutation. Blood 2006; 108: 2173–81.
89. Gattermann N, Billiet J, Kronenwett R et al. High frequency of the JAK2 V617F mutation in patients with thrombocytosis (platelet count > 600 × 109/L) and ringed sideroblasts more than 15% considered as MDS/MPD, unclassifiable. Blood 2007; 109: 1334–5.
90. Pardanani A, Akin C, Valent P. Pathogenesis, clinical features, and treatment advances in mastocytosis. Best Pract Res Clin Haematol 2006; 19: 595–615.
91. Heinrich MC, Blanke CD, Druker BJ et al. Inhibition of KIT tyrosine kinase activity: a novel approach to the treatment of KIT-positive malignancies. J Clin Oncol 2002; 20: 1692–703.
92. Siddiqui MA, Scott LJ. Imatinib: a review of its use in the management of gastrointestinal stromal tumours. Drugs 2007; 67: 805–20.
93. Growney JD, Clark JJ, Adelsperger J et al. Activation mutations of human c-KIT resistant to imatinib mesylate are sensitive to the tyrosine kinase inhibitor PKC412. Blood 2005; 106: 721–4.
94. Schittenhelm MM, Shiraga S, Schroeder A et al. Dasatinib (BMS-354825), a dual SRC/ABL kinase inhibitor, inhibits the kinase activity of wild-type, juxtamembrane, and activation loop mutant KIT isoforms associated with human malignancies. Cancer Res 2006; 66: 473–81.
95. von Bubnoff N, Gorontla SH, Kancha RK et al. The systemic mastocytosis-specific activating cKit mutation D816V can be inhibited by the tyrosine

kinase inhibitor AMN107. Leukemia 2005; 19: 1670–1.

96. Cogswell PC, Morgan R, Dunn M et al. Mutations of the ras protooncogenes in chronic myelogenous leukemia: a high frequency of ras mutations in bcr/abl rearrangement-negative chronic myelogenous leukemia. Blood 1989; 74: 2629–33.
97. Hirsch-Ginsberg C, LeMaistre AC, Kantarjian H et al. RAS mutations are rare events in Philadelphia chromosome-negative/bcr gene rearrangement-negative chronic myelogenous leukemia, but are prevalent in chronic myelomonocytic leukemia. Blood 1990; 76: 1214–19.
98. Flotho C, Valcamonica S, Mach-Pascual S et al. RAS mutations and clonality analysis in children with juvenile myelomonocytic leukemia (JMML). Leukemia 1999; 13: 32–7.
99. Matsuda K, Shimada A, Yoshida N et al. Spontaneous improvement of hematologic abnormalities in patients having juvenile myelomonocytic leukemia with specific RAS mutations. Blood 2007; 111: 966–7.
100. Tartaglia M, Niemeyer CM, Fragale A et al. Somatic mutations in PTPN11 in juvenile myelomonocytic leukemia, myelodysplastic syndromes and acute myeloid leukemia. Nat Genet 2003; 34: 148–50.
101. Side LE, Emanuel PD, Taylor B et al. Mutations of the NF1 gene in children with juvenile myelomonocytic leukemia without clinical evidence of neurofibromatosis, type 1. Blood 1998; 92: 267–72.
102. Tono C, Xu G, Toki T et al. JAK2 Val617Phe activating tyrosine kinase mutation in juvenile myelomonocytic leukemia. Leukemia 2005; 19: 1843–4.
103. Kurzrock R, Bueso-Ramos CE, Kantarjian H et al. BCR rearrangement-negative chronic myelogenous leukemia revisited. J Clin Oncol 2001; 19: 2915–26.
104. von Bubnoff N, Sandherr M, Schlimok G et al. Myeloid blast crisis evolving during imatinib treatment of an FIP1L1-PDGFR alpha-positive chronic myeloproliferative disease with prominent eosinophilia. Leukemia 2005; 19: 286–7.
105. Lierman E, Folens C, Stover EH et al. Sorafenib (BAY43–9006) is a potent inhibitor of FIP1L1-PDGFRα and the imatinib resistant FIP1L1-PDGFRα T674I mutant. Blood 2006; 108: 1374–6.
106. Cools J, Stover EH, Boulton CL et al. PKC412 overcomes resistance to imatinib in a murine model of an FIP1L1-PDGFR alpha-positive chronic myeloproliferative disease. Cancer Cell 2003; 3: 459–69.
107. von Bubnoff N, Gorantla SP, Thone S et al. The FIP1L1-PDGFRA T674I mutation can be inhibited by the tyrosine kinase inhibitor AMN107 (nilotinib). Blood 2006; 107: 4970–1.
108. Chen J, DeAngelo DJ, Kutok JL et al. PKC412 inhibits the zinc finger 198-fibroblast growth factor receptor 1 fusion tyrosine kinase and is active in treatment of stem cell myeloproliferative disorder. Proc Natl Acad Sci U S A 2004; 101: 14479–84.
109. Chase A, Grand FH, Cross NC. Activity of TKI258 against primary cells and cell lines with FGFR1 fusion genes associated with the 8p11 myeloproliferative syndrome. Blood 2007; 110: 3729–34.
110. Talpaz M, Shah NP, Kantarjian H et al. Dasatinib in imatinib-resistant Philadelphia-chromosome-positive leukemias. N Engl J Med 2006; 354: 2531–41.
111. Kantarjian H, Giles F, Wunderle L et al. Nilotinib in imatinib-resistant CML and Philadelphia chromosome-positive ALL. N Engl J Med 2006; 354: 2542–51.
112. Stover EH, Chen J, Lee BH et al. The small molecule tyrosine kinase inhibitor AMN107 inhibits TEL-PDGFRbeta and FIP1L1-PDGFRalpha in vitro and in vivo. Blood 2005; 106: 3206–13.

Systemic mastocytosis

13

Animesh Pardanani, Ayalew Tefferi

INTRODUCTION

Mast cells originate from CD34+/c-KIT+/CD13+ pluripotent hematopoietic cells in the bone marrow and are released into the circulation in the immature state before they undergo terminal maturation/differentiation in different tissues.[1–4] The interaction between the cytokine stem cell factor (SCF) and its cognate receptor, c-KIT (KIT) plays a key role in regulating mast cell growth and differentiation. c-*KIT* is the cellular homolog of the v-*KIT* oncogene of the Hardy-Zuckerman 4 feline sarcoma virus (HZ4-FeSV),[5] and encodes for KIT, which belongs to the type III subfamily of receptor tyrosine kinases (RTK). KIT is expressed on hematopoietic progenitors and is downregulated upon their differentiation into mature cells of all lineages, except mast cells, which retain high levels of cell surface KIT expression.[6] Soluble SCF exists as a homodimer in plasma and can crosslink two KIT receptors on the cell surface, thereby leading to activation of KIT, as well as downstream signal transduction.[7]

Mast cells are ubiquitous, but are most numerous at anatomic sites that are in contact with the environment, such as in the mucosa of airways and gut, as well as in the skin. Although mast cells have long been identified as key cellular mediators of the allergic inflammatory response,[8–12] they have other physiological functions, including a role in innate immunity.[13–16] Mast cells mediate 'early-phase' (e.g. anaphylaxis, acute asthma) and 'late-phase' allergic responses, as well as non-type I hypersensitivity reactions through release of mediators (*vide infra*).[17] Furthermore, mast cells mediate upregulation of Th2-responses and allergen-specific IgE biosynthesis, which contribute to host defenses against parasitic infections.[18,19]

Mast cells undergo activation, classically following cross-linking of FcεRI-bound IgE by multivalent allergen in sensitized individuals. Non-IgE triggers for mast cell mediator release include anaphylatoxins of the complement system (C3a and C5a), neuropeptides (e.g. vasoactive intestinal peptide, somatostatin, substance P), lipopolysaccharides (LPS), chemokines (e.g. CCL3/MIP1α), and Toll-like receptors (TLR).[13,14,16] Upon activation by either IgE-dependent or -independent mechanisms, the following mediators are released: (1) vasoactive amines, particularly histamine; (2) several distinct tryptases (α, β, and δ) that comprise the principal protein component of mast cells; (3) anionic proteoglycans (e.g. heparin, chondroitin sulphate) that confer metachromasia upon staining with toluidine blue; (4) various lipid mediators, these arachidonic acid-derived eicosanoids, which include leukotriene C_4, leukotriene B_4, and prostaglandin D_2, mediate vasodilation, vasopermeability, smooth muscle constriction, mucus secretion, as well as other proinflammatory processes; (5) other proteases (e.g. chymase, carboxypeptidase A); and (6) specific cytokines.[9,20–30] The latter recruit and activate specific cells, including basophils (IL-3), eosinophils (IL-5), neutrophils (tumor necrosis factor (TNF)-α/IL-8), and lymphocytes (IL-4/IL-13).

MASTOCYTOSIS

Mast cell disease/mastocytosis is characterized by the abnormal growth and accumulation of morphologically and immunophenotypically abnormal mast cells in one or more organs in the body.

Pathogenesis

Furitsu *et al.* initially showed that KIT expressed on HMC-1 cells, an immature mast cell line established from a patient with mast cell leukemia,[31] was constitutively phosphorylated and activated in the absence of SCF.[32] Sequencing of c-*KIT* in these cells revealed two point mutations, one each in the juxtamembrane (V560G) and tyrosine kinase (D816V) domains. Soon after this report, Nagata *et al.* published the first report of the *KIT* D816V mutation in human mastocytosis.[33] Since then, other *KIT* mutations, either involving D816 or an adjacent amino acid residue (e.g. D816Y,[34–36] D816F,[34] D816H,[37] I817V or VI815-816,[38] and D820G[39]), or other domains (extracellular,[40] transmembrane,[41,42] or juxtamembrane[43,44]) have also been identified in mastocytosis. The juxtamembrane mutations include V560G, K509I, and V559A; some are rare alleles detected in germline DNA in cohorts with familial mastocytosis.[45]

While activating *KIT* mutations are clearly associated with human mastocytosis, they do not occur universally,[46] and the question as to whether individual mutations are necessary and sufficient to cause mast cell transformation remains to be determined. Although introduction of human *KIT* D816V (or its murine homologs) into IL-3-dependent cell lines (e.g. Ba/F3) can induce cytokine-independent growth,[47–49] such experiments do not provide direct confirmation of the neoplastic transformation potential of activating *KIT* mutations since these cell lines are immortalized and have acquired, *a priori*, the capacity to self-renew by unknown events.

Systemic mastocytosis (SM) patients may exhibit eosinophilia,[50–53] and in some cases, harbor the *FIP1L1-PDGFRA* oncogene, which results from an interstitial deletion in chromosome 4q12, leading to constitutively active platelet-derived growth factor receptor *A* (PDGFRA) tyrosine kinase activity, that is uniquely sensitive to inhibition by imatinib mesylate.[54] However, the revised WHO criteria for the classification of myeloid neoplasms categorize *FIP1L1-PDGFRA*-associated eosinophilia and bone marrow mastocytosis in a group different from SM.

Classification

The WHO classification incorporates recent advances in our understanding of mastocytosis, including the role of c-*KIT* mutations, aberrant expression of cell surface immunophenotypic markers on neoplastic mast cells, and the utility of mast cell mediators as surrogate measures of mast cell burden.[55,56] It classifies mastocytosis into seven variants (Table 13.1):

Table 13.1 World Health Organization variants of mastocytosis[56]

Cutaneous mastocytosis (CM)
Maculopapular CM
Diffuse CM
Mastocytoma of skin
Indolent systemic mastocytosis (ISM)
Smoldering systemic mastocytosis (SSM)
Isolated bone marrow mastocytosis
Systemic mastocytosis with an associated clonal hematological non-mast cell lineage disease (SM-AHNMD)
SM-MDS
SM-MPD
SM-CEL
SM-CMML
SM-NHL
Aggressive systemic mastocytosis (ASM)
With eosinophilia (SM-eo)
Mast cell leukemia (MCL)
Aleukemic MCL
Mast cell sarcoma
Extracutaneous mastocytoma

MDS, myelodysplastic syndrome; MPD, myeloproliferative disorder; CEL, chronic eosinophilic leukemia; CMML, chronic myelomonocytic leukemia; NHL, non-Hodgkin lymphoma.

cutaneous mastocytosis (CM), indolent systemic mastocytosis (ISM), systemic mastocytosis with an associated clonal hematological non-mast cell disorder (SM-AHNMD), aggressive systemic mastocytosis (ASM), mast cell leukemia (MCL), mast cell sarcoma, and extracutaneous mastocytoma. In addition, two relatively rare variants of mastocytosis with characteristic clinicopathological features have also been described: 'well-differentiated systemic mastocytosis' (WDSM) and 'systemic mastocytosis without skin involvement associated with recurrent anaphylaxis' (SM-ana).[38]

The WHO classification system mandates a number of staging investigations to define the exact subtype of disease.[56] Identification of 'B' findings (Table 13.2) alone such as >30% mast cells in the bone marrow or serum tryptase >200 ng/ml are indicative of a high systemic mast cell burden (i.e. 'smoldering SM'), while the additional presence of 'C' findings (Table 13.3) such as cytopenias, pathological fractures, hypersplenism, etc., indicate impaired organ function directly attributable to mast cell infiltration, and are diagnostic for the presence of 'aggressive' disease (i.e. ASM).

Clinical features

Urticaria pigmentosa (UP) is the commonest manifestation of mastocytosis. The skin lesions are typically yellow tan to reddish brown macules, and generally involve the extremities, trunk, and abdomen, but spare sun-exposed areas, including the palms, soles, and scalp. The lesions commonly exhibit an urticarial response to mechanical stimulation such as stroking or scratching (Darier's sign).[58,59] Biopsies of UP lesions demonstrate multifocal mast cell aggregates mainly around blood vessels and around skin appendages in the papillary dermis.[59,60] Children account for nearly two-thirds of all reported cases of cutaneous mastocytosis, with the majority of cases arising before the age of 2 years.[61–63] In contrast, most adult mastocytosis patients with UP have systemic disease at presentation, that is most commonly revealed by a bone marrow biopsy done as part of the diagnostic work-up.[64]

Another major manifestation of SM is referred to as 'mast cell degranulation symptoms': pruritus, urticaria, angioedema, flushing, bronchoconstriction, neuropsychiatric manifestations, and hypotension.[65] Gastrointestinal features such as nausea, vomiting, abdominal pain, diarrhea, and malabsorption may be prominent in some patients. Histamine receptor stimulation increases gastric acid production, which may cause peptic ulcer disease with potential morbidity from a bleeding peptic ulcer and/or perforation.[66,67] Presyncope, episodic vascular collapse, and sudden death represent the more dramatic clinical presentations of mast cell mediator release.[68]

Other manifestations include musculoskeletal symptoms (bone pain, diffuse osteoporosis or osteopenia, myalgias, arthralgias, pathological

Table 13.2 'B' findings: indication of high mast cell burden[57]

Infiltration grade (mast cells) in >30% in bone marrow in histology and serum total tryptase levels >200 ng/ml
Hypercellular marrow with loss of fat cells, discrete signs of dysmyelopoiesis without substantial cytopenias or WHO criteria for an MDS or MPD
Organomegaly: palpable hepatomegaly, splenomegaly, or lymphadenopathy (on computed tomography or ultrasound) >2 cm without impaired organ function

MDS, myelodysplastic syndrome; MPD, myeloproliferative disorder.

Table 13.3 'C' findings: indication of impaired organ function attributable to mast cell infiltration[56]

Cytopenia(s): absolute neutrophil count <1000/μl, or hemoglobin <10 g/dl, or platelets <100 000/μl
Hepatomegaly with ascites and impaired liver function
Palpable splenomegaly with hypersplenism
Malabsorption with hypoalbuminemia and weight loss
Skeletal lesions: large-sized osteolysis or severe osteoporosis causing pathological fractures
Life-threatening organopathy in other organ systems that definitively is caused by an infiltration of the tissue by neoplastic mast cells

fractures, skeletal deformities, and/or compression radiculopathies), hepatosplenomegaly (with or without liver dysfunction, ascites, or hypersplenism), lymphadenopathy, and malabsorption with hypoalbuminemia and weight loss. Extensive marrow involvement may result in anemia and eventually to pancytopenia.

Diagnosis

The WHO criteria for diagnosis of systemic mastocytosis are enumerated in Table 13.4.[56] The bone marrow is virtually always involved in adults and shows characteristic histologic features; in contrast, histological criteria for non-bone marrow organ involvement have not been clearly defined. A bone marrow examination also allows determination of whether an associated clonal non-mast cell lineage hematological disorder is present. The pathognomonic lesion, which represents the WHO major diagnostic criterion, is presence of multifocal, dense mast cell aggregates, frequently in perivascular and/or paratrabecular locations (Figure 13.1). These aggregates may be relatively monomorphic, composed mainly of fusiform mast cells, or may be polymorphic with mast cells admixed with lymphocytes, eosinophils, neutrophils, histiocytes, endothelial cells, and fibroblasts.[69] Eosinophils are most commonly observed at the periphery of mast cell aggregates (often focally).[70] While irregular trabecular thickening is commonly noted, other cases may be characterized by a marked thinning of bone marrow trabeculae and osteopenia. In some cases, mast cell infiltrates may be associated with a dense network of reticulin fibers.

Table 13.4 World Health Organization criteria for diagnosis of systemic mastocytosis[56]

Major
Multifocal dense infiltrates of mast cells in bone marrow or other extracutaneous organ sections (>15 mast cells aggregating)
Minor
≥25% mast cells in tissue sections or bone marrow aspirate smear are spindle shaped or have atypical morphology
c-KIT point mutation at codon 816V
Expression of CD2 and/or CD25 by mast cells
Baseline serum tryptase persistently >20 ng/ml (not valid in presence of another non-mast cell clonal disorder)

Major plus one minor or three minor criteria are needed to diagnose systemic mastocytosis.

The most frequent non-mast cell disorders associated with mastocytosis are the chronic myeloproliferative disorders (except *BCR-ABL*-positive chronic myeloid leukemia (CML)), acute myeloid leukemia (AML), and myelodysplastic syndromes (MDS).[71–73] Mast cell leukemia (MCL) is characterized by increased numbers of mast cells in bone marrow (>20% in aspirate smear) and peripheral blood (>10%), with associated bone marrow failure manifest as peripheral cytopenias. The mast cells are immature, sometimes blastic, and often have sparse metachromatic granules, and hence may be missed on routine staining unless tryptase[74,75] and/or immunophenotyping studies are performed.[76,77]

In general, mast cells may not be readily recognized by standard dyes such as Giemsa, particularly when associated with significant hypogranulation or with abnormal nuclear morphology.[69,78] Among the immunohistochemical markers, staining for tryptase is considered the most sensitive, being able to detect even small-sized mast cell infiltrates (Figure 13.1).[79,80] Given that virtually all mast cells, irrespective of their stage of maturation, activation status, or tissue of localization express tryptase, staining for this marker detects even those infiltrates that are primarily composed of immature, poorly granulated mast cells.[76] Neither tryptase, nor other immunohistochemical markers such as chymase, KIT/CD117, or CD68 can distinguish between normal and neoplastic mast cells.[81] In contrast, immunohistochemical detection of aberrant CD25 expression on bone marrow mast cells appears to be a reliable diagnostic tool in systemic mastocytosis, given its ability to detect abnormal mast cells in all mastocytosis subtypes.[76]

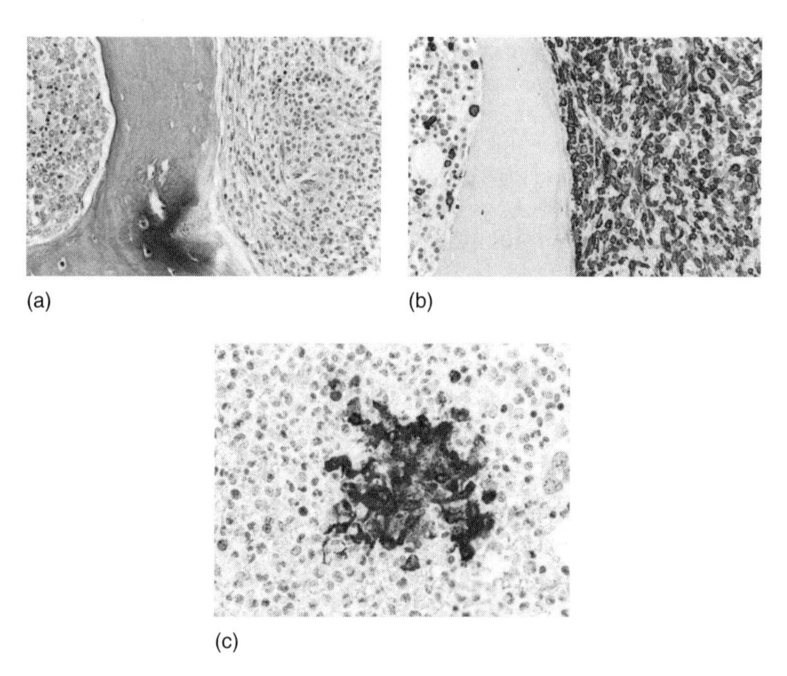

Figure 13.1 Bone marrow trephine biopsy showing paratrabecular mast cell infiltrate comprising morphologically atypical (fusiform) mast cells, as shown by (a) hematoxylin-eosin stain, and (b) tryptase immunostain. (c) Pathognomonic mast cell aggregate as shown by tryptase immunostain.

Mast cell immunophenotyping by multiparametric flow cytometry can be extremely useful in distinguishing normal bone marrow mast cells from their pathological counterparts.[82] Normal mast cells typically express KIT/CD117 and FcεRI, and their typical profile is CD117++/FcεRI+/CD34–/CD38–/CD33+/CD45+/CD11c+/CD71+. Neoplastic mast cells typically express CD25 and/or CD2, and the abnormal expression of at least one of these two antigens counts as a minor criterion towards the diagnosis of systemic mastocytosis as defined by the WHO system.[56] In general, the detection of CD25 on mast cells, by either flow cytometry or immunohistochemistry, appears to be the more reliable marker (relative to CD2).[76,83] Other immunophenotypic features of neoplastic mast cells include abnormally high expression of complement-related markers such as CD11c,[84] CD35,[85] CD59,[85] and CD88,[85] as well as increased expression of the CD69 early-activation antigen,[86] and the CD63 lysosomal-associated protein.[87]

Measurement of serum tryptase (a mast cell enzyme) has proven to be a useful disease-related marker in SM, and is included as a minor criterion for diagnosing the condition per WHO guidelines.[56,88] The total tryptase level ranges from 1 to 15 ng/ml in healthy individuals, but is increased in most patients with SM (>20 ng/ml). An elevated serum tryptase level may also, however, be observed in patients with non-mast cell myeloid malignancies, including AML,[89,90] MDS,[91] and CML,[92] which mandates exclusion of these conditions before reaching a diagnosis of SM. Furthermore, the serum tryptase level is frequently elevated in the setting of anaphylaxis or severe allergic reaction.[88] Total tryptase levels may be useful for monitoring treatment response in mastocytosis patients, although the levels may vary considerably (e.g. with use of radiocontrast agents or narcotics).

Molecular studies in mastocytosis patients are important from the diagnostic standpoint and, increasingly, from the therapeutic standpoint as well. The rate of detection of *KIT* D816V is correlated to the proportion of lesional/clonal cells in the sample, as well as to the sensitivity of the screening method employed.[45] The specimen mast cell content may be enriched by laser capture microdissection, or magnetic bead- or flow cytometry-based cell sorting.[93–95] Furthermore, use of allele-specific polymerase chain reaction (PCR),[96] or PCR with peptide nucleic acid (PNA) probes to 'clamp' the wild-type allele, dramatically enhance the probability of mutation detection in bulk cells (sensitivity 10^{-3}).[36,38] Using the latter method, the D816V mutation has been detected in virtually all patients with ISM or ASM (93%).[38]

MANAGEMENT OF PATIENTS WITH SYSTEMIC MASTOCYTOSIS

An algorithm illustrating our general approach for treating patients with SM is presented in Figure 13.2. Management of mast cell degranulation symptoms includes measures to prevent mast cell degranulation, with use of medications for symptom relief. In all cases, avoidance of triggers for mast cell degranulation (e.g. animal venoms, extremes of temperature, mechanical irritation, alcohol, and emotional and physical stress) remains the cornerstone of therapy. Some patients cannot tolerate certain agents such as opioid analgesics, alcohol, aspirin/other non-steroidal anti-inflammatory medications, and contrast dyes; the patient history often provides useful clues in this regard. Furthermore, appropriate precautionary measures during anesthesia and surgery are recommended in these patients.[97–100]

Non-cytoreductive therapy of mast cell degranulation symptoms includes the use of oral H-1 (e.g. hydroxyzine, diphenhydramine, fexofenadine, cetirizine, cyproheptadine, chlorpheniramine) and H-2 (e.g. ranitidine, famotidine) antihistaminics for pruritus and peptic symptoms, respectively, and orally administered cromolyn sodium for nausea, abdominal pain, and diarrhea. Use of the latter is supported by level I evidence.[101,102] Corticosteroids are occasionally used for treating recurrent or refractory symptoms, and it is recommended that patients with a propensity towards vasodilatory shock wear a medical alert bracelet and carry an Epi-Pen injector for self-administration of subcutaneous epinephrine.[103] In the rare case of a patient with severe and/or recurrent life-threatening degranulation-related events that are refractory to the aforementioned agents, cautious consideration may be given to the use of cytostatic or cytoreductive

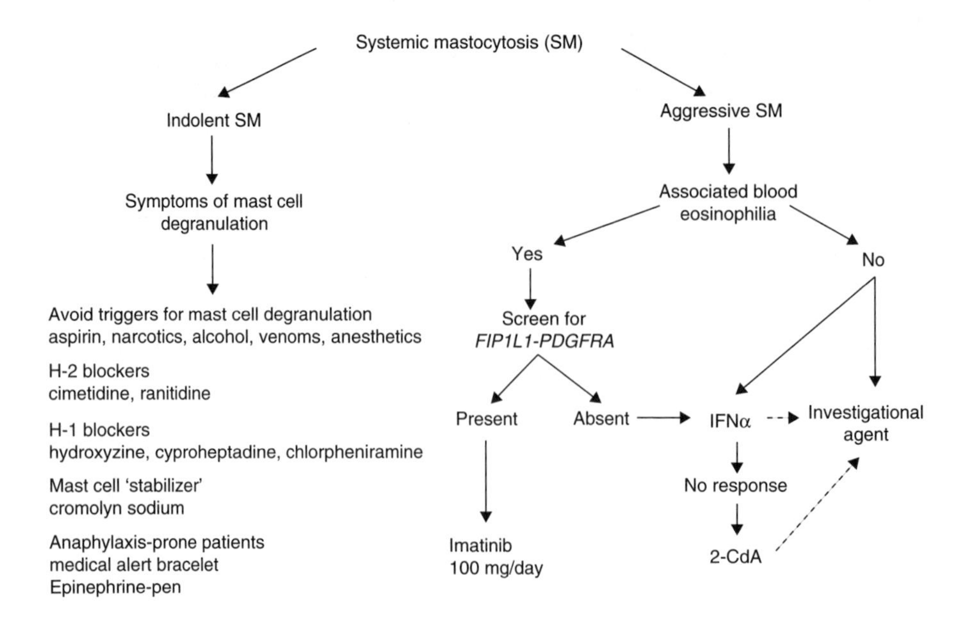

Figure 13.2 A treatment algorithm for systemic mastocytosis.

agents; one must keep in mind, however, the potential adverse effects, including potentially mutagenic effects of the such agents.

Cytoreductive treatment in systemic mastocytosis

Cytoreductive therapy in SM is generally reserved for patients with progressive symptomatic disease and organopathy ('C' findings) that is directly related to tissue mast cell infiltration.

Interferon alfa

Interferon alfa (IFNα) is often considered the first-line cytoreductive therapy in SM.[104] IFNα is generally started at the dose of 1 million units (MU) subcutaneously three times per week, followed by gradual escalation to 3–5 MU three to five times per week, if tolerated. IFNα (with or without concomitant corticosteroids for synergistic effect) has been reported to improve symptoms of mast cell degranulation,[105] decrease bone marrow mast cell infiltration,[106–111] and ameliorate mastocytosis-related ascites/hepatosplenomegaly,[106,107,112] cytopenias,[113] skin findings,[104,108,114] and osteoporosis.[109,110,115,116] The optimal dose and duration of IFNα therapy for SM remain uncertain. The time to best response may be a year or longer[113] and delayed responses to therapy have been described.[117] IFNα treatment is frequently (up to 50%) complicated by toxicities, including flu-like symptoms, bone pain, fever, worsening cytopenias, depression, and hypothyroidism.[105,107] Consequently, the adverse dropout rate with IFNα treatment is not trivial and must be factored into the treatment strategy. Finally, a significant proportion of patients will relapse within several months of IFNα treatment being discontinued, outlining the largely 'cytostatic' effect of IFNα on neoplastic mast cells.[105,107]

2-Chlorodeoxyadenosine/cladribine

Single-agent 2-chlorodeoxyadenosine (2-CdA) has therapeutic activity in the setting of IFNα refractory/intolerant mastocytosis.[118–122] In a prospective multicenter pilot study of ten patients, 2-CdA was found to be therapeutically active in all mastocytosis subsets.[122] While all patients had a clinical response, and bone marrow mast cell cytoreduction was also noted in nine of ten patients, no complete remissions were observed. Myelosuppression was the major adverse effect in this study. Wider use of single-agent 2-CdA has been restrained by the relatively limited experience in this setting; additional data are awaited to clarify the optimal dose/schedule of administration, response rates in specific mastocytosis subtypes, and durability of treatment responses. Given the potential for prolonged bone marrow aplasia and lymphopenia and associated risk of opportunistic infections, its use is probably best restricted to select cases with IFNα refractory disease.

Imatinib mesylate (Gleevec®)

Imatinib is an orally bioavailable small molecule inhibitor of KIT, ABL, ARG, and PDGFR tyrosine kinases. Clinically meaningful responses have been observed in the rare mastocytosis patient with KIT juxtamembrane mutations (e.g. F522C, K509I).[42,44] Furthermore, patients who harbor *FIP1L1-PDGFRA* also uniformly achieve complete clinical, histological, and molecular/cytogenetic responses with 'low-dose' imatinib therapy, in the absence of mutations that confer imatinib resistance (*PDGFRA*-T764I), which may be acquired with clonal evolution.[123–127] Finally, imatinib is predicted to be effective in SM with specific mutations such as V560G[128] and del419,[40] although clinically proof is lacking to date. It is currently recommended that patients with primary eosinophilia, particularly in the presence of increased bone marrow mast cells/increased serum tryptase level (i.e. SM-CEL/CEL) be screened for presence of *FIP1L1-PDGFRA* (Figure 13.2). Imatinib mesylate, generally at the 100 mg daily dose level, is considered to be first-line therapy for this group of patients.[129–131] Initiation of imatinib therapy in patients with clonal eosinophilia harboring *FIP1L1-PDGFRA* can rarely lead to cardiogenic shock resulting from rapid onset of eosinophil lysis/degranulation in the endomyocardium.[132,133] Consequently, consideration may be given to starting imatinib concurrently with corticosteroids, particularly in the presence of either an abnormal echocardiogram or an elevated serum troponin level prior to treatment. Consistent with predictions from *in vitro* data,[134,135] currently available data suggest that mastocytosis patients harboring *KIT* D816V are refractory to imatinib therapy.[136,137] This mutation maps to the KIT enzymatic site and disrupts the imatinib binding site.[138] For patients harboring D816V, or those without detectable imatinib-sensitive mutations, IFNα may represent an attractive initial treatment option. While a modest clinical benefit may be observed with imatinib at 400 mg daily in some patients without either *KIT* D816V or *FIP1L1-PDGFRA*,[139] the use of imatinib in this setting is considered investigational.

Investigational therapies

Tyrosine kinase inhibitors

PKC412 is a n-benzoyl-staurosporine, with inhibitory activity against protein kinase C (PKC), FLT3 (FMS-like tyrosine kinase), KIT, vascular endothelial growth factor receptor-2 (VEGFR-2), PDGFR, and fibroblast growth factor receptor (FGFR) tyrosine kinases.[140,141] PKC412 potently inhibits growth of cell lines harboring *KIT* D816V,[142,143] and early data suggest activity in patients with advanced SM;[144,145] preliminary data from the latter phase II study indicated that six of nine patients responded to PKC412 therapy. PKC412 has limited efficacy as a single agent for treatment of AML,[146] but may be active against constitutively activated ZNF198-FGFR1 for the treatment of 8p11 myeloproliferative syndrome (EMS).[147]

Dasatinib (BMS354825) is an orally bioavailable, thiazolecarboxamide that is structurally unrelated to imatinib. It is a dual BRC-ABL kinase inhibitor that is more potent than imatinib, and demonstrates inhibitory activity against a number of BCR-ABL mutations linked to imatinib resistance in CML, but not T315I.[148] Dasatinib inhibits cell lines harboring *KIT* WT or *KIT* D816V at nanomolar concentrations.[149,150] In contrast to imatinib, dasatinib binds to the ABL and KIT ATP-binding sites irrespective of the activation-loop conformation.[151,152] Preliminary data indicate modest activity in SM mastocytosis; in one report, although 30% had symptomatic benefit, only two of 24 patients achieved significant mast cell cytoreduction (both patients were *KIT* D816V-negative and achieved complete remission).[153]

Non-tyrosine kinase inhibitors

17-(allylamino)-17-demethoxygeldanamycin (17-AAG) is a geldanamycin derivative that binds to heat shock protein 90 (hsp90), thus enhancing the proteasomal degradation of several hsp90 client kinases, including mutant KIT. In one report, a dose-dependent decrease in phosphorylation of KIT, AKT, and STAT3 was observed in both human mast cell line (HMC) 1.1 and HMC 1.2 cells.[154] Furthermore, 17-AAG inhibited patient-derived neoplastic mast cells *ex vivo*, relative to mononuclear cells. 17-AAG is currently in phase II clinical trials for the treatment of mastocytosis.

REFERENCES

1. Kirshenbaum AS, Kessler SW, Goff JP et al. Demonstration of the origin of human mast cells from CD34+ bone marrow progenitor cells. J Immunol 1991; 146: 1410–15.
2. Kirshenbaum AS, Goff JP, Semere T et al. Demonstration that human mast cells arise from a progenitor cell population that is CD34(+), c-KIT(+), and expresses aminopeptidase N (CD13). Blood 1999; 94: 2333–42.
3. Mitsui H, Furitsu T, Dvorak AM et al. Development of human mast cells from umbilical cord blood cells by recombinant human and murine c-KIT ligand. Proc Natl Acad Sci U S A 1993; 90: 735–9.
4. Toru H, Eguchi M, Matsumoto R et al. Interleukin-4 promotes the development of tryptase and chymase double-positive human mast cells accompanied by cell maturation. Blood 1998; 91: 187–95.
5. Besmer P, Murphy JE, George PC et al. A new acute transforming feline retrovirus and relationship of its oncogene v-KIT with the protein kinase gene family. Nature 1986; 320: 415–21.
6. Scheijen B, Griffin JD. Tyrosine kinase oncogenes in normal hematopoiesis and hematological disease. Oncogene 2002; 21: 3314–33.

7. Lennartsson J, Jelacic T, Linnekin D et al. Normal and oncogenic forms of the receptor tyrosine kinase KIT. Stem Cells 2005; 23: 16–43.
8. Marone G, Triggiani M, Genovese A et al. Role of human mast cells and basophils in bronchial asthma. Adv Immunol 2005; 88: 97–160.
9. Metcalfe DD, Baram D, Mekori YA. Mast cells. Physiol Rev 1997; 77: 1033–79.
10. Gurish MF, Austen KF. The diverse roles of mast cells. J Exp Med 2001; 194: F1–5.
11. Galli SJ, Zsebo KM, Geissler EN. The KIT ligand, stem cell factor. Adv Immunol 1994; 55: 1–96.
12. Kawakami T, Galli SJ. Regulation of mast-cell and basophil function and survival by IgE. Nat Rev Immunol 2002; 2: 773–86.
13. Galli SJ, Kalesnikoff J, Grimbaldeston MA et al. Mast cells as "tunable" effector and immunoregulatory cells: recent advances. Annu Rev Immunol 2005; 23: 749–86.
14. Galli SJ, Nakae S, Tsai M. Mast cells in the development of adaptive immune responses. Nat Immunol 2005; 6: 135–42.
15. Grimbaldeston MA, Metz M, Yu M et al. Effector and potential immunoregulatory roles of mast cells in IgE-associated acquired immune responses. Curr Opin Immunol 2006; 18: 751–60.
16. Bischoff SC. Role of mast cells in allergic and nonallergic immune responses: comparison of human and murine data. Nat Rev Immunol 2007; 7: 93–104.
17. Williams CM, Galli SJ. The diverse potential effector and immunoregulatory roles of mast cells in allergic disease. J Allergy Clin Immunol 2000; 105: 847–59.
18. King CL, Xianli J, Malhotra I et al. Mice with a targeted deletion of the IgE gene have increased worm burdens and reduced granulomatous inflammation following primary infection with Schistosoma mansoni. J Immunol 1997; 158: 294–300.
19. Lantz CS, Boesiger J, Song CH et al. Role for interleukin-3 in mast-cell and basophil development and in immunity to parasites. Nature 1998; 392: 90–3.
20. Stevens RL, Austen KF. Recent advances in the cellular and molecular biology of mast cells. Immunol Today 1989; 10: 381–6.
21. Bienenstock J, Befus AD, Denburg J. Mast cell heterogeneity: basic questions and clinical implications. In: Befus AD, Bienenstock J, Denburg J, eds. Mast Cell Differentiation and Heterogeneity. New York: Raven Press, 1986: 391–402.
22. Costa JJ, Galli SJ. Mast cells and basophils. In: Rich RR, ed. Clinical Immunology Principles and Practice, 1st edn. St Louis: Mosby, 1996: 408–30.
23. Schwartz LB, Huff TF. Biology of mast cells and basophils. In: Middleton EJ, Reed CE, Ellis EF, Adkinson NFJ, Yunginger JW, Busse WW, eds. Allergy: Principles and Practice, 4th edn. St Louis: Mosby, 1993; 1: 135–68.
24. Valone FH, Boggs JM, Goetzl EJ. Lipid mediators of hypersensitivity and inflammation. In: Middleton EJ, Reed CE, Ellis EF, Adkinson NFJ, Yunginger JW, Busse WW, eds. Allergy: Principles and Practice, 4th edn. St Louis: Mosby, 1993: 302–19.
25. Galli SJ, Costa JJ. Mast-cell-leukocyte cytokine cascades in allergic inflammation. Allergy 1995; 50: 851–62.
26. Galli SJ, Lichtenstein LM. Biology of mast cells and basophils. In: Middleton EJ, Reed CE, Ellis EF, Adkinson NFJ, Yunginger JW, eds. Allergy: Principles and Practice, 3rd edn. St Louis: Mosby, 1988: 106–34.
27. Galli SJ. Mast cells and basophils. Curr Opin Hematol 2000; 7: 32–9.
28. Gordon JR, Burd PR, Galli SJ. Mast cells as a source of multifunctional cytokines. Immunol Today 1990; 11: 458–64.
29. Gordon JR, Galli SJ. Mast cells as a source of both preformed and immunologically inducible TNF-alpha/cachectin. Nature 1990; 346: 274–6.
30. Holgate ST, Robinson C, Church MK. Mediators of immediate hypersensitivity. In: Middleton EJ, Reed CE, Ellis EF, Adkinson NFJ, Yunginger JW, Busse WW, eds. Allergy: Principles and Practice, 4th edn. St Louis: Mosby, 1993: 267–301.
31. Butterfield JH, Weiler D, Dewald G et al. Establishment of an immature mast cell line from a patient with mast cell leukemia. Leuk Res 1988; 12: 345–55.
32. Furitsu T, Tsujimura T, Tono T et al. Identification of mutations in the coding sequence of the protooncogene c-KIT in a human mast cell leukemia cell line causing ligand- independent activation of c-KIT product. J Clin Invest 1993; 92: 1736–44.
33. Nagata H, Worobec AS, Oh CK et al. Identification of a point mutation in the catalytic domain of the protooncogene c-KIT in peripheral blood mononuclear cells of patients who have mastocytosis with an associated hematologic disorder. Proc Natl Acad Sci U S A 1995; 92: 10560–4.
34. Longley BJ Jr, Metcalfe DD, Tharp M et al. Activating and dominant inactivating c-KIT catalytic domain mutations in distinct clinical forms of human mastocytosis. Proc Natl Acad Sci U S A 1999; 96: 1609–14.
35. Beghini A, Cairoli R, Morra E et al. In vivo differentiation of mast cells from acute myeloid leukemia blasts carrying a novel activating ligand-independent C-KIT mutation. Blood Cells Mol Dis 1998; 24: 262–70.
36. Sotlar K, Escribano L, Landt O et al. One-step detection of c-KIT point mutations using peptide nucleic acid-mediated polymerase chain reaction clamping and hybridization probes. Am J Pathol 2003; 162: 737–46.
37. Pullarkat VA, Pullarkat ST, Calverley DC et al. Mast cell disease associated with acute myeloid leukemia: detection of a new c-KIT mutation Asp816His. Am J Hematol 2000; 65: 307–9.
38. Garcia-Montero AC, Jara-Acevedo M, Teodosio C et al. KIT mutation in mast cells and other bone marrow haematopoietic cell lineages in systemic mast cell disorders. A prospective study of the Spanish Network

on Mastocytosis (REMA) in a series of 113 patients. Blood 2006; 108: 2366–72.
39. Pignon JM, Giraudier S, Duquesnoy P et al. A new c-KIT mutation in a case of aggressive mast cell disease. Br J Haematol 1997; 96: 374–6.
40. Hartmann K, Wardelmann E, Ma Y et al. Novel germline mutation of KIT associated with familial gastrointestinal stromal tumors and mastocytosis. Gastroenterology 2005; 129: 1042–6.
41. Tang X, Boxer M, Drummond A et al. A germline mutation in KIT in familial diffuse cutaneous mastocytosis. J Med Genet 2004; 41: e88.
42. Akin C, Fumo G, Yavuz AS et al. A novel form of mastocytosis associated with a transmembrane c-KIT mutation and response to imatinib. Blood 2004; 103: 3222–5.
43. Beghini A, Tibiletti MG, Roversi G et al. Germline mutation in the juxtamembrane domain of the KIT gene in a family with gastrointestinal stromal tumors and urticaria pigmentosa. Cancer 2001; 92: 657–62.
44. Zhang LY, Smith ML, Schultheis B et al. A novel K509I mutation of KIT identified in familial mastocytosis – in vitro and in vivo responsiveness to imatinib therapy. Leuk Res 2006; 30: 373–8.
45. Akin C. Molecular diagnosis of mast cell disorders: a paper from the 2005 William Beaumont Hospital Symposium on Molecular Pathology. J Mol Diagn 2006; 8: 412–19.
46. Valent P, Akin C, Sperr W et al. Mastocytosis: Pathology, genetics, and current options for therapy. Leuk Lymphoma 2005; 46: 35–48.
47. Piao X, Bernstein A. A point mutation in the catalytic domain of c-KIT induces growth factor independence, tumorigenicity, and differentiation of mast cells. Blood 1996; 87: 3117–23.
48. Kitayama H, Kanakura Y, Furitsu T et al. Constitutively activating mutations of c-KIT receptor tyrosine kinase confer factor-independent growth and tumorigenicity of factor-dependent hematopoietic cell lines. Blood 1995; 85: 790–8.
49. Hashimoto K, Tsujimura T, Moriyama Y et al. Transforming and differentiation-inducing potential of constitutively activated c-KIT mutant genes in the IC-2 murine interleukin-3-dependent mast cell line. Am J Pathol 1996; 148: 189–200.
50. Mutter RD, Tannenbaum M, Ultmann JE. Systemic mast cell disease. Ann Intern Med 1963; 59: 887–906.
51. Lawrence JB, Friedman BS, Travis WD et al. Hematologic manifestations of systemic mast cell disease: a prospective study of laboratory and morphologic features and their relation to prognosis. Am J Med 1991; 91: 612–24.
52. Travis WD, Li CY, Bergstralh EJ et al. Systemic mast cell disease. Analysis of 58 cases and literature review. Medicine (Baltimore) 1988; 67: 345–68.
53. Pardanani A, Baek JY, Li CY et al. Systemic mast cell disease without associated hematologic disorder: a combined retrospective and prospective study. Mayo Clin Proc 2002; 77: 1169–75.
54. Cools J, DeAngelo DJ, Gotlib J et al. A tyrosine kinase created by fusion of the PDGFRA and FIP1L1 genes as a therapeutic target of imatinib in idiopathic hypereosinophilic syndrome. N Engl J Med 2003; 348: 1201–14.
55. Valent PHH, Li CY, Longley JB et al. Mastocytosis (Mast cell disease). World Health Organization (WHO) Classification of Tumors. Pathology & Genetics. Tumors of the Haematopoietic and Lymphoid Tissues. Lyon: IARC, 2001; 1.
56. Valent P, Horny HP, Escribano L et al. Diagnostic criteria and classification of mastocytosis: a consensus proposal. Leuk Res 2001; 25: 603–25.
57. Valent P. Diagnostic evaluation and classification of mastocytosis. Immunol Allergy Clin North Am 2006; 26: 515–34.
58. Hartmann K, Henz BM. Cutaneous mastocytosis – clinical heterogeneity. Int Arch Allergy Immunol 2002; 127: 143–6.
59. Hartmann K, Henz BM. Classification of cutaneous mastocytosis: a modified consensus proposal. Leuk Res 2002; 26: 483–484; author reply 485–6.
60. Soter NA. Mastocytosis and the skin. Hematol Oncol Clin North Am 2000; 14: 537–555, vi.
61. Kettelhut BV, Metcalfe DD. Pediatric mastocytosis. J Invest Dermatol 1991; 96: 15S–8S.
62. Azana JM, Torrelo A, Mediero IG et al. Urticaria pigmentosa: a review of 67 pediatric cases. Pediatr Dermatol 1994; 11: 102–6.
63. Middelkamp Hup MA, Heide R, Tank B et al. Comparison of mastocytosis with onset in children and adults. J Eur Acad Dermatol Venereol 2002; 16: 115–20.
64. Czarnetzki BM, Kolde G, Schoemann A et al. Bone marrow findings in adult patients with urticaria pigmentosa. J Am Acad Dermatol 1988; 18: 45–51.
65. Castells M, Austen KF. Mastocytosis: mediator-related signs and symptoms. Int Arch Allergy Immunol 2002; 127: 147–52.
66. Cherner JA, Jensen RT, Dubois A et al. Gastrointestinal dysfunction in systemic mastocytosis. A prospective study. Gastroenterology 1988; 95: 657–67.
67. Cherner JA. Gastric acid secretion in systemic mastocytosis. N Engl J Med 1989; 320: 1562.
68. Horan RF, Austen KF. Systemic mastocytosis: retrospective review of a decade's clinical experience at the Brigham and Women's Hospital. J Invest Dermatol 1991; 96: 5S–13S; discussion 13S–14S.
69. Brunning RD, McKenna RW, Rosai J et al. Systemic mastocytosis. Extracutaneous manifestations. Am J Surg Pathol 1983; 7: 425–38.
70. Horny HP, Parwaresch MR, Lennert K. Bone marrow findings in systemic mastocytosis. Hum Pathol 1985; 16: 808–14.
71. Horny HP, Ruck M, Wehrmann M et al. Blood findings in generalized mastocytosis: evidence of

frequent simultaneous occurrence of myeloproliferative disorders. Br J Haematol 1990; 76: 186–93.
72. Travis WD, Li CY, Yam LT et al. Significance of systemic mast cell disease with associated hematologic disorders. Cancer 1988; 62: 965–72.
73. Stevens EC, Rosenthal NS. Bone marrow mast cell morphologic features and hematopoietic dyspoiesis in systemic mast cell disease. Am J Clin Pathol 2001; 116: 177–82.
74. Horny HP, Valent P. Diagnosis of mastocytosis: general histopathological aspects, morphological criteria, and immunohistochemical findings. Leuk Res 2001; 25: 543–51.
75. Sperr WR, Escribano L, Jordan JH et al. Morphologic properties of neoplastic mast cells: delineation of stages of maturation and implication for cytological grading of mastocytosis. Leuk Res 2001; 25: 529–36.
76. Sotlar K, Horny HP, Simonitsch I et al. CD25 indicates the neoplastic phenotype of mast cells: a novel immunohistochemical marker for the diagnosis of systemic mastocytosis (SM) in routinely processed bone marrow biopsy specimens. Am J Surg Pathol 2004; 28: 1319–25.
77. Noack F, Sotlar K, Notter M et al. Aleukemic mast cell leukemia with abnormal immunophenotype and c-KIT mutation D816V. Leuk Lymphoma 2004; 45: 2295–302.
78. Li CY. Diagnosis of mastocytosis: value of cytochemistry and immunohistochemistry. Leuk Res 2001; 25: 537–41.
79. Horny HP, Sillaber C, Menke D et al. Diagnostic value of immunostaining for tryptase in patients with mastocytosis. Am J Surg Pathol 1998; 22: 1132–40.
80. Horny HP, Valent P. Histopathological and immunohistochemical aspects of mastocytosis. Int Arch Allergy Immunol 2002; 127: 115–17.
81. Jordan JH, Walchshofer S, Jurecka W et al. Immunohistochemical properties of bone marrow mast cells in systemic mastocytosis: evidence for expression of CD2, CD117/KIT, and bcl-x(L). Hum Pathol 2001; 32: 545–52.
82. Escribano L, Garcia Montero AC, Nunez R et al. Flow cytometric analysis of normal and neoplastic mast cells: role in diagnosis and follow-up of mast cell disease. Immunol Allergy Clin North Am 2006; 26: 535–47.
83. Pardanani A, Kimlinger T, Reeder T et al. Bone marrow mast cell immunophenotyping in adults with mast cell disease: a prospective study of 33 patients. Leuk Res 2004; 28: 777–83.
84. Escribano L, Diaz-Agustin B, Lopez A et al. Immunophenotypic analysis of mast cells in mastocytosis: When and how to do it. Proposals of the Spanish Network on Mastocytosis (REMA). Cytometry B Clin Cytom 2004; 58: 1–8.
85. Nunez-Lopez R, Escribano L, Schernthaner GH et al. Overexpression of complement receptors and related antigens on the surface of bone marrow mast cells in patients with systemic mastocytosis. Br J Haematol 2003; 120: 257–65.
86. Diaz-Agustin B, Escribano L, Bravo P et al. The CD69 early activation molecule is overexpressed in human bone marrow mast cells from adults with indolent systemic mast cell disease. Br J Haematol 1999; 106: 400–5.
87. Escribano L, Orfao A, Diaz Agustin B et al. Human bone marrow mast cells from indolent systemic mast cell disease constitutively express increased amounts of the CD63 protein on their surface. Cytometry 1998; 34: 223–8.
88. Schwartz LB, Metcalfe DD, Miller JS et al. Tryptase levels as an indicator of mast-cell activation in systemic anaphylaxis and mastocytosis. N Engl J Med 1987; 316: 1622–6.
89. Sperr WR, Jordan JH, Baghestanian M et al. Expression of mast cell tryptase by myeloblasts in a group of patients with acute myeloid leukemia. Blood 2001; 98: 2200–9.
90. Sperr WR, Hauswirth AW, Valent P. Tryptase a novel biochemical marker of acute myeloid leukemia. Leuk Lymphoma 2002; 43: 2257–61.
91. Sperr WR, Stehberger B, Wimazal F et al. Serum tryptase measurements in patients with myelodysplastic syndromes. Leuk Lymphoma 2002; 43: 1097–105.
92. Samorapoompichit P, Kiener HP, Schernthaner GH et al. Detection of tryptase in cytoplasmic granules of basophils in patients with chronic myeloid leukemia and other myeloid neoplasms. Blood 2001; 98: 2580–3.
93. Sotlar K, Fridrich C, Mall A et al. Detection of c-KIT point mutation Asp-816—> Val in microdissected pooled single mast cells and leukemic cells in a patient with systemic mastocytosis and concomitant chronic myelomonocytic leukemia. Leuk Res 2002; 26: 979–84.
94. Pardanani A, Reeder T, Li CY et al. Eosinophils are derived from the neoplastic clone in patients with systemic mastocytosis and eosinophilia. Leuk Res 2003; 27: 883–5.
95. Yavuz AS, Lipsky PE, Yavuz S et al. Evidence for the involvement of a hematopoietic progenitor cell in systemic mastocytosis from single-cell analysis of mutations in the c-KIT gene. Blood 2002; 100: 661–5.
96. Lawley W, Hird H, Mallinder P et al. Detection of an activating c-KIT mutation by real-time PCR in patients with anaphylaxis. Mutat Res 2005; 572: 1–13.
97. Greenblatt EP, Chen L. Urticaria pigmentosa: an anesthetic challenge. J Clin Anesth 1990; 2: 108–15.
98. Lerno G, Slaats G, Coenen E et al. Anaesthetic management of systemic mastocytosis. Br J Anaesth 1990; 65: 254–7.
99. Scott HW Jr, Parris WC, Sandidge PC et al. Hazards in operative management of patients with systemic mastocytosis. Ann Surg 1983; 197: 507–14.
100. Rosenbaum KJ, Strobel GE. Anesthetic considerations in mastocytosis. Anesthesiology 1973; 38: 398–401.

101. Horan RF, Sheffer AL, Austen KF. Cromolyn sodium in the management of systemic mastocytosis. J Allergy Clin Immunol 1990; 85: 852–5.
102. Frieri M, Alling DW, Metcalfe DD. Comparison of the therapeutic efficacy of cromolyn sodium with that of combined chlorpheniramine and cimetidine in systemic mastocytosis. Results of a double-blind clinical trial. Am J Med 1985; 78: 9–14.
103. Turk J, Oates JA, Roberts LJ 2nd. Intervention with epinephrine in hypotension associated with mastocytosis. J Allergy Clin Immunol 1983; 71: 189–92.
104. Petit A, Pulik M, Gaulier A et al. Systemic mastocytosis associated with chronic myelomonocytic leukemia: clinical features and response to interferon alfa therapy. J Am Acad Dermatol 1995; 32: 850–3.
105. Casassus P, Caillat-Vigneron N, Martin A et al. Treatment of adult systemic mastocytosis with interferon-alpha: results of a multicentre phase II trial on 20 patients. Br J Haematol 2002; 119: 1090–7.
106. Kluin-Nelemans HC, Jansen JH, Breukelman H et al. Response to interferon alfa-2b in a patient with systemic mastocytosis. N Engl J Med 1992; 326: 619–23.
107. Butterfield JH. Response of severe systemic mastocytosis to interferon alpha. Br J Dermatol 1998; 138: 489–95.
108. Kolde G, Sunderkotter C, Luger TA. Treatment of urticaria pigmentosa using interferon alpha. Br J Dermatol 1995; 133: 91–4.
109. Lehmann T, Beyeler C, Lammle B et al. Severe osteoporosis due to systemic mast cell disease: successful treatment with interferon alpha-2B. Br J Rheumatol 1996; 35: 898–900.
110. Weide R, Ehlenz K, Lorenz W et al. Successful treatment of osteoporosis in systemic mastocytosis with interferon alpha-2b. Ann Hematol 1996; 72: 41–3.
111. Butterfield JH, Tefferi A, Kozuh GF. Successful treatment of systemic mastocytosis with high-dose interferon-alfa: long-term follow-up of a case. Leuk Res 2005; 29: 131–4.
112. Takasaki Y, Tsukasaki K, Jubashi T et al. Systemic mastocytosis with extensive polypoid lesions in the intestines; successful treatment with interferon-alpha. Intern Med 1998; 37: 484–8.
113. Hauswirth AW, Simonitsch-Klupp I, Uffmann M et al. Response to therapy with interferon alpha-2b and prednisolone in aggressive systemic mastocytosis: report of five cases and review of the literature. Leuk Res 2004; 28: 249–57.
114. Kluin-Nelemans HC, Jansen JH, Breukelman H et al. Response to interferon alfa-2b in a patient with systemic mastocytosis. N Engl J Med 1992; 326: 619–23.
115. Weide R, Ehlenz K, Lorenz W et al. Successful treatment of osteoporosis in systemic mastocytosis with interferon alpha-2b. Ann Hematol 1996; 72: 41–3.
116. Lehmann T, Lammle B. IFNalpha treatment in systemic mastocytosis. Ann Hematol 1999; 78: 483–4.
117. Lippert U, Henz BM. Long-term effect of interferon alpha treatment in mastocytosis. [comment]. Br J Dermatol 1996; 134: 1164–5.
118. Tefferi A, Li CY, Butterfield JH et al. Treatment of systemic mast-cell disease with cladribine. N Engl J Med 2001; 344: 307–9.
119. Pardanani A, Hoffbrand AV, Butterfield JH et al. Treatment of systemic mast cell disease with 2-chlorodeoxyadenosine. Leuk Res 2004; 28: 127–31.
120. Escribano L, Perez de Oteyza J, Nunez R et al. Cladribine induces immunophenotypical changes in bone marrow mast cells from mastocytosis. Report of a case of mastocytosis associated with a lymphoplasmacytic lymphoma. Leuk Res 2002; 26: 1043–6.
121. Schleyer V, Meyer S, Landthaler M et al. "Smoldering systemic mastocytosis". Successful therapy with cladribine. Hautarzt 2004; 55: 658–62.[in German]
122. Kluin-Nelemans HC, Oldhoff JM, Van Doormaal JJ et al. Cladribine therapy for systemic mastocytosis. Blood 2003; 102: 4270–6.
123. Pardanani A, Ketterling RP, Li CY et al. FIP1L1-PDGFRA in eosinophilic disorders: prevalence in routine clinical practice, long-term experience with imatinib therapy, and a critical review of the literature. Leuk Res 2006; 30: 965–70.
124. Pardanani A, Brockman SR, Paternoster SF et al. FIP1L1-PDGFRA fusion: prevalence and clinicopathologic correlates in 89 consecutive patients with moderate to severe eosinophilia. Blood 2004; 104: 3038–45.
125. Pardanani A, Ketterling RP, Brockman SR et al. CHIC2 deletion, a surrogate for FIP1L1-PDGFRA fusion, occurs in systemic mastocytosis associated with eosinophilia and predicts response to imatinib mesylate therapy. Blood 2003; 102: 3093–6.
126. Klion AD, Robyn J, Akin C et al. Molecular remission and reversal of myelofibrosis in response to imatinib mesylate treatment in patients with the myeloproliferative variant of hypereosinophilic syndrome. Blood 2004; 103: 473–8.
127. Klion AD, Noel P, Akin C et al. Elevated serum tryptase levels identify a subset of patients with a myeloproliferative variant of idiopathic hypereosinophilic syndrome associated with tissue fibrosis, poor prognosis, and imatinib responsiveness. Blood 2003; 101: 4660–6.
128. Frost MJ, Ferrao PT, Hughes TP et al. Juxtamembrane mutant V560GKIT is more sensitive to Imatinib (STI571) compared with wild-type c-KIT whereas the kinase domain mutant D816VKIT is resistant. Mol Cancer Ther 2002; 1: 1115–24.
129. Tefferi A, Pardanani A. Systemic mastocytosis: current concepts and treatment advances. Curr Hematol Rep 2004; 3: 197–202.
130. Tefferi A, Pardanani A. Imatinib therapy in clonal eosinophilic disorders, including systemic mastocytosis. Int J Hematol 2004; 79: 441–7.
131. Tefferi A, Pardanani A. Clinical, genetic, and therapeutic insights into systemic mast cell disease. Curr Opin Hematol 2004; 11: 58–64.

132. Pardanani A, Reeder T, Porrata LF et al. Imatinib therapy for hypereosinophilic syndrome and other eosinophilic disorders. Blood 2003; 101: 3391–7.
133. Pitini V, Arrigo C, Azzarello D et al. Serum concentration of cardiac Troponin T in patients with hypereosinophilic syndrome treated with imatinib is predictive of adverse outcomes. Blood 2003; 102: 3456–7; author reply 3457.
134. Ma Y, Zeng S, Metcalfe DD et al. The c-KIT mutation causing human mastocytosis is resistant to STI571 and other KIT kinase inhibitors; kinases with enzymatic site mutations show different inhibitor sensitivity profiles than wild-type kinases and those with regulatory-type mutations. Blood 2002; 99: 1741–4.
135. Akin C, Brockow K, D'Ambrosio C et al. Effects of tyrosine kinase inhibitor STI571 on human mast cells bearing wild-type or mutated c-KIT. Exp Hematol 2003; 31: 686–92.
136. Pardanani A, Elliott M, Reeder T et al. Imatinib for systemic mast-cell disease. Lancet 2003; 362: 535–6.
137. Musto P, Falcone A, Sanpaolo G et al. Inefficacy of imatinib-mesylate in sporadic, aggressive systemic mastocytosis. Leuk Res 2004; 28: 421–2.
138. Mol CD, Dougan DR, Schneider TR et al. Structural basis for the autoinhibition and STI-571 inhibition of c-KIT tyrosine kinase. J Biol Chem 2004; 279: 31655–63.
139. Pardanani AD, Elliott MA, Reeder TL et al. Imatinib therapy for systemic mast cell disease. Lancet 2003; 362: 535–6.
140. Weisberg E, Boulton C, Kelly LM et al. Inhibition of mutant FLT3 receptors in leukemia cells by the small molecule tyrosine kinase inhibitor PKC412. Cancer Cell 2002; 1: 433–43.
141. Fabbro D, Ruetz S, Bodis S et al. PKC412 – a protein kinase inhibitor with a broad therapeutic potential. Anticancer Drug Des 2000; 15: 17–28.
142. Gleixner KV, Mayerhofer M, Aichberger KJ et al. PKC412 inhibits in vitro growth of neoplastic human mast cells expressing the D816V-mutated variant of KIT: comparison with AMN107, imatinib, and cladribine (2CdA) and evaluation of cooperative drug effects. Blood 2006; 107: 752–9.
143. Growney JD, Clark JJ, Adelsperger J et al. Activation mutations of human c-KIT resistant to imatinib mesylate are sensitive to the tyrosine kinase inhibitor PKC412. Blood 2005; 106: 721–4.
144. Gotlib J, Berube C, Growney JD et al. Activity of the tyrosine kinase inhibitor PKC412 in a patient with mast cell leukemia with the D816V KIT mutation. Blood 2005; 106: 2865–70.
145. Gotlib J, George TI, Linder A et al. Phase II trial of the tyrosine kinase inhibitor PKC412 in advanced systemic mastocytosis: Preliminary results. Blood (ASH Annual Meeting Abstracts) 2006; 108, abstract 3609.
146. Stone RM, DeAngelo DJ, Klimek V et al. Patients with acute myeloid leukemia and an activating mutation in FLT3 respond to a small-molecule FLT3 tyrosine kinase inhibitor, PKC412. Blood 2005; 105: 54–60.
147. Chen J, Deangelo DJ, Kutok JL et al. PKC412 inhibits the zinc finger 198-fibroblast growth factor receptor 1 fusion tyrosine kinase and is active in treatment of stem cell myeloproliferative disorder. Proc Natl Acad Sci U S A 2004; 101: 14479–84.
148. Shah NP, Tran C, Lee FY et al. Overriding imatinib resistance with a novel ABL kinase inhibitor. Science 2004; 305: 399–401.
149. Shah NP, Lee FY, Luo R et al. Dasatinib (BMS-354825) inhibits KIT^{D816V}, an imatinib-resistant activating mutation that triggers neoplastic growth in the majority of patients with systemic mastocytosis. Blood 2006; 108: 286–91.
150. Schittenhelm MM, Shiraga S, Schroeder A et al. Dasatinib (BMS-354825), a dual SRC/ABL kinase inhibitor, inhibits the kinase activity of wild-type, juxtamembrane, and activation loop mutant KIT isoforms associated with human malignancies. Cancer Res 2006; 66: 473–81.
151. Lombardo LJ, Lee FY, Chen P et al. Discovery of N-(2-chloro-6-methyl-phenyl)-2-(6-(4-(2-hydroxyethyl)-piperazin-1-yl)-2-methylpyrimidin-4-ylamino)thiazole-5-carboxamide (BMS-354825), a dual Src/Abl kinase inhibitor with potent antitumor activity in preclinical assays. J Med Chem 2004; 47: 6658–61.
152. Tokarski JS, Newitt JA, Chang CY et al. The structure of Dasatinib (BMS-354825) bound to activated ABL kinase domain elucidates its inhibitory activity against imatinib-resistant ABL mutants. Cancer Res 2006; 66: 5790–7.
153. Verstovsek S, Kantarjian H, Cortes J et al. Dasatinib (Sprycel) therapy for patients with systemic mastocytosis. Blood (ASH Annual Meeting Abstracts) 2006; 108, abstract 3627.
154. Fumo G, Akin C, Metcalfe DD et al. 17-Allylamino-17-demethoxygeldanamycin (17-AAG) is effective in down-regulating mutated, constitutively activated KIT protein in human mast cells. Blood 2004; 103: 1078–84.

Polycythemia vera

14

Tiziano Barbui, Guido Finazzi

Polycythemia vera (PV) is characterized by clonal proliferation of bone marrow progenitors leading to abnormal production of erythroid cell line that is independent of physiological growth factor erythropoietin (EPO). This notion led investigators to examine downstream receptors events and pathogenesis. The diagnosis of this disease has advanced considerably with the recent discovery of acquired mutations of Janus kinase 2 (*JAK2*) gene in the vast majority of patients.[1–6]

Early studies in untreated patients found a high incidence of thrombotic events and a life expectancy of about 18 months after diagnosis.[7] Cytoreductive treatments of blood hyperviscosity by phlebotomy or chemotherapy as well as antithrombotic therapy have been shown to dramatically reduce the number of vascular events, though hematological transformations to post-polycythemic myelofibrosis (MF) and acute leukemia still represent a major cause of death.[8]

In this chapter, we undertake a short review of the seminal studies contributing to the status quo up to the year 2000; challenges and unanswered questions at the beginning of this century; and discuss the most recent developments in the current state-of-the-art and some speculations for the future.

SEMINAL STUDIES UP TO THE YEAR 2000

Pathogenesis

Clonality and EPO independence of erythroid colonies are the defining features of PV and the necessary background for appreciating the clinical significance of the discovery of *JAK2* mutations.

The original studies of clonality in PV used a rare polymorphism in the glucose-6-phosphate dehydrogenase *(G6PD)* gene that gives rise to identifiably distinct protein products. Red blood cells, platelets, granulocytes, and bone marrow buffy coat showed predominant expression of a single allele, whereas both alleles were expressed in skin or bone marrow fibroblasts.[9] Then, clonality assays underwent progressive refinement to be useful in a larger proportion of patients and to truly reflect X-chromosome inactivation of genes. Some investigators differentiated between the active and inactive X-chromosomes by examining the methylation status of various genes such as the human androgen receptor gene (*HUMARA*).[10] Other groups developed a method based on direct measurement of X-chromosome mRNA transcripts so as to truly differentiate between genes located on the active versus inactive X-chromosome.[11] Using these approaches, >90% of informative females with the full PV phenotype showed clonal reticulocytes, granulocytes, platelets, and, at times, B lymphocytes.[12]

In 1974 the key observation was made that cultures of PV bone marrow cells yielded *in vitro* erythroid colonies even when no exogenous EPO was added to the culture media.[13] These have been termed endogenous (or EPO-independent) erythroid colonies (EEC). It was subsequently shown that the EEC from a given patient all expressed the same G6PD allele, and that this was the same allele that was expressed in granulocytes and platelets.[14] By contrast, colonies grown in the presence of added EPO were mixed, with some colonies expressing one parental G6PD allele and the remainder expressing the other.[14] Several studies showed that EEC provided a useful diagnostic tool and were found in almost all PV patients.[15,16] However, the mechanism(s) responsible for EEC remained obscure. An important clue was the reported hypersensitivity of PV progenitors to several different growth factors including stem cell factor (SCF), interleukin-3 (IL-3), granulocyte-monocyte colony-stimulating factor (GM-CSF), and insulin-like growth factor-1 (IGF-1).[17,18] These findings were consistent with a model in which the acquired pathogenetic lesion in PV was not restricted to the EPO receptor molecule. Thus, the search for a defect in a downstream signal transduction pathway common to multiple different receptors was started.

Diagnosis

The Polycythemia Vera Study Group (PVSG) was the first to formulate a set of diagnostic criteria for PV,[19] initially aimed at enrolling a uniform patient population with overt disease for studies on therapeutic intervention. Consequently, if these stringent criteria are adopted, patients in the initial stages of the disease may be excluded from this diagnosis. For such individuals, more specific techniques including cytogenetic studies, endogenous colony formation, and serum EPO assay were developed.[20] A revision of the PVSG criteria that also takes into account these latter findings was proposed by the WHO and is reported in Table 14.1.[21] The WHO retained the PVSG concept of distinguishing major and minor diagnostic criteria but it should be recognized that robust tools for the diagnosis of PV were still lacking. The available tests were expensive, not universally available, and lacking in sensitivity and specificity. This uncomfortable situation prompted several investigators to look for a molecular diagnostic marker.

Table 14.1 World Health Organization criteria for polycythemia vera[21]

Major criteria
Elevated red cell mass >25% above mean normal predicted value, or hemoglobin >18.5 g/dl in men, 16.5 g/dl in women, or >99th centile of method-specific reference range for age, sex, and altitude of residence
No cause of secondary erythrocytosis, including:
absence of familial erythrocytosis
no elevation of erythropoietin owing to:
hypoxia (arterial pO_2 ≤92%)
high oxygen affinity hemoglobin
truncated erythropoietin receptor
inappropriate erythropoietin production by tumor
Splenomegaly
Clonal genetic abnormality other than Philadelphia chromosome or *BCR-ABL* fusion gene in marrow cells
Endogenous erythroid colony formation *in vitro*
Minor criteria
Thrombocytosis $>400\times10^9$/l
Leukocytosis $>12\times10^9$/l
Bone marrow biopsy showing panmyelosis with prominent erythroid and megakaryocytic proliferation
Low serum erythropoietin levels

Diagnosis requires the presence of the first two major criteria together with either any one other major criterion or two minor criteria.

The first molecular marker described for PV was a reduced expression of the thrombopoietin (TPO) receptor, c-Mpl. Moliterno *et al.*[22] reported that c-Mpl expression was markedly reduced on platelets of 34 of 34 PV patients as well as 13 of 14 MF patients but not in patients with chronic myeloid leukenia (CML) or secondary erythrocytosis (SE). These authors also demonstrated the feasibility of using Western blotting to quantify c-Mpl protein for the diagnosis of PV: in a cohort of 27 PV and 19 SE patients, this assay showed a sensitivity of 96% and a specificity of 95% for the distinction of PV from SE.[23] However, these promising findings were not confirmed by other studies.[24] Technical differences may in large part account for the discrepancies, emphasizing the logistic difficulties involved in using Western blotting as a diagnostic tool. Soon after, another molecular marker of PV was proposed, that is quantification of polycythemia rubra vera-1 (PRV-1) receptor.[25] The PRV-1 mRNA was found to be 8- to 64-fold overexpressed in granulocytes from PV patients compared with patients with SE and healthy controls. A quantitative reverse transcriptase polymerase chain reaction (RT-PCR) assay was developed and validation of this assay on 48 PV patients, 34 healthy controls, and eight patients with SE revealed a sensitivity and specificity of 100%.[26] Further experiences with this assay were less favorable[27,28] and its current role in the diagnosis of PV is marginal, if any.[20] Nevertheless, the way was opened for a molecularly based identification of the disease.

Therapy

The modern therapy of PV started with the PVSG studies. In the first trial,[19] 431 patients were randomized to one of the following treatments: phlebotomy alone, radiophosphorus (^{32}P) plus phlebotomy, and chlorambucil plus phlebotomy. Patients treated with phlebotomy alone had a better median survival time (13.9 years) than those receiving ^{32}P (11.8 years) or chlorambucil (8.9 years). Causes of death were different in the three groups. Phlebotomized patients showed an excess of mortality within the first 2–4 years, principally caused by thrombotic complications. Those in the two myelosuppression arms suffered higher rates of acute leukemia and other malignancies developing later during the follow-up. The incidence of MF was virtually identical in the three arms.

In the late 1970s, the search for a nonmutagenic myelosuppressive agent led the PVSG to investigate hydroxyurea, an antimetabolite that prevents DNA synthesis by inhibiting the enzyme ribonucleoside reductase. At that time, it was assumed that this agent would not be leukemogenic or carcinogenic. In the 1997 PVSG report,[29] 51 PV patients treated with hydroxyurea were followed for a median and maximum of 8.6 and 15.3 years, respectively. The incidence of acute leukemia, myelofibrosis, and death were compared with the incidence in 134 patients treated only with phlebotomy in the PVSG-01 protocol. There were no significant differences in any of the three parameters, although the hydroxyurea group showed a tendency to more acute leukemias (9.8% versus 3.7%), less myelofibrosis (7.8% versus 12.7%), and fewer total deaths (39.2% versus 55.2%).

Based on these studies, the PVSG produced the following recommendations. Phlebotomy was suggested in all patients to keep the hematocrit below 0.45. Stable patients at low risk for thrombosis (age <60 years, no history of thrombosis) might not require additional therapy. In patients at high risk of thrombosis or with a very high phlebotomy requirement or progressive splenomegaly, the choice of a myelosuppressive agent was age adapted. Older patients could be managed with ^{32}P, busulfan, or pipobroman, whereas hydroxyurea was considered the agent of choice in younger patients.

In a small nandomized controlled trial, the PVSG evaluated the role of aspirin in PV.[30] A group of 166 patients were randomly assigned to the combination of high-dose aspirin (900 mg daily) plus phlebotomy and dypiridamole versus ^{32}P. The trial was stopped because of an excess of major bleeding without the demonstration of efficacy in thrombosis prevention. This study had a significant impact on clinical practice: in a recent survey among American physicians it was reported that the use of aspirin was reserved to a minority of PV patients owing to the concern of safety.[31]

CHALLENGES AT THE BEGINNING OF THIS CENTURY

Factors to be determined include:

(1) Pathogenic mechanism(s) underlying clonal and EPO-independent hematopoiesis in PV;
(2) Molecular markers of the disease to be used as a sound diagnostic tool;

(3) Impact of the therapeutic PVSG recommendations on survival and major clinical complications;
(4) Efficacy and safety of low-dose aspirin in preventing thrombosis.

IMPORTANT DEVELOPMENTS SINCE THE YEAR 2000

Pathogenesis

One approach to identifying genetic mutations associated with PV was to screen PV patients using microsatellite markers and search for loss of heterozygosity. Loss of heterozygosity signifies loss of an allele in a gene pair. Using this approach, loss of heterozygosity in the short arm of chromosome 9 was found in six of 20 PV patients screened.[32] This finding provided a starting point for later investigators, who more closely examined the short arm of chromosome 9 for pathogenic mutations.

A second approach relied on the loss of erythropoietic functions owing to various inhibitors. EPO exerts its effect on erythropoiesis through the EPO receptor. Binding of EPO to the homodimer receptor results in a conformational change with consequent phosphorylation and activation of JAK2. The activated JAK2 then initiates a cascade of intracellular signalling promoting erythroid proliferation and differentiation. A role for JAK2 in the pathogenesis of PV was first suggested by experiments in which inhibition of the JAK2 pathway by a short inhibitory RNA prevented the formation of EPO-independent colonies and the erythroid differentiation of PV cells.[33] These experiments prompted a closer examination of the *JAK2* gene for any mutations.

Using either loss of heterozygosity or function strategies to screen for genetic mutations, in 2005 several groups of investigators described the V617F mutation.[1–6] JAK2 V617F, resulting from a G to T somatic mutation at nucleotide 1849 in exon 14, causes the substitution of valine with phenylalanine at position 617 of the JAK2 protein. This residue is located in the JH2, or pseudokinase, domain, which negatively regulates the kinase domain. This change in a single amino acid renders the JAK2 enzyme constitutively active. Biochemical studies have shown that the *JAK2* V617F mutation causes cytokine-independent activation of JAK-STAT and other pathways, all of which are implicated in intracellular EPO-receptor signaling.[1,2,5]

In mice, *JAK2* V617F induces a PV-like disease with erythrocytosis, low serum EPO level, splenomegaly, extramedullary hematopoiesis, granulocytosis, megakaryocytic hyperplasia, and delayed-onset bone marrow fibrosis and anemia.[1] Primary blood and spleen cells from mice with *JAK2* V617F-induced 'PV' display constitutive STAT5 activation and endogenous and EPO-hypersensitive erythroid colony formation.[34]

In man, the mutation occurs in about 95% of patients with PV and in approximately 50% of those with essential thrombocythemia (ET) and primary myelofibrosis.[1–6] Conversely, *JAK2* V617F was found in <3% of *de novo* patients with myelodysplastic syndrome or acute myeloid leukemia and is virtually absent in patients with chronic myeloid leukemia.[35] Interestingly, the remaining 5% of patients with V617F-negative PV may have other *JAK2* mutations with functional effects similar to those of V617F. Scott *et al.* have recently described four in-frame deletions or tandem point mutations in exon 12 of the *JAK2* gene.[36] As for V617F, the exon 12 *JAK2* mutations induce cytokine-independent proliferation of cell lines that express EPO receptor and cause these cells to become hypersensitive to cytokines.

Overall, the V617F (and exon 12) *JAK2* mutations provide a unifying explanation for many features of the myeloproliferative disorders and are now regarded as a major breakthrough in the understanding of the pathogenesis of these disorders and as a target for the development of new treatments.[37,38] However, it is becoming increasingly evident that *JAK2* mutations are not an essential component for MPD other than PV and might not be the initial clonogenic event even in PV.[39]

Future studies should be addressed to identify the molecular mechanism(s) underlying *JAK2*-negative ET and MF and to establish whether cooperating mutations occur at an early stage of *JAK2*-positive MPD even predating the *JAK2* mutation.

Diagnosis

The discovery of *JAK2* mutations provides an excellent molecular marker for the diagnosis of PV, since virtually all patients with PV carry *JAK2* mutations, whereas those with secondary polycythemia do not. Testing for the *JAK2* V617F mutation is now widely available and allows simplification of the diagnostic work-up.

Allele-specific PCR assay, pyrosequencing, restriction-enzyme digestion, and real-time PCR are all sufficiently sensitive to detect the presence of heterozygous mutation in as few as 5–10% of cells.[37] These assays have low false-positive rates, making them useful diagnostic tools. However, it should be recognized that the current *JAK2*-mutation screening tests are not standardized and quality control is not guaranteed, so that molecular testing should not be substituted for sound clinical judgment.[40] It is important to consider not only that highly sensitive assays can detect low levels of *JAK2* V617F in healthy people, but also that inadequately sensitive assays lead to false-negative results in patients with a low allele burden.[40] In general, quantitative PCR assays are preferred, because they enable accurate assessment of allele burden as well as molecular monitoring of treatment response and residual disease.

Recently, the WHO's committee on hematological cancers revised the diagnostic criteria for diagnosis of PV including information on *JAK2* mutations, as outlined in Table 14.2.[41] Most of the previous major and minor WHO criteria (Table 14.1) were considered no longer necessary and replaced by adding 'presence of *JAK2* V617F or other functionally similar *JAK2* mutation' as a major criterion (Table 14.2). Accordingly, two 'major' criteria have been proposed: laboratory evidence of increased hemoglobin, hematocrit, or red cell mass (RCM); and the presence of a *JAK2* mutation.

Similarly, three biologically relevant 'minor' criteria have been suggested: MPD-consistent bone marrow histology; decreased serum erythropoietin level; and presence of endogenous erythroid colonies. Diagnosis of PV under the new proposed criteria will require either the presence of both major criteria and at least one minor criterion or the presence of the first major criterion and at least two minor criteria (Table 14.2).

In the first major criterion, a documented increase of hemoglobin or hematocrit has been added to help bypass the need for

Table 14.2 Proposed revised World Health Organization criteria for polycythemia vera.[41] Diagnosis requires the presence of both major criteria and one minor criterion *or* the presence of the first major criterion together with two minor criteria

Major criteria
Hemoglobin >18.5 g/dl in men, 16.5 g/dl in women *or* another evidence of increased red cell volume*
Presence of *JAK2* V617F or other functionally similar mutation such as *JAK2* exon 12 mutation
Minor criteria
Bone marrow biopsy showing hypercellularity with trilineage hyperplasia (panmyelosis) with prominent erythroid, granulocytic, and megakaryocytic proliferation
Low serum erythropoietin level
Endogenous erythroid colony formation *in vitro*

*Hemoglobin or hematocrit >99th centile of method-specific reference range for age, sex, and altitude of residence, or hemoglobin >17 g/dl in men, 15 g/dl in women if associated with a documented and sustained increase of at least 2 g/dl from an individual's baseline value that cannot be attributed to correction of iron deficiency, *or* elevated red cell mass >25% above mean normal predicted value.

RCM measurement. This assay is a technically demanding procedure that is difficult to standardize and many laboratories have greatly reduced or abandoned the test.[20] Nevertheless, the diagnostic relevance of RCM measurement is still a matter of debate[20,42] and it was considered wise, for the moment, to maintain this test in the revised criteria.

Other proposals for diagnosis of PV including *JAK2* mutations have been put forward.[38] Which of these diagnostic combinations will become the standard of practice is a challenge for the future.

Therapy

European Collaboration on Low-dose Aspirin in Polycythemia Vera study

The long-term effect of the management recommendations proposed by the PVSG investigators, as well as the role of low-dose aspirin in the prevention of thrombosis in PV patients, have been investigated in a large, prospective collaborative study carried out in Europe called European Collaboration on Low-dose Aspirin in Polycythemia Vera (ECLAP).[8,43]

General design

The ECLAP study included a network of 94 hematological centers from 12 countries and an international coordinating center in Italy (Consorzio Mario Negri Sud). Overall, 1638 PV patients were included in the study. In all, 518 (32%) of these patients were entered into a parallel, double-blind, placebo-controlled, randomized clinical trial aimed at assessing the efficacy and safety of low-dose aspirin.[43] The remaining 1120 (68%) were registered into an observational, prospective, cohort study.[8] The main reasons for excluding the patients from the randomized trial were the need for antithrombotic therapy (66%), contraindication to aspirin (24%), and patients' unwillingness (18%).

Diagnosis of PV was based upon the criteria established by the PVSG[19] and patients were asked to adhere to the treatment recommended by the hematologist in charge of their care. The procedures in the study were planned to mimic the routine care of patients with PV. Data collection was specifically recorded at follow-up visits at 12, 24, 36, 48, and 60 months, respectively. The mean duration of follow-up was 2.7 years (0–5.3 years).

The main outcome measures were fatal, major, and minor thrombosis. Major thrombosis included cerebral ischemic stroke, myocardial infarction, peripheral arterial thrombosis, and venous thromboembolism. All fatal and major events were objectively documented and validated by an ad-hoc committee of expert clinicians blinded to patients' treatment assignment. Hematological evolution to myelofibrosis or acute leukemia and overall mortality were also evaluated. Standard statistical methods were used for analysis.

Clinical course of patients

Of the 1638 enrolled patients 35% had been newly diagnosed or diagnosed in the 2 years before registration, whereas in 27% and 38% of cases the diagnosis of PV had been made between 2 and 5 years, and more than 5 years prior to registration, respectively. Median age at diagnosis and at registration was 60 and 65 years, respectively. Thrombotic events before registration were documented in 633 (38.4%) cases. The median duration of follow-up from registration was 2.8 years (range 0–5.3 years) and the median time elapsed from diagnosis was 6.3 years (range 1–18 years). Overall mortality during follow-up was 3.5 deaths/100 persons per year. As compared with the general Italian population standardized for age and sex, the excess of mortality of PV patients was 2.1 times. Cardiovascular events, hematological transformation (mainly acute leukemia), and major bleeding were responsible for 41%, 13% and 4% of deaths, respectively.

During follow-up, non-fatal major thromboses were observed in 122 patients (7.4%), of which 87 were arterial (53 cerebral ischemia, 14 acute myocardial infarction, and 20 peripheral arterial thrombosis) and 50 (3%) were venous. Progression to MF occurred in

38 patients (2.3%), with an incidence rate of approximately 1% per patient-year. Transformation in acute leukemia during 2.7 years follow-up was registered in 22 cases (1.3%) with a median time lapse from diagnosis of 6.3 years.

Risk stratification

In the ECLAP study, the incidence of cardiovascular complications was higher in patients aged more than 65 years (5.0% per patient-year, hazard ratio 2.0, 95% confidence interval (CI) 1.22–3.29, $p<0.006$) or with a history of thrombosis (4.93% per patient-year, hazard ratio 1.96, 95% CI 1.29–2.97, $p = 0.0017$) than in younger subjects with no history of thrombosis (2.5% per patient-year, reference category). Patients with both a history of thrombosis and age >65 years had the highest risk of cardiovascular events during follow-up (10.9% per patient-year, hazard ratio 4.35, 95% CI 2.95–6.41, $p<0.0001$). These data confirm previous findings that increasing age and a history of thrombosis are the two most important prognostic factors for the development of vascular complications.[19] Other significant predictors of survival and cardiovascular morbidity were smoking, diabetes mellitus, and congestive heart failure.

In a more recent re-evaluation of the predictors of thrombosis in the patients enrolled in the ECLAP study, a relevant role for the white blood cell (WBC) count has been reported. Patients with a WBC count $>15 \times 10^9$/l, compared with those with a WBC count $<10 \times 10^9$/l, had a significant increase in the risk of thrombosis (hazard ratio 1.71, 95% CI 1.10–2.65, $p = 0.017$), mainly deriving from an increased risk of myocardial infarction (hazard ratio 2.84, 95% CI 1.25–6.46, $p = 0.013$).[44] This finding has been confirmed also in patients with ET.[45,46]

Overall, patients with PV should be stratified into different risk categories on the basis of their probability of developing thrombotic complications. Young age and no prior thrombosis define a low-risk category, whereas age >65 years or prior thrombosis define a 'high-risk' category. This classification forms the rationale for a risk-adapted therapy.[47]

The aspirin trial

The efficacy and safety of low-dose aspirin (100 mg daily) has been formally assessed in a nested double-blind, placebo-controlled, randomized clinical trial carried out in the frame of the ECLAP project.[43] A total of 518 patients (32% of the total ECLAP study population) without a clear indication or contraindication to aspirin were enrolled. Median age at recruitment was 61 years and 59% of patients were males. Previous cardiovascular events were reported in only 10% of cases, so that this trial included mainly an asymptomatic, low-risk population. Median follow-up was 2.8 years. Aspirin lowered significantly the risk of a primary combined end-point including cardiovascular death, non-fatal myocardial infarction, non-fatal stroke, and major venous thromboembolism (relative risk 0.4, 95% CI 0.18–0.91, $p = 0.0277$). Total and cardiovascular mortality were also reduced by 46% and 59%, respectively. Major bleeding was only slightly increased by aspirin (relative risk 1.6, 95% CI 0.27–9.71). Thus, the results of this trial have eliminated the concern raised by the PVSG about the benefit–risk ratio of aspirin in PV.

In other studies, aspirin at different doses (30–500 mg/day) has been found to control microvascular symptoms, such as erythromelalgia, and transient neurological and ocular disturbances including dysarthria, hemiparesis, scintillating scotomas, amaurosis fugax, migraine, and seizures.[48]

Current treatment recommendations (Figure 14.1)

Based on the PVSG seminal randomized controlled trial,[19] phlebotomy is recommended in all patients with PV and should represent the only cytoreductive treatment in patients at low-risk for vascular complications. The target hematocrit of 45% in males and 42% in females was suggested by this study group,

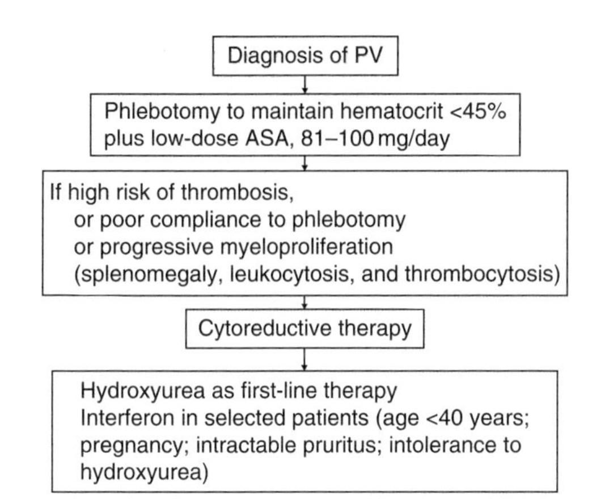

Figure 14.1 Flow-chart of recommended treatment for patients with polycythemia vera (PV).

although not supported by solid data. This recommendation was taken by Pearson and Wetherley-Main,[49] who showed in univariate analysis a correlation between thrombosis and hematocrit when this was >45%. In the ECLAP study, despite the recommendation of maintaining the hematocrit values at <45%, only 48% of patients had hematocrit values below this threshold, while 39% and 13% had values between 45% and 50% and >50%, respectively, and no correlation was found between hematocrit level and thrombotic complications or mortality.[50] Thus, an appropriate controlled study to establish the real hematocrit target in PV is needed.

Given the results of the ECLAP trial,[43] low-dose aspirin (100 mg daily) is recommended in all PV patients without a history of major bleeding, gastric intolerance, or extreme values of thrombocytosis. However, previous gastrointestinal bleeding is not an absolute contraindication to the prophylactic use of aspirin since the use of proton pump inhibitors may overcome the risk of gastric bleeding owing to aspirin.[51]

Hydroxyurea

Hydroxyurea is highly effective in patients with myeloproliferative disorders (MPD) at high risk of thrombosis and should be considered as first-line therapy; however, concerns regarding its leukemogenic potential should be carefully considered.[52–54]

To date there are no randomized studies with sufficient power to assess the relative risk of malignant transformation in MPD patients given hydroxyurea. These disorders have an inherent tendency to evolve into acute leukemia, even in the absence of specific therapy. Thus, studies that enrolled patients in need of therapy automatically selected patients with more active disease and a higher propensity to malignant transformation. Furthermore, leukemic transformation occurs after a lead time of several years and only long-term studies with a large number of patients are suitable to assess this issue.[55]

The 1638 patients prospectively enrolled in the ECLAP study, with a median disease duration of 6.3 years, represent an appropriate population to reach this goal. In a recent analysis of the leukemogenic risk in these patients, hydroxyurea alone did not enhance the risk of leukemia in comparison with patients treated with phlebotomy only (hazard ratio 0.86, 95% CI 0.26–2.88, $p=0.8$).[56] During the same period, the risk was significantly increased by exposure to radiophosphorus, busulfan or pipobroman (hazard ratio 5.46, 95% CI 1.84–16.25, $p=0.002$). The use of hydroxyurea in patients already treated with alkylating agents or radiophosphorus also enhanced the leukemic risk (hazard ratio 7.58, 95% CI 1.85–31, $p=0.0048$) and this was seen also in ET.[56,57]

Thus, the bulk of evidence does not support a leukemogenic risk for hydroxyurea but the debate on whether acute leukemia is part of the natural history of PV or is a consequence of therapy is still matter of discussion. It is wise to adopt a cautionary principle and to consider carefully the use of this agent in young subjects and in those previously treated with other myelosuppressive agents or carrying cytogenetic abnormalities.

Interferon alfa

The use of interferon alfa (IFNα) in PV was pioneered by Silver.[58] IFNα suppresses the proliferation of hematopoietic progenitors, has a direct inhibiting effect on bone marrow fibroblast progenitor cells, and antagonizes the action of platelet-derived growth factor, transforming growth factor-β and other cytokines, which may be involved in the development of myelofibrosis.[59]

Published reports concern small consecutive series of patients in whom hematological response and side-effects were evaluated. One review analyzed the cumulative experience with IFNα in 279 patients from 16 studies.[60] Overall responses were 50% for reduction of hematcrit to <0.45% without concomitant phlebotomies, 77% for reduction in spleen size, and 75% for reduction of pruritus. Results from single-institution studies with long-term follow-up were similar.[61,62]

In a review article, Silver updated his experience on the long-term use (median 13 years) of IFNα in 55 patients with PV.[63] Complete responses, defined by phlebotomy free, hematocrit <45%, and platelet number below 600 000/μl, were reached in the great majority of cases after 1–2 years of treatment and the maintenance dose could be decreased in half of the patients. Noteworthy is the absence of thrombohemorrhagic events during this long follow-up.

The main problem with IFNα therapy, apart from its costs and parenteral route of administration, is the incidence of side-effects. Fever and flu-like symptoms are experienced by most patients and usually require treatment with paracetamol. Signs of chronic IFNα toxicity, such as weakness, myalgia, weight and hair loss, severe depression, and gastrointestinal and cardiovascular symptoms, make it necessary to discontinue the drug in about one-third of patients.[60] Overall, the role of IFNα in PV therapy requires controlled clinical trials evaluating long-term clinical endpoints.

Future scenarios

The description of the V617F point mutation in the JAK2 kinase of patients with PV has generated great interest in determining if patients would be sensitive to small molecular agents specific to the pseudokinase domain of JAK2 or to other tyrosine kinase inhibitors.

Pilot clinical studies have explored whether imatinib may have a role in PV. Silver *et al.* have reported responses in a small group of PV patients at doses up to 800 mg/day.[64] Imatinib was effective in reducing phlebotomy requirements, lowering abnormal platelet counts, and reducing spleen size. The relation of imatinib treatment and *JAK2* mutation was evaluated by Jones *et al.* in nine PV patients for whom pretreatment samples were available.[65] They reported two cases who achieved complete hematological remission and a 2–3-fold reduction in the percentage of V617F alleles. However, the clinical experience with this drug is still very limited and we do not recommend imatinib for the current treatment of patients with PV.

Recently, semisynthetic pegylated forms of IFNα (peg-IFNα) have been used to treat MPD, which in a limited number of studies have been shown to be superior to unmodified IFN as related to its adverse event profile and efficacy.[66] In one study, the use of peg-IFNα-2a was able to decrease the percentage of mutated JAK2 allele in 24 of 27 treated PV patients from a mean of 49% to a mean of 27%.[67] A more limited effect of other forms of peg-IFNα-2b on *JAK2* mutational status has been reported.[68,69] Further studies are needed to establish whether the reduction of *JAK2* V617F allele burden is clinically relevant and whether its monitoring during therapy is of any value.

A series of more specific *JAK2* V617F inhibitors with promising potency and pharmaceutical properties for utility in the therapy of PV have been recently synthesized.[70–72] Preliminary data indicated that at least some of these small molecules inhibit cell growth that is dependent on constitutive JAK2/STAT signaling and preferentially suppress growth of progenitors carrying JAK-activating mutations, Thus, these drugs hold promise as molecularly targeted agents for the therapy of patients with PV.

REFERENCES

1. James C, Ugo V, Le Couedic JP et al. A unique clonal JAK2 mutation leading to constitutive signaling causes polycythemia vera. Nature 2005; 434: 1144–8.
2. Levine RL, Wadleigh M, Cools J et al. Activating mutation of the tyrosine kinase JAK2 in polycythemia vera, essential thrombocythemia, and myeloid metaplasia with myelofibrosis. Cancer Cell 2005; 7: 387–97.
3. Baxter EJ, Scott LM, Campbell PJ et al. Acquired mutation of the tyrosine kinase JAK2 in human myeloproliferative diseases. Lancet 2005; 365: 1054–61.
4. Kralovics R, Passamonti F, Buser AS et al. A gain-of-function mutation of JAK2 in myeloproliferative disorders. N Engl J Med 2005; 352: 1779–90.
5. Zhao R, Xing S, Li Z et al. Identification of an acquired JAK2 mutation in polycythemia vera. J Biol Chem 2005; 280: 22788–92.
6. Jones AV, Kreil S, Zoi K et al. Widespread occurrence of the JAK2 V617 mutation in chronic myeloproliferative disorders. Blood 2005; 106: 2162–8.
7. Chievitz E, Thiede T. Complications and causes of death in polycythemia vera. J Intern Med 1962; 2: 513–23.
8. Marchioli R, Finazzi G, Landolfi R et al. Vascular and neoplastic risk in a large cohort of patients with polycythemia vera. J Clin Oncol 2005; 23: 2224–32.
9. Adamson JW, Fialkow PJ, Murphy S et al. Polycythemia vera: stem cell and probable clonal origin of the disease. N Engl J Med 1976; 295: 913–16.
10. Gilliland DG, Blanchard KL, Levy J et al. Clonality in myeloproliferative disorders: analysis by means of the polymerase chain reaction. Proc Natl Acad Sci U S A 1991; 88: 6848–52.
11. Prchal JT, Guan YT, Prchal JF et al. Transcriptional analysis of the active X-chromosome in normal and clonal hematopoiesis. Blood 1993; 81: 269–71.
12. Liu E, Jelinek J, Pastore YD et al. Discrimination of polycythemias and thrombocytosis by novel, simple, accurate clonality assays and BFU-E response to erythropoietin. Blood 2003; 101: 3294–301.
13. Prchal JF, Axelrad AA. Bone marrow responses in polycythemia vera. N Engl J Med 1974; 290: 1382.
14. Bench AJ, Green AR, Huntly BJP et al. The cellular and genetic pathology of polycythemia vera. Hematology Am Soc Hematol Educ Progr Book 2000: 56–61.
15. Hinshelwood S, Bench AJ, Green AR. Pathogenesis of polycythemia vera. Blood Rev 1997; 11: 224–32.
16. Kralovics R, Prchal JT. Hematopoietic progenitors and signal transduction in polycythemia vera and essential thrombocythemia. Baillieres Clin Hematol 1998; 11: 803–18.
17. Dai CH, Krants SB, Green WF et al. Polycythemia vera III. Burst-forming units-erythroid (BFU-E) response to stem cell factor and c-kit receptor expression. Br J Haematol 1994; 86: 12–21.
18. Correa PN, Eskinazi D, Axelrad AA. Circulating erythroid progenitors in polycythemia vera are hypersensitive to insulin-like growth factor-1 in vitro: studies in an improved serum-free medium. Blood 1994; 83: 99–112.
19. Berk PD, Goldberg JD, Donovan PB et al. Therapeutic recommendations in polycythemia vera based on Polycythemia Vera Study Group protocols. Semin Hematol 1986; 23: 132–43.
20. Tefferi A. The diagnosis of polycythemia vera: new tests and old dictums. Best Pract Res Clin Hematol 2006; 19: 455–69.
21. Pierre R, Imbert M, Thiele J et al. Polycythaemia vera. In: Jaffe ES, Harris NL, Stein H, Vardiman JW, eds. World Health Organization Classification of Tumours. Pathology and Genetics of Tumours of Hematopoietic and Lymphoid Tissues. Lyon: IARC Press, 2001: 32–4.
22. Moliterno AR, Hankins D, Spivak JL. Impaired expression of the thrombopoietin receptor by platelets from patients with polycythemia vera. N Engl J Med 1998; 338: 572–80.
23. Moliterno AR, Silver RT, Spivak JL. A diagnostic assay for polycythemia vera. Blood 2000; 96: 512a.
24. Le Blanc K, Andersson P, Samuelsson J. Marked heterogeneity in protein levels and functional integrity of the thrombopoietin receptor c-mpl in polycythemia vera. Br J Haematol 2000; 108: 80–5.
25. Temerinac S, Klippel S, Strunck E et al. Cloning of PRV-1, a novel member of the uPAR receptor superfamily, which is overexpressed in polycythemia rubra vera. Blood 2000; 95: 2569–76.
26. Klippel S, Strunck E, Temerinac S et al. Quantification of PRV-1 expression, a molecular marker for the diagnosis of polycythemia vera. Blood 2001; 98: 470a.
27. Passamonti F, Pietra D, Malabarba L et al. Clinical significance of neutrophil CD177 mRNA expression in Ph-negative chronic myeloproliferative disorders. Br J Haematol 2004; 126: 650–6.
28. Zhang J, Pellagatti A, Campbell L et al. Neutrophil PRV-1 gene expression in myeloproliferative, myelodysplastic and reactive bleed disorders. Br J Haematol 2004; 125: 17a.
29. Fruchtman SM, Mack K, Kaplan ME et al. From efficacy to safety: a polycythemia vera study group report on hydroxyurea in patients with polycythemia vera. Semin Hematol 1997; 34: 17–23.
30. Tartaglia AP, Goldberg JD, Berk PD et al. Adverse effects of antiaggregating platelet therapy in the treatment of polycythemia vera. Semin Hematol 1986; 23: 172–6.
31. Streiff MB, Smith B, Spivak JL. The diagnosis and management of polycythemia vera in the era since the Polycythemia Vera Study Group: a survey of the American Society of Hematology members' practice patterns. Blood 2002; 99: 1144–9.

32. Kralovics R, Guan Y, Prchal JT. Acquired uniparental disomy of chromosome 9p is a frequent stem cell defect in polycythemia vera. Exp Hematol 2002; 30: 229–36.
33. Ugo V, Marzac C, Teyssandier I et al. Multiple signaling pathways are involved in erythropoietin-independent differentiation of erythroid progenitors in polycythemia vera. Exp Hematol 2004; 32: 179–87.
34. Wernig G, Mercher T, Okabe R et al. Expression of JAK2 V617F causes a polycythemia vera-like disease with associated myelofibrosis in a murine bone marrow transplant model. Blood 2006; 107: 4274–81.
35. Steensma DP, Dewald GW, Lasho TL et al. The JAK2 V617F activating tyrosine kinase mutation is an infrequent event both in "atypical" myeloproliferative disorders and myelodysplastic syndromes. Blood 2005; 106: 1207–9.
36. Scott LM, Tong W, Levine RL et al. JAK2 exon 12 mutations in polycythemia vera and idiopathic erythrocytosis. N Engl J Med 2007; 356: 459–68.
37. Tefferi A. Classification, diagnosis and management of myeloproliferative disorders in the JAK2 V617F era. Hematology Am Soc Hematol Educ Prog Book 2006: 240–5.
38. Campbell PJ, Green AR. The myeloproliferative disorders. N Engl J Med 2006; 355: 2452–66.
39. Nussenzveig RH, Swierczek SI, Jelinek J et al. Polycythemia vera is not initiated by JAK2V617F mutation. Exp Hematol 2007; 35: 32–8.
40. Tefferi A. JAK2 mutations in polycythemia vera – molecular mechanisms and clinical applications. N Engl J Med 365: 444–5.
41. Tefferi A, Thiele J, Orazi A et al. Proposals for revision of the World Health Organization diagnostic criteria for polycythemia vera, essential thrombocythemia, and primary myelofibrosis: from an ad hoc international expert panel. Blood 2007; 110: 1092–7.
42. Spivak JL. Polycythemia vera: myths, mechanisms and management. Blood 2002; 100: 4272–90.
43. Landolfi R, Marchioli R, Kutti J et al. Efficacy and safety of low-dose aspirin in polycythemia vera. N Engl J Med 2004; 350: 114–24.
44. Landolfi R, Di Gennaro L, Barbui T et al. Leukocytosis as a major thrombotic risk factor in patients with polycythemia vera. Blood 2007; 109: 2446–52.
45. Carobbio A, Finazzi G, Guerini V et al. Leukocytosis is a risk factor for thrombosis in essential thrombocythemia: interaction with treatment, standard risk factors and Jak 2 mutation status. Blood 2007; 109: 2310–13.
46. Wolanskyj AP, Schwager SM, McClure RF et al. Essential thrombocythemia beyond the first decade: life expectancy, long-term complication rates, and prognostic factors. Mayo Clin Proc 2006; 81: 159–66.
47. Finazzi G, Barbui T. How we treat patients with polycythemia vera. Blood 2007; 109: 6104–11.
48. Van Genderen PJJ, Prins F, Michiels JJ et al. Thromboxane-dependent platelet activation in vivo precedes arterial thrombosis in thrombocythaemia: a rationale for the use of low-dose aspirin as an antithrombotic agent. Br J Haematol 1999; 104: 438–41.
49. Pearson TC, Wetherley-Mein G. Vascular occlusive episodes and venous haematocrit in primary proliferative polycythaemia. Lancet 1978; 2: 1219–22.
50. Di Nisio M, Barbui T, Di Gennaro L et al. The haematocrit and platelet target in polycythemia vera. Br J Haematol 2007; 136: 249–59.
51. Patrono C, Garcia-Rodriguez LA, Landolfi R et al. Low-dose aspirin for the prevention of atherothrombosis. N Engl J Med 2005; 353: 2373–83.
52. Nand S, Stock W, Godwin J et al. Leukemogenic risk of hydroxyurea therapy in polycythemia vera, essential thrombocythemia and myeloid metaplasia with myelofibrosis. Am J Hematol 1996; 52: 42–6.
53. Sterkers Y, Preudhomme C, Lai J-L et al. Acute myeloid leukemia and myelodyslastic syndromes following essential thrombocythemia treated with hydroxyurea: high proportion of cases with 17p deletion. Blood 1998; 91: 616–22.
54. Hanft VN, Fruchtman SR, Pickens CV et al. Acquired DNA mutations associated with in vivo hydroxyurea exposure. Blood 2000; 95: 3589–93.
55. Marchioli R, Finazzi G, Marfisi RM et al. Clinical trials in myeloproliferative disorders: looking forward. Semin Hematol 2005; 42: 259–65.
56. Finazzi G, Caruso V, Marchioli R et al. Acute leukemia in polycythemia vera. An analysis of 1,638 patients enrolled in a prospective observational study. Blood 2005; 105: 2664–70.
57. Finazzi G, Ruggeri M, Rodeghiero F et al. Second malignancies in patients with essential thrombocythemia treated with busulphan and hydroxyurea: long-term follow-up of a randomized clinical trial. Br J Haematol 2000; 110: 577–83.
58. Silver RT. Interferon alpha2b: a new treatment for polycythemia vera. Ann Intern Med 1993; 119: 1091–2.
59. Martyre MC. Critical review of pathogenetic mechanisms in myelofibrosis with myeloid metaplasia. Curr Hematol Rep 2003; 2: 257–63.
60. Lengfelder E, Berger U, Hehlmann R. Interferon alpha in the treatment of polycythemia vera. Ann Hematol 2000; 79: 103–9.
61. Heis N, Rintelen C, Gisslinger B et al. The effect of interferon alpha on myeloproliferation and vascular complications in polycythemia vera. Eur J Haematol 1999; 62: 27–31.
62. Gilbert HS. Long term treatment of myeloproliferative disease with interferon alpha-2b: feasibility and efficacy. Cancer 1998; 83: 1205–13.
63. Silver RT. Long-term effects of the treatment of polycythemia vera with recombinant interferon-alpha. Cancer 2006; 107: 451–8.

64. Silver RT, Fruchtman SM, Feldman EJ et al. Imatinib mesylate (Gleevec) is effective in the treatment of polycythemia vera: a multi-institutional clinical trial. Blood 2004; 104: 89a.
65. Jones AV, Silver RT, Waghorn K et al. Minimal molecular response in polycythemia vera patients treated with imatinib or with interferon alpha. Blood 2006; 107: 3339–41.
66. Quintas-Cardama A, Kantarjian HM, Giles F et al. Pegylated interferon therapy for patients with Philadelphia chromosome-negative myeloproliferative disorders. Semin Thromb Hemost 2006; 32: 409–16.
67. Kiladjian JJ, Cassinat B, Turlure P et al. High molecular response rate of polycythemia vera patients treated with pegylated interferon alpha-2a. Blood 2006; 108: 2037–40.
68. Jones AV, Silver RT, Waghorn K et al. Minimal molecular response in polycythemia vera patients treated with imatinib or with interferon alpha. Blood 2006; 107: 3339–41.
69. Samuelsson J, Mutschler M, Birgegard G et al. Limited effects on JAK2 mutational status after pegylated interferon alpha-2b therapy in polycythemia vera and essential thrombocythemia. Haematologica 2006; 91: 1281–2.
70. Pardanani A, Hood J, Lasho T et al. TG101209, a selective JAK2 kinase inhibitor, suppressess endogenous and cytokine-supported colony formation from hematopoietic progenitors carrying JAK2V617F or MPLW515K/L mutations. Blood 2006; 108: 758a.
71. Gaikwad AS, Prchal JT. Efficacy of tyrosine kinase inhibitors in polycythemia vera. Blood 2006; 108: 762a.
72. Hood J, Cao J, Hanna E et al. JAK2 inhibitors for the treatment of myeloproliferative disorders. Blood 2006; 108: 1038a.

Chronic idiopathic myelofibrosis 15

Srdan Verstovsek, Jorge Cortes

INTRODUCTION

Myelofibrosis is a term that is applied to both clonal, primary disorders of the bone marrow and secondary, reactive processes. The disease phenotype that is currently referred to as chronic idiopathic myelofibrosis (CIMF) includes both *de novo* disease presentation (also referred to as myelofibrosis with myeloid metaplasia (MMM) or agnogenic myeloid metaplasia (AMM)), and disease developing in the setting of polycythemia vera (PV; post-polycythemic mylofibrosis, post-PV MF) or essential thrombocythemia (ET; post-thrombocythemic myelofibrosis, post-ET MF), usually at a rate 10–15% after 10–20 years of follow-up.[1] In either case it represents stem cell-derived clonal myeloproliferation that is accompanied by intense bone marrow stromal reaction including collagen fibrosis, osteosclerosis, and angiogenesis.[1] These entities have been recently reclassified and renamed by the International Working Group for Myelofibrosis Research and Treatment (IWG-MRT).[2] This group has recommended standardizing the nomenclature referring to CIMF and made the following suggestions: (1) the term primary myelofibrosis (PMF) should be used to refer to this entity, and is preferable to others such as CIMF, AMM, and MMM; (2) myelofibrosis that develops in the setting of either PV or ET should be referred to as post-PV MF and post-ET MF, respectively; and (3) 'leukemic' transformation should be referred to as blast phase (e.g. PMF-BP, post-PV/ET MF in blast phase). This nomenclature clarification is awaiting formal acceptance by the Steering Committee for Revisions of the World Health Organization (WHO) Classification of Hematopoietic and Lymphoid Neoplasms. In this chapter we refer to patients with myelofibrosis, whether primary or secondary, and to ET or PV, as patients with CIMF.

CLINICAL FEATURES

CIMF is a heterogeneous disorder with variable age of onset, presenting features, phenotypic manifestations, and prognosis. It is estimated that 701 patients were diagnosed with myelofibrosis in 2003 in the US, the only year for which statistics are available to date.[3] However, it is widely believed that this represents an underestimation of the actual incidence. The incidence increases with age, with the median age at diagnosis being 67 years,[4] although patients may present in the 3rd to 5th decades of life.[5] Average life expectancy is approximately 5–7 years, although younger patients with good prognostic features may have a life expectancy of 15 years or more.[4,5]

Clinical presentation of patients diagnosed with CIMF may range from being asymptomatic, with their disease discovered on investigation for occult causes of leukocytosis or splenomegaly, to being severely debilitating. Myeloproliferation is one of the major features of the disease and can lead to a spectrum of clinical problems ranging from asymptomatic mild leukocytosis and/or thrombocytosis to severe organ damage. Clinical consequences of myeloproliferation can lead to morbidity and mortality from either a direct effect owing to increases in circulating cells or indirectly owing to organ damage resulting from sequestration of immature cells and production of blood cells in sites other than the bone marrow, a phenomenon known as extramedullary hematopoiesis (EMH). This is commonly manifested as marked hepatosplenomegaly, with associated pain, early satiety, sequestration of erythrocytes and platelets, and portal hypertension.[6] In addition, non-hepatosplenic EMH might cause symptoms in various other organs including the lungs (e.g. respiratory distress and pulmonary hypertension), peritoneum (e.g. ascites), spine (e.g. paralysis), and pericardium (e.g. tamponade).[7] Current evidence suggests that sequestration of circulating myeloid progenitors is the underlying cause of EMH in CIMF.[8] Although most frequently leukocytosis by itself is asymptomatic, extreme elevations of leukocytes (i.e. $>100 \times 10^9/l$), particularly when a large percentage of them are immature (increasing myeloblasts as opposed to mature neutrophils), may be associated with leukostasis. This latter phenomenon is not common in CIMF and when it occurs is more likely in the setting of leukemic transformation. Thrombocytosis is more common and may lead to vascular events (i.e. thrombosis or bleeding).

Cytopenias of varying severity also are characteristic of CIMF and are frequently multifactorial. Anemia is the most common cytopenia resulting from factors such as ineffective hematopoiesis, decreased marrow reserve as a direct result of collagen fibrosis and osteosclerosis, splenic sequestration, myelosuppression owing to cytoreductive therapy, hemolysis, bleeding from the gastrointestinal tract including variceal bleeding, and occasionally coexistent deficiencies of iron, vitamin B_{12} or folate. Thrombocytopenia in CIMF might be secondary to ineffective hematopoiesis, splenic sequestration, and increased consumption from disseminated intravascular coagulation (DIC). Leukopenia occurs less frequently and is rarely severe.

Constitutional symptoms can be quite debilitating in CIMF and include significant fatigue, weight loss, night sweats, fever, and pruritus.[9] These symptoms can dominate the clinical presentation and frequently do not respond to most of the medical interventions currently being employed in the disorder.[1] It has been postulated that the constitutional symptoms may be caused at least in part to tumor necrosis factor-α (TNF-α). Interestingly, in a pilot study involving 22 patients with CIMF, treatment with etanercept (TNF-α antagonist) produced an improvement in constitutional symptoms in 60% of patients.[10]

Among the most feared complications of CIMF is leukemic transformation, occurring in 10–20% of patients in the first 10 years after diagnosis.[11] This transformation is nearly always to a myeloid phenotype, most frequently M7 (megakaryocytic). Cytogenetic abnormalities are identified in approximately 90% of patients at the time of transformation. The outcome after transformation is very poor, with a median survival of only approximately 3 months.[11] Other causes of death for patients with CIMF include infection, bleeding, organ failure, and portal hypertension.

PATHOGENETIC INSIGHTS AND NOVEL DIAGNOSTIC CRITERIA FOR CHRONIC IDIOPATHIC MYELOFIBROSIS

Approximately 30–50% of patients with CIMF have cytogenetic abnormalities identified.[12] The most frequently encountered cytogenetic abnormalities include 13q–, 20q–, trisomy 8, and abnormalities of chromosomes 1, 7, and 9. A recent study reported that those with no cytogenetic abnormalities and those with interstitial deletions of chromosomes 13 or 20 have a similar outcome, while those with other abnormalities have a significantly worse outcome.[13]

Until recently, the molecular underpinnings of *BCR-ABL*-negative myeloproliferative disorders (MPD) have remained elusive. However, several groups recently described almost simultaneously a novel activating somatic point mutation in the gene encoding the cytoplasmic Janus kinase 2 (JAK2), characterized by the replacement of valine by phenylalanine at codon 617 (*JAK2* V617F) in exon 14.[14] In these reports, this mutation was identified in 37–57% of patients with CIMF.[15] Interestingly, the same mutation is identified in patients with other MPD, most prominently in PV where it is present in >90% of patients. Not surprisingly, mutated JAK2 is found in over 90% of patients with post-PV MF.[16] Since identical *JAK2* mutations can be found in patients with other MPD (PV and ET), it is unclear how the same molecular abnormality evolves into different phenotypes. It is possible that additional events, such as germline genetic variation or other mutations may affect the phenotype. Also, mutations may be homozygous or heterozygous, although homozygous mutations are rarely seen in patients with myelofibrosis, in contrast to PV where heterozygous mutations represent approximately 20% of all mutations.[17] Those with homozygous mutations may have more splenomegaly and more frequently have pruritus.

The discovery of the *JAK2* V617F was a watershed moment in the understanding of the pathogenesis of the *BCR-ABL*-negative MPD. More recently similar discoveries have started to unravel the molecular pathophysiology of CIMF, emphasizing its complexity and heterogeneity. Other molecular events recently identified are mutations in c-*MPL* (c-*MPL* W515L/K), and additional mutations in exon 12 of *JAK2* among patients not expressing the *JAK2* V617F mutation.[18,19] Although the currently identified molecular defects do not fully explain many issues of MPD pathogenesis, they provide a deeper insight into its molecular pathogenesis, provide an additional diagnostic and monitoring tool, and offer the hope of a potential fruitful therapeutic target.

With this in mind, the international expert panel recently suggested revisions of the diagnostic criteria for MPD, including CIMF, to members of the Clinical Advisory Committee for the revision of the WHO Classification of Myeloid Neoplasms who endorsed the document and recommended its adoption.[20] Under the newly proposed revised criteria (Table 15.1), three major and four minor criteria are enlisted. The first major criterion underscores histology as a critical diagnostic criterion for PMF. The other two major criteria underline the need to exclude either myelofibrosis associated with another myeloid neoplasm or reactive bone marrow fibrosis. In order to reinforce diagnostic accuracy, the revised WHO diagnostic criteria for CIMF require the presence of at least two of four CIMF-characteristic peripheral blood or clinical features: leukoerythroblastosis, increased serum lactate dehydrogenase level, anemia, and palpable splenomegaly.

In addition to ineffective erythropoiesis, CIMF is characterized by prominent bone marrow stromal reaction that occurs in early stages of the disease and has been associated with increased marrow expression of profibrogenic and proangiogenic cytokines such as transforming growth factor-β (TGF-β), platelet derived growth factor (PDGF), tumor necrosis factor-α (TNF-α), basic fibroblast growth factor (bFGF), and vascular endothelial growth factor (VEGF).[21] Therapies aimed at molecular targets involved in the aforementioned pathogenetic pathways represent the foundation of current clinical trials in CIMF.

MANAGEMENT OF PATIENTS WITH MYELOFIBROSIS

The management of patients with myelofibrosis has been challenging in many ways. Lack of known molecular abnormality that uniformly defined CIMF has made the development of specific therapeutic agents for this disease difficult. Thus, symptomatic improvement has traditionally been the primary endpoint of most therapeutic attempts. For the same reason therapeutic intervention has been traditionally reserved for CIMF patients with more advanced disease, judged by the presence of prognostic factors known to affect the survival.[22] Adverse prognostic factors for survival include older age and anemia (hemoglobin <10 g/dl), leukocytosis, leukopenia, circulating blasts, increased numbers of granulocyte precursors, thrombocytopenia, abnormal karyotype, and hypercatabolic symptoms.[22] Various prognostic models have been devised, with the Lille system being perhaps the most frequently used.[23] This score relies on only two variables; adverse prognostic factors are hemoglobin <10 g/dl, and white blood cell (WBC) count $<4 \times 10^9$ or $>30 \times 10^9$/l. Risk groups are defined

Table 15.1 Proposed revised World Health Organization criteria for primary myelofibrosis. Diagnosis requires meeting all three major criteria and two minor criteria

Major criteria

Presence of megakaryocyte proliferation and atypia,* usually accompanied by either reticulin and/or collagen fibrosis, *or* in the absence of significant reticulin fibrosis, the megakaryocyte changes must be accompanied by an increased bone marrow cellularity characterized by granulocytic proliferation and often decreased erythropoiesis (i.e. prefibrotic cellular-phase disease)

Not meeting WHO criteria for polycythemia vera,† chronic myelogenous leukemia,‡ myelodysplastic syndrome,** or other myeloid neoplasm

Demonstration of *JAK2* V617F or other clonal marker (e.g. *MPL* W515L/K), *or* in the absence of a clonal marker, no evidence of bone marrow fibrosis owing to underlying inflammatory or other neoplastic diseases††

Minor criteria

Leukoerythroblastosis‡‡

Increase in serum lactate dehydrogenase level‡‡

Anemia‡‡

Palpable splenomegaly‡‡

*Small to large megakaryocytes with an aberrant nuclear/cytoplasmic ratio and hyperchromatic, bulbous, or irregularly folded nuclei and dense clustering.
†Requires the failure of iron replacement therapy to increase hemoglobin level to the polycythemia vera range in the presence of decreased serum ferritin. Exclusion of polycythemia vera is based on hemoglobin and hematocrit levels. Red cell mass measurement is not required.
‡Requires the absence of BCR-ABL.
**Requires absence of dyserythropoiesis and dysgranulopoiesis.
††Secondary to infection, autoimmune disorder or other chronic inflammatory condition, hairy cell leukemia or other lymphoid neoplasm, metastatic malignancy, or toxic (chronic) myelopathies. It should be noted that patients with conditions associated with reactive myelofibrosis are not immune to primary myelofibrosis and the diagnosis should be considered in such cases if other criteria are met.
‡‡Degree of abnormality could be borderline or marked.

as low risk, no adverse risk factors; intermediate risk, one risk factor; and high risk, two risk factors; reported median survival time for the three groups was 93, 26, and 13 months, respectively.[23] It is expected that the International Working Group on Myelofibrosis Research and Treatment (IWG-MRT) will publish an international prognostic scoring system that will become a universal tool for assessing patient risk of disease progression and early death.

The identification of mutations in JAK2 and c-MPL opens the possibility for more effective therapies and means of monitoring the extent of the response. Whether changes in the status of these molecular abnormalities can be used as surrogate markers of a changing natural history of the disease in response to therapy remains to be seen. In addition, no uniform criteria for response to therapy are yet available. Recently, the IWG-MRT has proposed consensus criteria for response to treatment in CIMF (Table 15.2).[24] Although these criteria may need to be adjusted as new therapies are developed, it is an important first step in trying to make the evaluation of responses more objective and comparable across different studies. Several treatment strategies have been used for patients with CIMF. Here we describe some of those that are used as standard therapy and some of the new and promising investigational agents.

Cytotoxic therapy

Hydroxyurea is an oral, well-tolerated, nonspecific myelosuppressive agent which can reliably control the leukocytosis as well as thrombocytosis associated with CIMF.[25] Some studies have suggested that cytoreductive therapy may decrease the risk of recurrent

Table 15.2 International Working Group (IWG) consensus criteria for treatment response in chronic idiopathic myelofibrosis

Complete remission (CR)
Complete resolution of disease-related symptoms and signs including palpable hepatosplenomegaly

Peripheral blood count remission defined as hemoglobin level at ≥110 g/l, platelet count at ≥100 × 10^9/l, and absolute neutrophil count (ANC) at ≥1.0 × 10^9/l. In addition, all 3 blood counts should be no higher than the upper normal limit

Normal leukocyte differential including disappearance of nucleated red blood cells, blasts, and immature myeloid cells in the peripheral smear, in the absence of splenectomy*

Bone marrow histological remission defined as the presence of age-adjusted normocellularity, ≤5% myeloblasts, and an osteomyelofibrosis grade no higher than 1†

Partial remission (PR) – requires all of the above criteria for CR except the requirement for bone marrow histological remission. However, a repeat bone marrow biopsy is required in the assessment of PR and may or may not show favorable changes that do not fulfill criteria for CR

Clinical improvement (CI) – requires one of the following in the absence of both disease progression (as outlined below) and CR/PR assignment (CI response is validated only if it lasts for no fewer than 8 weeks)

A ≥20.0-g/l increase in hemoglobin level or becoming transfusion independent (applicable only for patients with baseline hemoglobin level of <100 g/l)

Either a ≥50% reduction in palpable splenomegaly of a spleen that is ≥10 cm at baseline or a spleen that is palpable at ≥5 cm at baseline becomes not palpable‡

A ≥100% increase in platelet count and an absolute platelet count of ≥50× 10^9/l (applicable only for patients with baseline platelet count <50 × 10^9/l)

A ≥100% increase in ANC and an ANC of ≥0.5 × 10^9/l (applicable only for patients with baseline ANC <1.0 × 10^9/l)

Progressive disease (PD) – requires one of the following:**

Progressive splenomegaly that is defined by the appearance of a previously absent splenomegaly that is palpable at ≥5 cm below the left costal margin or a ≥100% increase in palpable distance for baseline splenomegaly of 5–10 cm or a ≥50% increase in palpable distance for baseline splenomegaly of >10 cm

Leukemic transformation confirmed by a bone marrow blast count of ≥20%

An increase in peripheral blood blast percentage of ≥20% that lasts for at least 8 weeks

Stable disease (SD) – none of the above

Relapse – loss of CR, PR, or CI. In other words, a patient with CR or PR is considered to have undergone relapse when he or she no longer fulfills the criteria for even CI. However, changes from either CR to PR or CR/PR to CI should be documented and reported

*Because of subjectivity in peripheral blood smear interpretation, CR does not require absence of morphological abnormalities of red cells, platelets, and neutrophils.

†In patients with CR, a complete cytogenetic response is defined as failure to detect a cytogenetic abnormality in cases with a pre-existing abnormality. A partial cytogenetic response is defined as ≥50% reduction in abnormal metaphases. In both cases, at least 20 bone marrow- or peripheral blood-derived metaphases should be analyzed. A major molecular response is defined as the absence of a specific disease-associated mutation in peripheral blood granulocytes of previously positive cases. In the absence of a cytogenetic/molecular marker, monitoring for treatment-induced inhibition of endogenous myeloid colony formation is encouraged. Finally, baseline and post-treatment bone marrow slides are to be stained at the same time and interpreted at one sitting by a central review process.

‡Transfusion dependency is defined by a history of at least 2 units of red blood cell transfusions in the past month for a hemoglobin level of <85 g/l that was not associated with clinically overt bleeding. Similarly, during protocol therapy, transfusions for a hemoglobin level of ≥85 g/l is discouraged unless it is clinically indicated. In splenectomized patients, palpable hepatomegaly is substituted with the same measurements.

**It is acknowledged that worsening cytopenia might represent progressive disease, but its inclusion as a formal criterion was avoided because of the difficulty distinguishing disease-associated from drug-induced myelosuppression. However, a decrease in hemoglobin level of ≥20 g/l a 100% increase in transfusion requirement, and new development of transfusion dependency, each lasting for >3 months after the discontinuation of protocol therapy, can be considered disease progression.

thrombosis in patients with PV and ET. It is less clear whether the same is true for patients with CIMF. However, by controlling the leukocytosis, thrombocytosis and, in some instances, splenomegaly, hydroxyurea can improve the symptoms and quality of life of some patients. Alkylating agents (e.g. melphalan) have activity in CIMF by causing a direct, non-specific, myelosuppression and, therefore, may potentially palliate symptoms associated with myeloproliferation.[26] However, it has been suggested that the risk of leukemic transformation may be increased in treated patients.

Erythropoietin

Erythropoietin (EPO) may help to alleviate the anemia that may be the main cause of symptoms in some patients. In a meta-analysis of published data on the use of EPO in CIMF, Rodriguez *et al.* reported a response rate of 33%.[27] Patients with endogenous serum EPO levels of <125 mU/ml had the highest likelihood of response. More recent reports confirmed that EPO treatment should be restricted to patients with anemia and inadequate EPO levels.[28]

Interferon alfa

Therapy with interferon alfa (IFNα) has been utilized in patients with CIMF based on its cytoreductive properties. IFNα can control leukocytosis and/or thrombocytosis in patients exhibiting hyperproliferative features, and there have been sporadic reports of bone marrow fibrosis regression.[29] Clinical trials of IFNα, including long-acting preparations, in CIMF have been generally disappointing.[30] One recent publication reported that one of 11 patients treated with pegylated IFNα-2b achieved a complete hematological response, with no responses in all other patients.[31]

Stem cell transplantation

Curative therapy in CIMF is currently possible only with allogeneic hematopoietic stem cell transplantation (alloSCT). Unfortunately, alloSCT is associated with a relatively high risk of mortality as well as morbidity that undermines its broad application. Currently both fully myeloablative[32] and non-myeloablative[33] alloSCT approaches have been described for CIMF. The precise role of alloSCT, the optimal candidate, and which conditioning regimen should be chosen is a complex and evolving problem for CIMF patients. Essential to the decision-making process in determining the appropriateness of low intensity or high intensity therapies for CIMF patients is the issue of prognosis.[34] The prognosis for CIMF patients is quite variable, with various prognostic features being used to predict the suspected outcomes in CIMF patients. There are also anecdotal reports of successful autologous stem cell transplantation for patients with CIMF, but the experience is very limited and, thus, this is not an option that is considered as widely applicable.[35]

Immunomodulatory inhibitory drugs: lenalidomide and pomalidomide

Thalidomide has antiangiogenic and immunomodulatory properties that made it attractive for investigation in CIMF. When used at low dose (50 mg/day) thalidomide is relatively well tolerated and leads to improvement of anemia and splenomegaly in one-third of patients and thrombocytopenia in a higher proportion.[36] The addition of prednisone to low-dose thalidomide appears to be more efficacious as well as better tolerated than thalidomide alone.[37]

The group of inhibitory cytokine and antiangiogenic agents collectively known as immunomodulatory inhibitory drugs (IMID), have shown great promise in CIMF. These agents have been developed as analogs of thalidomide, in order to improve the efficacy and diminish the toxicity seen with this agent.[38] Lenalidomide is a second generation IMID with pleiotropic cytokine modulating activity, which is significantly more potent than thalidomide in modulating the cytokines previously mentioned as important in the pathogenesis of the disease such as TNF-α, and it has no known teratogenicity or neurotoxicity. Based upon the benefits observed with thalidomide, the clinical activity of lenalidomide has been evaluated in two phase II trials involving 68 patients with symptomatic CIMF.[39] Lenalidomide therapy (10 mg/day PO) resulted in the overall response rates of 22% for anemia, 33% for splenomegaly, and 50% for thrombocytopenia. Remarkably, normalization of hemoglobin levels was observed in eight (17%) of 46 patients who were either transfusion dependent or had a baseline hemoglobin of <10 g/dl. In addition, four of these patients also displayed resolution of leukoerythroblastosis. Notably, two patients had resolution of intramedullary features of fibrosis and angiogenesis, and one patient with a del5(q) had cytogenetic remission. Although these latter responses were in a very small subset, they represent the first time that such responses have been possible in CIMF without stem cell transplantation. In aggregate, although the initial response rates to lenalidomide do not appear to differ from the prior experience with thalidomide, the nature of the responses seem more profound. Two large-scale trials have recently been completed, and results are eagerly awaited, evaluating whether combining this agent with corticosteroids will further improve upon responses observed with single-agent lenalidomide. Another promising IMID, pomalidomide, is 20 000-fold more potent than thalidomide in inhibiting TNF-α, although cross-resistance with the latter does not appear to occur.[38] Owing to its excellent oral absorption and adequate pharmacokinetics, pomalidomide is suitable for once-daily administration. In phase I trials in patients with multiple myeloma, the main side-effects associated with pomalidomide therapy were related to myelosuppression and deep vein thrombosis.[40] Given the promising results obtained with lenalidomide, a randomized, placebo-controlled, international clinical study to determine the activity of pomalidomide (with or without a prednisone taper) in CIMF is currently under way.

JAK2 inhibitors

JAK2 inhibitors represent probably the most promising class of agents in view of the discovery of the pathophysiological importance of JAK-STAT pathway in MPD in general, and CIMF in particular. There are currently numerous agents in development that have demonstrated the ability *in vitro* to inhibit the aberrant *JAK2* V617F as well as the wild-type *JAK2*. These agents include TG101209,[41] Go6976,[42] MK0457,[43] CEP-701,[44] and Z3.[45] Several JAK2 inhibitors are currently in clinical trials, and others will be soon. Intriguingly, in primary cells from patients with wild-type JAK2 disease that have c-*MPL* W515L/K, growth inhibition can similarly be accomplished by JAK2 inhibitors, such as TG101209.[41] This observation suggests that even in patients with wild-type *JAK2* MPD there is growth dependency on the JAK-STAT pathway. Thus, agents targeting this pathway may be active regardless of the *JAK2* mutation status. This hypothesis is further supported by the continual discovery of other aberrations in this pathway, such as in exon 12 of *JAK2* in patients with *JAK2* V617F-negative PV.[19]

Antiangiogenic agents (angiogenesis inhibitors)

Vatalanib (PTK787/ZK 222584), an oral inhibitor of the VEGF receptor-1 (VEGFR-1) and VEGFR-2 tyrosine kinases, has been used in clinical trials in patients with MPD because of its antiangiogenic activity.[46] PTK/ZK also inhibits a broad array of additional tyrosine kinases including PDGF receptor, c-KIT, and c-FMS. Despite the potential clinical value of PTK/ZK in patients with CIMF based on its mechanism of action, the responses observed in a recent clinical trial were quite modest with mainly clinical improvement (according to IWG-MRT criteria[24]) seen.[46] Twenty-nine patients with MF received a continuous dosing schedule of PTK/ZK of 500 or 750 mg twice daily. One (3%) patient achieved a complete remission and five (17%) had clinical improvement.

Significant decrease in intramedullary angiogenesis was not observed, while only modest reductions in marrow hypercellularity were described. Intriguingly, one patient did experience a complete remission (according to IWG-MRT criteria[24]) suggesting a particularly sensitive target (not identified) in this individual.

The results of the PTK/ZK trial parallel the modest results reported with another VEGFR inhibitor SU5416 in MF.[47] SU5416 is a synthetic inhibitor of VEGFR-2, KIT, and FLT-3. In a multicenter phase II study, intravenous SU5416 145 mg/m^2 was given twice weekly for a median of three 4-week cycles to 32 adult MPD patients, including three with CIMF. One of the patients attained a partial response. However, the overall clinical activity was marginal and the tolerability was poor.[47] Sunitinib (SU11248) is an orally bioavailable, multitargeted kinase inhibitor with selectivity for PDGF receptors, VEGF receptors, KIT, and FLT-3.[48] Sunitinib has been recently reported to be active in a phase I/II study of patients with acute myeloid leukemia[49] and a phase II study of this agent in CIMF is underway.

Fibrogenesis inhibitors

TGF-β_1 plays a central role in the prominent bone marrow stromal reaction observed in patients with CIMF. Several compounds, originally designed for the treatment of other profibrotic conditions inhibit TGF-β_1-mediated signaling.[50] GC-1008, a pan-specific human anti-TGF-β_1 antibody, is one such agent. GC-1008 is currently undergoing clinical evaluation for several indications, including pulmonary fibrosis, renal cancer, and melanoma of the skin. Current evidence suggests that spontaneous activation of the nuclear factor kappa beta (NF-κB) pathway with secretion of the fibrogenic cytokine TGF-β_1 takes place in megakaryocytes, monocytes, and CD34+ cells from patients with CIMF.[51] Rameshwar *et al.* reported that monocytes from patients with CIMF had spontaneous activation of the NF-κB transduction pathway and that NF-κB inhibition by antisense oligonucleotides decreased TGF-β_1 secretion.[52] Data in a murine model of myelofibrosis suggest that the proteasome inhibitor bortezomib inhibits activation of the NF-κB pathway and decreases plasma concentration of TGF-β_1, thus inhibiting the development of myelofibrosis.[53] Based on these latter findings clinical trials of bortezomib in patients with CIMF have been initiated.

Tyrosine kinase inhibitors

Imatinib mesylate is an inhibitor of the tyrosine kinase activity of ABL, PDGFR, c-KIT and ARG.[54] The employment of imatinib for the therapy of patients with CIMF was based on its inhibitory activity against PDGF-mediated signaling and the reduction of bone marrow fibrosis and microvessel density observed in patients with chronic myeloid leukemia (CML), for which imatinib is standard therapy.[55] Results from phase II trials of imatinib in patients with CIMF reported to date are modest.[56] Dasatinib (BMS-354825) is a dual SRC- and ABL-kinase inhibitor, and 300-fold more potent as an ABL kinase inhibitor than imatinib.[57] In addition, dasatinib effectively inhibits PDGFR-β (IC_{50} 28 nM). Based on these preclinical data and on the results obtained with imatinib, a clinical trial of dasatinib in patients with CIMF has been initiated; unfortunately, preliminary results reported in 11 patients with CIMF identified no responders.[58]

Farnesyl transferase inhibitors

RAS gene mutations are commonly encountered in hematological malignancies and are present in 6% of patients with CIMF.[59] Attachment of RAS to the cellular membrane is critical for its activation and this is accomplished through a post-translational modification termed prenylation. Prenylation occurs through the action of one of two enzymes, farnesyltransferase and, to a lesser extent, geranylgeranyl-protein transferases. Inhibition of these enzymes has been investigated as a means of interfering with RAS signaling, which led to the development of farnesyl transferase inhibitors (FTI). Their activity, however, appears to extend beyond

RAS inhibition and may be mediated through inhibition of other prenylation-dependent proteins, such as RHOB, CENP-E, and CENP-F. In one clinical trial tipifarnib (R115777), a non-peptidomimetic FTI, was administered at 600 mg orally twice daily for 4 weeks out of every 6 weeks to eight patients with CIMF.[60] Two of them had a significant decrease in splenomegaly, one had normalization of white blood cell count and differential, and one became transfusion independent. Notably, responders had markedly higher pretreatment plasma VEGF concentrations than non-responders during therapy.

In parallel efforts, *in vitro* testing of tipifarnib demonstrated that aberrant myeloid colony formation was reduced by 50% at concentrations of 34 nM and 2.7 nM for myeloid and megakaryocytic colonies from CIMF patients, respectively. Since these concentrations seemed quite achievable at tolerable dose levels (i.e. 300 mg twice daily) a phase II trial was undertaken.[61] Eligible patients had histologically confirmed CIMF and were symptomatic, defined by anemia (hemoglobin <10 g/dl or transfusion dependent) or palpable hepatosplenomegaly. Patients received 300 mg of tipifarnib orally twice daily for the first 21 days of a 28-day cycle. The primary endpoint was response, as defined by improvement in either anemia or organomegaly. Median time to discontinuation of protocol therapy was 4.6 months; reasons for early termination ($n = 19$; 56%) included disease progression (21%) and adverse drug effects (18%). Toxicities (≥grade 3) included myelosuppression ($n = 16$), neuropathy ($n = 2$), fatigue ($n = 1$), rash ($n = 1$), and hyponatremia ($n = 1$). Response rate was 33% for hepatosplenomegaly and 38% for transfusion-requiring anemia. No favorable changes occurred in bone marrow fibrosis, angiogenesis or cytogenetic status. Pre- and post-treatment patient sample analysis for *in vitro* myeloid colony growth revealed substantial reduction in the latter. Clinical response did not correlate with either degree of colony growth, measurable decrease in quantitative JAK2 mutation levels or tipifarnib IC_{50} values (median 11.8 nM) seen in pretreatment samples. Additional MPD patients were treated on a broad phase II trial (15 unclassified MPD patients),[62] and similar to the CIMF trial, the response was a non-specific decrease in leukocytosis. These studies suggest that there is moderate tipifarnib activity in CIMF.

Other novel investigational agents

Other approaches with potential clinical activity in patients with CIMF are being investigated. GX15-070 is a synthetic small molecule that inhibits the binding of the anti-apoptotic proteins BCL-2, BCL-XL, BCL-W, and MCL-1 to the pro-apoptotic proteins BAX and BAK, thus re-instituting programmed cell death in transformed cells. In a phase I study of GX15-070 in patients with chronic lymphocytic leukemia (CLL), two of four patients who were anemic at baseline (one of whom was transfusion dependent) showed significant sustained elevations in their hemoglobin levels.[63] Based on this preliminary data, GX15-070 is being investigated in other hematological malignancies, including CIMF, to determine whether this compound might improve cytopenias.

Aberrant CpG island hypermethylation in regulatory areas of tumor suppressor genes leading to inactivation is commonly encountered in human cancer.[64] Aberrant methylation of $p15^{INK4B}$, $p16^{INK4A}$, and the retinoic acid receptor β has been observed in advanced-stage CIMF.[65] Azacitidine and decitabine are DNA methyltransferase inhibitors that induce reactivation of methylated genes. Both agents are approved by the Food and Drug Administration in the USA for the treatment of patients with MDS, and are currently being investigated in phase II studies in CIMF. Preliminary results of one study of azacitidine in 34 CIMF patients were recently reported.[66] Responses were observed in ten (29%) patients, including complete response in one, partial response in seven, and hematological improvement in two. The median time to best response was 20 weeks (range 3–26). Azacitidine was generally well tolerated: ten patients (29%) had grade 3 or 4 toxicity, and neutropenia was the only grade 4 toxicity (in four patients).

CONCLUSION

The development of novel therapies for MPD patients has been historically hampered by limited progress regarding the molecular pathogenesis of this disease. However, great strides have been made in this regard over the past decade, culminating in the recent discovery of the gain-of-function *JAK2* V617F mutation. A challenge for the near future will be the development of targeted agents with an acceptable toxicity profile able to interfere with the JAK-STAT signaling pathway. The hope is that such intervention may result not only in clinical responses for patients, but also that it may change the natural history of the disease. Clinical trials with such agents have been initiated. In recent years, a number of other agents with various mechanisms of action have been tested in clinical studies for CIMF patients, with disappointing results, including pirfenidone, imatinib, tipifarnib, vatalanib, and SU5416. However, promising results have been obtained with thalidomide, which has encouraged clinicians and researchers to pursue the development of novel, more potent IMID, such as lenalidomide and pomalidomide. Ideally, all patients with CIMF should be included in clinical trials with any of the new agents being developed for this indication, such as IMID, novel antiangiogenic agents, proteasome inhibitors, and novel signal transduction inhibitors, whether alone or in combination. Only through continued research in preclinical models and in clinical trials we will be able to reach the goal of specific and highly effective therapy for patients with CIMF. Fortunately, we appear to be much closer to this goal than ever before.

REFERENCES

1. Tefferi A. Myelofibrosis with myeloid metaplasia. N Engl J Med 2000; 342: 1255–65.
2. Mesa RA, Verstovsek S, Cervantes F et al. Primary myelofibrosis (PMF), post polycythemia vera myelofibrosis (post-PV MF), post essential thrombocythemia myelofibrosis (post-ET MF), blast phase PMF (PMF-BP): consensus on terminology by the international working group for myelofibrosis research and treatment (IWG-MRT). Leuk Res 2007; 31: 737–40.
3. Rollison DE, Hayat M, Smith M et al. First report of national estimates of the incidence of myelodysplastic syndromes and chronic myeloproliferative disorders from the US SEER Program. Blood 2006; 180: 77a, abstract 247.
4. Mesa RA, Silverstein MN, Jacobsen SJ et al. Population-based incidence and survival figures in essential thrombocythemia and agnogenic myeloid metaplasia: an Olmsted County Study, 1976–1995. Am J Hematol 1999; 61: 10–15.
5. Cervantes F, Barosi G, Hernandez-Boluda JC et al. Myelofibrosis with myeloid metaplasia in adult individuals 30 years old or younger: presenting features, evolution and survival. Eur J Haematol 2001; 66: 324–7.
6. Mesa RA, Nagorney DS, Schwager S et al. Palliative goals, patient selection, and perioperative platelet management: outcomes and lessons from 3 decades of splenectomy for myelofibrosis with myeloid metaplasia at the Mayo Clinic Cancer. Cancer 2006; 107: 361–70.
7. Koch CA, Li CY, Mesa RA et al. Nonhepatosplenic extramedullary hematopoiesis: associated diseases, pathology, clinical course, and treatment. Mayo Clin Proc 2003; 78: 1223–33.
8. Mesa RA, Li CY, Schroeder G et al. Clinical correlates of splenic histopathology and splenic karyotype in myelofibrosis with myeloid metaplasia. Blood 2001; 97: 3665–7.
9. Mesa RA, Niblack J, Wadleigh M et al. The burden of fatigue and quality of life in myeloproliferative disorders (MPDs): an international Internet-based survey of 1179 MPD patients. Cancer 2007; 109: 68–76.
10. Steensma DP, Mesa RA, Li CY et al. Etanercept, a soluble tumor necrosis factor receptor, palliates constitutional symptoms in patients with myelofibrosis with myeloid metaplasia: results of a pilot study. Blood 2002; 99: 2252–4.
11. Mesa RA, Li CY, Ketterling RP et al. Leukemic transformation in myelofibrosis with myeloid metaplasia: a single-institution experience with 91 cases. Blood 2005; 105: 973–7.
12. Tefferi A, Mesa RA, Schroeder G et al. Cytogenetic findings and their clinical relevance in myelofibrosis with myeloid metaplasia. Br J Haematol 2001; 113: 763–71.
13. Tefferi A, Dingli D, Li CY et al. Prognostic diversity among cytogenetic abnormalities in myelofibrosis with myeloid metaplasia. Cancer 2005; 104: 1656–60.
14. James C, Ugo V, Le Couedic JP et al. A unique clonal JAK2 mutation leading to constitutive signalling causes polycythaemia vera. Nature 2005; 434: 1144–8.
15. Tefferi A, Gilliland DG. The JAK2V617F tyrosine kinase mutation in myeloproliferative disorders: status

report and immediate implications for disease classification and diagnosis. Mayo Clin Proc 2005; 80: 947–58.
16. Tefferi A, Lasho TL, Schwager SM et al. The JAK2 tyrosine kinase mutation in myelofibrosis with myeloid metaplasia: lineage specificity and clinical correlates. Br J Haematol 2005; 131: 320–8.
17. Tefferi A, Lasho TL, Schwager SM et al. The clinical phenotype of wild-type, heterozygous, and homozygous JAK2V617F in polycythemia vera. Cancer 2006; 106: 631–5.
18. Pikman Y, Lee BH, Mercher T et al. MPLW515L is a novel somatic activating mutation in myelofibrosis with myeloid metaplasia. PLoS Med 2006; 3: e270.
19. Scott LM, Tong W, Levine RL et al. JAK2 exon 12 mutations in polycythemia vera and idiopathic erythrocytosis. N Engl J Med 2007; 356: 459–68.
20. Tefferi A, Thiele J, Orazi A et al. Proposals and rationale for revision of the World Health Organization diagnostic criteria for polycythemia vera, essential thrombocythemia, and primary myelofibrosis: recommendations from an ad hoc international expert panel. Blood 2007; 110: 1092–7.
21. Xu M, Bruno E, Chao J et al. The constitutive mobilization of bone marrow-repopulating cells into the peripheral blood in idiopathic myelofibrosis. Blood 2005; 105: 1699–705.
22. Cervantes F, Barosi G. Myelofibrosis with myeloid metaplasia: diagnosis, prognostic factors, and staging. Semin Oncol 2005; 32: 395–402.
23. Dupriez B, Morel P, Demory JL et al. Prognostic factors in agnogenic myeloid metaplasia: a report on 195 cases with a new scoring system. Blood 1996; 88: 1013–18.
24. Tefferi A, Barosi G, Mesa RA et al. International Working Group (IWG) consensus criteria for treatment response in myelofibrosis with myeloid metaplasia, for the IWG for Myelofibrosis Research and Treatment (IWG-MRT). Blood 2006; 108: 1497–503.
25. Lofvenberg E, Wahlin A. Management of polycythaemia vera, essential thrombocythaemia and myelofibrosis with hydroxyurea. Eur J Haematol 1988; 41: 375–81.
26. Petti MC, Latagliata R, Spadea T et al. Melphalan treatment in patients with myelofibrosis with myeloid metaplasia. Br J Haematol 2002; 116: 576–81.
27. Rodriguez JN, Martino ML, Dieguez JC et al. rHuEpo for the treatment of anemia in myelofibrosis with myeloid metaplasia. Experience in 6 patients and meta-analytical approach. Haematologica 1998; 83: 616–21.
28. Cervantes F, Alvarez-Larran A, Hernandez-Boluda JC et al. Erythropoietin treatment of the anaemia of myelofibrosis with myeloid metaplasia: results in 20 patients and review of the literature. Br J Haematol 2004; 127: 399–403.
29. Tefferi A, Elliot MA, Yoon SY et al. Clinical and bone marrow effects of interferon alfa therapy in myelofibrosis with myeloid metaplasia. Blood 2001; 97: 1896.
30. Heis-Vahidi-Fard N, Forberg E, Eichinger S et al. Ineffectiveness of interferon-gamma in the treatment of idiopathic myelofibrosis: a pilot study. Ann Hematol 2001; 80: 79–82.
31. Verstovsek S, Lawhorn K, Giles F et al. PEG-Intron for myeloproliferative diseases: an update of ongoing phase II study. Blood 2004; 104: abstract 633.
32. Deeg HJ, Gooley TA, Flowers ME et al. Allogeneic hematopoietic stem cell transplantation for myelofibrosis. Blood 2003; 102: 3912–18.
33. Rondelli D, Barosi G, Bacigalupo A et al. Allogeneic hematopoietic stem cell transplantation with reduced intensity conditioning in intermediate or high risk patients with myelofibrosis with myeloid metaplasia. Blood 2005; 105: 4115–9.
34. Dingli D, Schwager SM, Mesa RA et al. Prognosis in transplant-eligible patients with agnogenic myeloid metaplasia: a simple CBC-based scoring system. Cancer 2006; 106: 623–30.
35. van Besien K, Deeg HJ. Hematopoietic stem cell transplantation for myelofibrosis. Semin Oncol 2005; 32: 414–21.
36. Marchetti M, Barosi G, Balestri F et al. Low-dose thalidomide ameliorates cytopenias and splenomegaly in myelofibrosis with myeloid metaplasia: a phase II trial. J Clin Oncol 2004; 22: 424–31.
37. Mesa RA, Steensma DP, Pardanani A et al. A phase 2 trial of combination low-dose thalidomide and prednisone for the treatment of myelofibrosis with myeloid metaplasia. Blood 2003; 101: 2534–41.
38. Muller GW, Chen R, Huang SY et al. Amino-substituted thalidomide analogs: potent inhibitors of TNF-alpha production. Bioorg Med Chem Lett 1999; 9: 1625–30.
39. Tefferi A, Cortes J, Verstovsek S et al. Lenalidomide therapy in myelofibrosis with myeloid metaplasia. Blood 2006; 108: 1158–64.
40. Schey SA, Fields P, Bartlett JB et al. Phase I Study of an Immunomodulatory Thalidomide Analog, CC-4047, in Relapsed or Refractory Multiple Myeloma 10.1200/JCO.2004.10.052. J Clin Oncol 2004; 22: 3269–76.
41. Pardanani A, Hood J, Lasho T et al. TG101209, a Selective JAK2 Kinase Inhibitor, Suppresses Endogenous and Cytokine-Supported Colony Formation from Hematopoietic Progenitors Carrying JAK2V617F or MPLW515K/L Mutations. Blood 2006; 108: 11, abstract 2680.
42. Grandage VL, Everington T, Linch DC et al. Go6976 is a potent inhibitor of the JAK 2 and FLT3 tyrosine kinases with significant activity in primary acute myeloid leukemia cells. Br J Haematol 2006; 135: 303–16.
43. Giles F, Freedman SJ, Xiao A et al. MK-0457, a novel multikinase inhibitor, has activity in refractory AML, including transformed JAK2 positive myeloproliferative disease (MPD), and in

Philadelphia-Positive ALL. Blood 2006; 108: 11, abstract 1967.

44. Dobrzanski P, Hexner E, Serdikoff C et al. CEP-701 Is a JAK2 inhibitor which attenuates JAK2/STAT5 signaling pathway and the proliferation of primary cells from patients with myeloproliferative disorders. Blood 2006; 108: 11, abstract 3594.
45. Sayyah J, Ostrov D, Sayeski P. Identification and characterization of a novel Jak2 tyrosine kinase inhibitor. Blood 2006; 108: 11, abstract 3604.
46. Giles FJ, List AF, Carroll M et al. PTK787/ZK 222584, a small molecule tyrosine kinase receptor inhibitor of vascular endothelial growth factor (VEGF), has modest activity in myelofibrosis with myeloid metaplasia. Leuk Res 2007; 31: 891–7.
47. Giles FJ, Cooper MA, Silverman L et al. Phase II study of SU5416 – a small-molecule, vascular endothelial growth factor tyrosine-kinase receptor inhibitor – in patients with refractory myeloproliferative diseases. Cancer 2003; 97: 1920–8.
48. O'Farrell AM, Abrams TJ, Yuen HA et al. SU11248 is a novel FLT3 tyrosine kinase inhibitor with potent activity in vitro and in vivo. Blood 2003; 101: 3597–605.
49. Fiedler W, Serve H, Dohner H et al. A phase 1 study of SU11248 in the treatment of patients with refractory or resistant acute myeloid leukemia (AML) or not amenable to conventional therapy for the disease. Blood 2005; 105: 986–93.
50. Yingling JM, Blanchard KL, Sawyer JS. Development of TGF-beta signalling inhibitors for cancer therapy. Nat Rev Drug Discov 2004; 3: 1011–22.
51. Komura E, Tonetti C, Penard-Lacronique V et al. Role for the nuclear factor kappaB pathway in transforming growth factor-beta1 production in idiopathic myelofibrosis: possible relationship with FK506 binding protein 51 overexpression. Cancer Res 2005; 65: 3281–9.
52. Rameshwar P, Narayanan R, Qian J et al. NF-kappa B as a central mediator in the induction of TGF-beta in monocytes from patients with idiopathic myelofibrosis: an inflammatory response beyond the realm of homeostasis. J Immunol 2000; 165: 2271–7.
53. Wagner-Ballon O, Pisani DF, Gastinne T et al. Proteasome inhibitor bortezomib impairs both myelofibrosis and osteosclerosis induced by high thrombopoietin levels in mice. Blood 2007; 110: 345–53.
54. Kantarjian H, Sawyers C, Hochhaus A et al. Hematologic and cytogenetic responses to imatinib mesylate in chronic myelogenous leukemia. N Engl J Med 2002; 346: 645–652.
55. Kvasnicka HM, Thiele J. Bone marrow angiogenesis: methods of quantification and changes evolving in chronic myeloproliferative disorders. Histol Histopathol 2004; 19: 1245–60.
56. Tefferi A, Mesa RA, Gray LA et al. Phase 2 trial of imatinib mesylate in myelofibrosis with myeloid metaplasia. Blood 2002; 99: 3854–6.
57. Lombardo LJ, Lee FY, Chen P et al. Discovery of N-(2-chloro-6-methyl-phenyl)-2-(6-(4-(2-hydroxyethyl)-piperazin-1-yl)-2-methylpyrimidin-4-ylamino)thiazole-5-carboxamide (BMS-354825), a dual Src/Abl kinase inhibitor with potent antitumor activity in preclinical assays. J Med Chem 2004; 47: 6658–61.
58. Verstovsek S, Atallah E, Thomas D et al. Dasatinib therapy for patients with Philadelphia-negative (Ph-) myeloproliferative disorders (MPD's) including systemic mastocytosis. J Clin Oncol 2007; 25: 18S, abstract 7086.
59. Reilly JT. Pathogenesis of idiopathic myelofibrosis: present status and future directions. Br J Haematol 1994; 88: 1–8.
60. Cortes J, Albitar M, Thomas D et al. Efficacy of the farnesyl transferase inhibitor R115777 in chronic myeloid leukemia and other hematologic malignancies. Blood 2003; 101: 1692–7.
61. Mesa RA, Camoriano JK, Geyer SM et al. A phase II trial of tipifarnib in myelofibrosis: primary, post-polycythemia vera and post-essential thrombocythemia. Leukemia 2007; 21: 1964–70.
62. Gotlib J, Loh M, Lancet JE et al. Phase I/II study of tipifarnib (Zarnestra, farnesyltransferase inhibitor (FTI) R115777) in patients with myeloproliferative disorders (MPDs): interim results. Blood 2003; 102: a3425.
63. O'Brien S, Kipps TJ, Faderl S et al. A phase I trial of the small molecule pan-Bcl-2 family inhibitor GX15–070 administered intravenously (iv) every 3 weeks to patients with previously treated chronic lymphocytic leukemia (CLL). Blood 2005; 106: abstract 446.
64. Baylin SB, Herman JG, Graff JR et al. Alterations in DNA methylation: a fundamental aspect of neoplasia. Adv Cancer Res 1998; 72: 141–96.
65. Tefferi A. Pathogenesis of myelofibrosis with myeloid metaplasia. J Clin Oncol 2005; 23: 8520–30.
66. Quintas-Cardama A, Kantarjian H, Garcia-Manero G et al. A Phase II study of Azacitidine for patients with myelofibrosis. Blood 2006; 108: 11, abstract 2706.

Essential thrombocythemia

16

Peter J Campbell, Anthony R Green

INTRODUCTION

The Philadelphia-negative myeloproliferative disorders (MPD) are clonal hematological malignancies with three main members: polycythemia vera (PV), essential thrombocythemia (ET), and primary myelofibrosis (PMF).[1] They are thought to result from transformation of a multipotent stem cell[2,3] and are characterized by overactive hematopoiesis, with increased red cell mass and platelets being the defining features of PV and ET, respectively. The major complications are thrombosis, either arterial or venous, and hemorrhage, with a long-term risk of myelofibrotic or acute leukemic progression.[4]

This chapter focuses primarily on ET, although many of the recent advances in our understanding of the molecular biology, diagnosis, and management of these conditions apply across all the MPD. William Dameshek was the first to link the MPD as a spectrum of related diseases in 1951,[5] together with chronic myeloid leukemia (CML), recognizing the significant overlap in clinical and laboratory features, such as marrow hypercellularity, propensity to thrombosis and hemorrhage, and risk of leukemic or myelofibrotic transformation over time.

The past 3 years have seen tremendous progress in our understanding of both the molecular pathogenesis and the treatment of MPD. The discovery of a single, acquired mutation in the *JAK2* gene[6–10] in nearly all patients with PV and about half those with ET and PMF[6] represents a significant advance in our search for the causative molecular lesions.

EPIDEMIOLOGY

The incidence of MPD is generally low, although because ET and PV have a life expectancy not too dissimilar to the reference population,[11,12] the prevalence is considerably higher. ET has an annual incidence of 1–3 cases per 100000 population,[13–16] roughly equal to the incidence of PV[13,16,17] and about ten times higher than the incidence of PMF.[13,14,16] Most ET patients present in their 60s and 70s,[13–16] but there is a significant proportion of patients who are much younger,[18] including occasional cases of childhood disease.[19] In ET, women outnumber men by 2 : 1.[20]

Very few risk factors for the development of ET have been identified. There are occasional familial clusters of MPD in first-degree relatives, and the rates of this appear to be greater than would be expected by chance alone.[16,21] These familial clusters appear to be distinct from inherited forms of thrombocytosis, caused by alterations of thrombopoietin translation.[22] Ionizing radiation is a recognized risk factor for MPD, including ET, with a greater incidence in survivors of the Hiroshima and Nagasaki nuclear attacks and in military personnel exposed to nuclear weapon testing.[23]

MOLECULAR PATHOGENESIS

The *JAK2* V617F and *MPL* W515 mutations

In 2005, several groups reported a single, acquired point mutation in the *JAK2* gene in the majority of patients with Philadelphia-negative MPD.[6–10] JAK2, a cytoplasmic tyrosine kinase, is critical for instigating intracellular signaling by the receptors for erythropoietin, thrombopoietin, interleukin-3, granulocyte-colony-stimulating factor (G-CSF), and granulocyte-macrophage colony-stimulating factor (GM-CSF).[24,25] *JAK2*-null mice die at embryonic day 12.5, with complete absence of definitive erythropoiesis,[26,27] a finding that underscores the vital role of JAK2 as a transducer of signals evoked by the binding of erythropoietin to its receptor. JAK2 binds to the erythropoietin receptor in the endoplasmic reticulum and is required for its cell surface expression.[28] Binding to erythropoietin provokes a conformational change in the receptor[29–31] with consequent phosphorylation and activation of JAK2.[32] The activated JAK2 then phosphorylates the receptor's cytoplasmic domain, thereby promoting the docking of downstream effector proteins and the initiation of intracellular signaling cascades.[24,25]

The *JAK2* mutation in the MPD is acquired, and has never been found as an inherited change.[6–10] Sensitive methods demonstrate the mutation in >95% of patients with PV[6,33] and in 50–60% of patients with ET[6,33–37] or PMF.[6,33,37–39] A substantial proportion of patients with PV or PMF are homozygous for the *JAK2* mutation as a result of mitotic recombination affecting chromosome 9p,[6–9] but this phenomenon is rarely detected in ET.[40] The mutation is also found in a small minority of patients with primary hypereosinophilic syndrome, chronic myelomonocytic leukemia, chronic neutrophilic leukemia, myelodysplasia, and acute myeloid leukemia,[37,41–46] but not in lymphoid malignancies, other cancers, or in normal subjects.[6–9,42,43,45,47] The *JAK2* mutation is also found in approximately 50% of patients with otherwise unexplained Budd–Chiari syndrome,[48] suggesting a masked myeloproliferative disorder in these cases.

The mutation in *JAK2* substitutes a bulky phenylalanine for a conserved valine at position 617 of the JAK2 protein (V617F). This residue is located in the JH2, or pseudokinase, domain, which negatively regulates the kinase domain.[49] Biochemical studies have shown that the *JAK2* V617F mutation causes cytokine-independent activation of JAK-STAT, PI3K-AKT, and MAPK-ERK pathways,[7–10] all of which are implicated in erythropoietin receptor signaling.[32,50–52]

Recently, acquired activating mutations in the thrombopoietin receptor (*MPL*) gene have been demonstrated in approximately 10% of patients with V617F-negative ET and PMF.[53,54] The mutation is located in a motif that is important for maintaining receptor inactivity,[55] and loss of its inhibitory function leads to constitutive activation of the receptor.

Pathophysiology

Mouse models

Expression of the *JAK2* V617F mutation in murine hematopoietic cells by means of a retroviral vector recapitulates the features of PV.[7,56–59] The animals have erythrocytosis and leukocytosis, and there is evolution to post-polycythemic myelofibrosis.[56–59] Interestingly, thrombocytosis is not a reproducible feature in these mice, perhaps because high levels of mutant *JAK2* generated by the retroviral vector inhibit megakaryocyte differentiation.[57] Constitutive Stat5 activation, erythropoietin hypersensitivity, and cytokine independence are all present, as in the human disease. These results provide direct evidence of a causal link between the mutation and the disease.

Co-operating mutations

Four lines of evidence suggest that co-operating mutations occur at an early stage in V617F-positive MPD, and may even pre-date the *JAK2* mutation. First, deletions of 20q and other cytogenetic abnormalities occur in 5–10% of patients with MPD.[60] In one patient with ET and one with PV, 20q-deleted granulocytes outnumbered V617F-positive granulocytes,[61] suggesting the 20q-deletion occurred before the *JAK2* mutation. Consistent with a co-operating gene on 20q, patients with molecularly defined 20q deletions are almost exclusively V617F-positive.[62] Second, some women with PV or ET have more clonally derived granulocytes (estimated by X-chromosome inactivation patterns) than *JAK2*-positive granulocytes.[33,61,62] Although interpreted as evidence for a clonal proliferation that preceded the *JAK2* mutation, this conclusion remains controversial.[62] Third, in some patients with V617F-positive PV or ET that undergoes leukemic transformation, the leukemic cells lack the *JAK2* mutation.[62] This finding is consistent with the leukemia arising in a mutant clone that preceded the *JAK2* mutation, although other interpretations are possible.[62] Fourth, in familial clusters of MPD, the *JAK2* mutation is acquired,[21] demonstrating that the inherited predisposition is unrelated to the *JAK2* mutation.

V617F homozygosity

V617F homozygosity plays a key role in the MPD. Homozygosity in granulocytes can be detected in about 30% of patients with PV.[6–9] However, when individual hematopoietic progenitor cell colonies derived from such patients were studied, approximately 90% of them were homozygous for the V617F mutation. By contrast, homozygous progenitor colonies were rare in ET.[40] This observation suggests that V617F homozygosity promotes the development of PV.

Signaling

The mutant JAK2 protein activates multiple downstream signaling pathways with effects on gene transcription,[63] apoptosis, the cell cycle, and differentiation.[24,25] Effects on apoptosis include overexpression of the cell-survival protein BCL-X in erythroid precursor cells in PV,[64] probably as a result of enhanced JAK-STAT signaling.[51,65,66] There is also reduction of apoptosis induced by death receptors in *JAK2* V617F-positive erythroid progenitors, an effect mediated through PI3K-AKT and MAPK-ERK pathways.[67] With respect to the cell cycle, mutant JAK2 promotes G_1/S phase transition in hematopoietic cell lines, accompanied by upregulation of cyclin D2 and downregulation of the inhibitor p27Kip.[68] Effects on erythroid differentiation may be mediated by the transcription factor NF-E2, which is upregulated in PV[63,69] and plays an important role in erythroid differentiation.[70,71]

It has been suggested that, unlike other kinases associated with hematological malignancies, the V617F protein requires a type I cytokine receptor (EpoR, TpoR or G-CSFR) to act as a scaffold and docking site for downstream effector proteins. Such a mechanism may explain the involvement of the erythroid, megakaryocyte, and granulocyte lineages in the MPD,[72] but detailed structural and biochemical analyses are needed to explain why residue 617 is so critical for JAK2 activation.

CLINICAL FEATURES AND NATURAL HISTORY OF ESSENTIAL THROMBOCYTHEMIA

Overall survival

Most studies of prognosis in ET have shown an overall survival similar to the reference population.[12,73,74] However, these studies may be hampered by small numbers of patients followed for >10 years: one recent study showed worse survival only in the second decade after diagnosis.[75]

Thrombosis and microvascular ischemia

ET may present with complications of microvascular ischemia, macrovascular thrombosis or hemorrhage, or, increasingly, with an asymptomatic increased platelet count. Microvascular ischemic symptoms particularly affect the circulations of the digits and the brain. Digital ischemia covers a range of syndromes. These include erythromelalgia, a painful, burning erythema or cyanosis affecting the extremities,[76,77] Raynaud's phenomenon,[78] and frank digital infarction, which can cause ulceration or gangrene in its most extreme manifestations.[77,78] The microvascular effects in the brain include transient, non-focal visual or neurological disturbances, headaches, and migraines.[79] The pathogenesis of microvascular disturbances in the MPD is thought to relate to vasospasm and arteriolar inflammation caused by release of vasoactive and/or inflammatory mediators from activated platelets and white cells.[76] These syndromes are often exquisitely sensitive to aspirin therapy.[76,77]

Macrovascular complications in the MPD include both arterial and venous thrombosis. The clinical spectrum of arterial thrombosis matches that of the general population, with high rates of myocardial infarction, strokes, transient ischemic attacks, and peripheral vascular thromboses.[11,12] The most common venous thromboembolic diseases are lower limb deep venous thrombosis and pulmonary embolism, but both PV and ET are associated with an unusually high incidence of hepatic vein, portal vein, and intracerebral sinus thromboses.[11,20,80,81] In fact, half of all portal vein thromboses may be attributed to MPD,[80] with recent data suggesting that this may be a feature of *JAK2* V617F-positive MPD specifically.[34,48]

In ET, the correlation between raised platelet count and thrombosis is controversial. Undoubtedly, reducing the platelet count with cytoreduction improves thrombosis rates in high-risk patients,[82] but studies have consistently failed to reveal a correlation between platelet count and thrombosis risk.[83–86] This may reflect the small numbers of patients in the studies, and the fact that thrombosis rates in ET are not necessarily greatly increased over the reference population once treatment starts; thus, many of the events seen in treated patients may be unrelated to the ET, but related to conventional risk factors such as smoking, hypercholesterolemia, and previous thrombosis.[86]

Hemorrhage

Increased rates of hemorrhage are seen in ET. The bleeding manifestations particularly involve the skin and mucous membranes, with bruising, epistaxis, and gastrointestinal hemorrhage predominating.[87] Intra-articular, intramuscular, and retroperitoneal bleeds are not a feature of the MPD, unless treated with warfarin anticoagulation. The pattern of mucosal bleeding, with little increased risk of deep-seated bleeding, suggests dysfunction of platelets or von Willebrand factor as the pathogenesis. Indeed, there is evidence for both mechanisms. Platelet function disturbances are common in untreated MPD,[88–90] although do not necessarily correlate with risk of hemorrhage (or thrombosis).[88] There appears to be loss of large von Willebrand multimers from the plasma of patients with high platelet counts,[91,92] probably through the adsorption of the proteins onto the cell surface of the platelets through von Willebrand factor receptors. The major risk factor for hemorrhage in MPD patients is an elevated platelet count, with most bleeding occurring at platelet counts over $1500 \times 10^9/l$.[83,88,93]

Myelofibrotic transformation

Myelofibrosis can develop as a result of transformation from prior ET or PV. Myelofibrotic transformation has traditionally been difficult to define because a degree of increased reticulin is frequently present in the marrow of patients with chronic phase disease.[94] Modern definitions have relied on the demonstration of significantly increased bone marrow reticulin staining (usually grade 3–4 on a four point scale[95]) with or without new bone formation together with a clinical syndrome consisting of two or more of progressive splenomegaly, anemia, tear-drop red cells, leukoerythroblastosis, and constitutional symptoms[20] (Table 16.1).

With this definition, estimates of the rates of myelofibrotic transformation of ET and PV range from 5 to 15% at 10 years.[97–100] It is responsible for the deaths of a significant proportion of patients followed for >10 years,[100–103] particularly those who present while relatively young (<60 years of age). Myelofibrotic transformation is associated with increased risk of further evolution to acute leukemia, with 30% of cases of leukemia arising from preceding myelofibrosis.[104]

Leukemic transformation

All three classic MPD have a many-fold increased risk of transformation to acute leukemia compared with the reference population.[75,105,106] Because untreated ET has a high incidence of

Table 16.1 Criteria for myelofibrotic transformation of essential thrombocythemia (as used in the PT-1 study,[20] modified from the Italian Consensus Criteria[96]).

Necessary criteria
Grade 3 or more reticulin fibrosis on bone marrow trephine on a 0–4 point scale[95] (with an increase of at least one grade from diagnostic trephine if available)
Optional criteria
Increase in spleen size of ≥3 cm
Unexplained decrease in hemoglobin by ≥2 g/dl to below the sex-specific lower limit of normal
Two or more immature myeloid or nucleated erythroid cells in the peripheral blood smear
Tear-drop poikilocytes in the blood smear
One or more systemic symptoms:
drenching night sweats (requiring changing of bed linen or nightwear)
generalized and otherwise unexplained bone pain
weight loss (>10% of pre-transformation body weight in 6 months)

Diagnosis requires the necessary criterion + any two optional criteria

thrombosis in older patients, most patients receive cytoreductive therapy, meaning it is impossible to define the 'natural' incidence of acute leukemia in ET. Furthermore, different therapeutic modalities are clearly associated with vastly different rates of leukemic transformation.[107] In general, radioactive phosphorus and alkylating agents such as busulfan and chlorambucil appear to cause the highest risk of acute leukemia, with the PVSG-01 trial finding actuarial incidence rates of 18% at 10 years for the chlorambucil arm and 15% at 10 years for ^{32}P, compared with <5% for phlebotomy.[107]

The agents hydroxyurea and pipobroman appear to be much less leukemogenic than ^{32}P or alkylating agents when used *de novo*. Studies have consistently shown rates of 3–5% at 10 years, possibly continuing to rise thereafter,[97,105,108] but it is difficult to be sure whether these agents do increase leukemic transformation as the risk in untreated patients with ET is not defined. It is very likely, however, that the use of hydroxyurea after previous ^{32}P therapy (and possibly alkylating agents) increases the risk of leukemia substantially over either agent alone.[97,105] Leukemic transformation of ET has an extremely poor prognosis, with failure to achieve partial or complete remission with standard chemotherapy regimens being common.[110]

CLASSIFICATION AND DIAGNOSIS OF ESSENTIAL THROMBOCYTHEMIA

Classification

Analysis of patients with ET has consistently demonstrated that the presence or absence of the *JAK2* V617F mutation divides patients into two biologically distinct subgroups.[34–36,111] V617F-positive patients display multiple features resembling PV, with significantly higher hemoglobin levels, neutrophil counts, bone marrow erythropoiesis, and granulopoiesis (Figure 16.1a), more venous thromboses and a higher incidence of polycythemic transformation.[34] In addition, mutation-positive patients have lower serum erythropoietin and ferritin levels than V617F-negative patients with ET.[34] These results imply that V617F-positive thrombocythemia and polycythemia may be better viewed as a continuum, and not as two distinct entities (Figure 16.2). V617F-negative individuals with ET do nonetheless exhibit features characteristic of an MPD, including cytogenetic abnormalities, hypercellular bone marrow with abnormal megakaryocyte morphology (Figure 16.1b), *PRV1* overexpression, growth of erythropoietin-independent erythroid colonies, and a risk of myelofibrotic or leukemic transformation.[34] These facts suggest that ET should be subclassified as either V617F-positive or V617F-negative ET, both *bona fide* MPD, although future studies may prove V617F-negative ET to be biologically heterogeneous.

Diagnosis

Proposed diagnostic criteria for ET incorporating the *JAK2* V617F mutation are shown in Table 16.2. and a flowchart for the suggested investigation of a patient with a high platelet

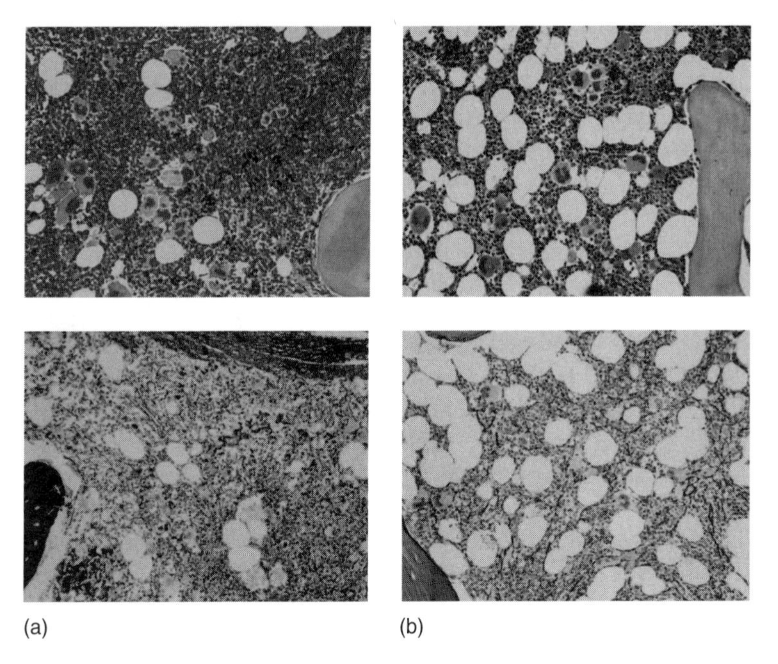

Figure 16.1 (a) Typical bone marrow trephine of a patient with *JAK2* V617F-positive thrombocythemia. H&E stain (40×) shows trilineage increase in cellularity, with clustered megakaryocytes, many of which are hyperlobated. The reticulin stain (40×) shows grade 1–2 reticulin levels. (b) Typical bone marrow trephine of a patient with *JAK2* V617F-negative essential thrombocythemia. The H&E stain (40×) is normocellular, with increased numbers of megakaryocytes, often showing nuclear hyperlobation. These have formed clusters in two locations. Upper panels, H&E; lower panels, reticulin.

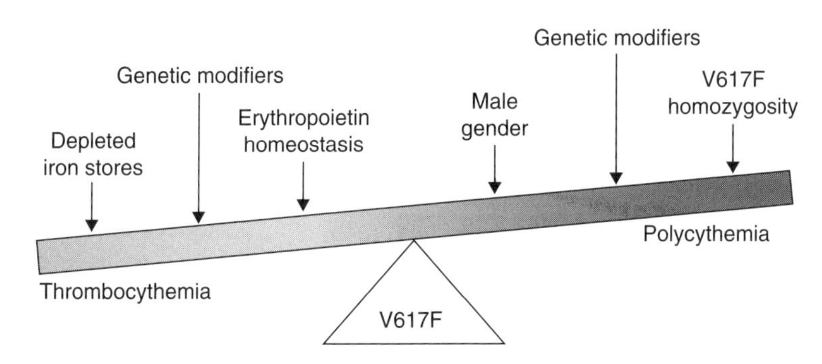

Figure 16.2 Continuum model for the relationship between *JAK2*-positive thrombocythemia and polycythemia. V617F-positive chronic phase disease forms a continuous spectrum, with several genetic and physiological factors affecting the phenotype. Male sex and especially V617F homozygosity[112] are associated with a polycythemic phenotype, whereas iron deficiency and erythropoietin homeostasis act to constrain the red cell mass within the normal range. Other acquired and constitutional genetic factors are likely to contribute to the phenotypic manifestations of the V617F mutation.

count in Figure 16.3. Testing for the *JAK2* V617F mutation is now widely available, and promises to simplify the diagnostic work-up. Allele-specific polymerase chain reaction (PCR),[6,34,113] pyrosequencing,[37,44] restriction enzyme digestion,[6,113] and real-time PCR[33] are all sufficiently sensitive to detect a heterozygous mutation when present in as little as 5–10% of cells. These assays have low false-positive rates, making them useful diagnostic tools.

An elevated platelet count in the presence of the *JAK2* V617F mutation has a very high positive predictive value for ET, reducing the need for exhaustive investigations to eliminate causes of reactive thrombocytosis. In such patients with *JAK2*-positive thrombocythemia, the major focus of the diagnostic evaluation is to differentiate ET from other myeloid disorders. A bone marrow aspirate and trephine will identify myelofibrosis and myelodysplasia (especially refractory anemia with ringed

Table 16.2 Diagnostic criteria for essential thrombocythemia incorporating testing for the *JAK2* V617F mutation[1]

JAK2*-positive thrombocythemia	
A1	Platelet count >450 × 10^9/l
A2	Mutation in *JAK2*
A3	No other myeloid malignancy, especially *JAK2*-positive polycythemia, myelofibrosis or myelodysplasia
***JAK2*-negative essential thrombocythemia**†	
A1	Platelet count >600 × 10^9/l‡ on two occasions at least one month apart
A2	Absence of mutation in *JAK2*
A3	No reactive cause for thrombocytosis
A4	Normal ferritin (>20 μg/l)
A5	No other myeloid malignancy, especially chronic myeloid leukemia, myelofibrosis, polycythemia vera or myelodysplasia

*Diagnosis requires all three criteria to be present.
†Diagnosis requires all five criteria.
‡This platelet threshold is preferred in patients lacking the *JAK2* mutation given the difficulty in excluding reactive thrombocytosis and the fact that 2.5% of normal individuals will have platelet counts above the normal range.

sideroblasts and thrombocythemia, which is commonly *JAK2*-positive). An elevated hematocrit will identify patients with PV.

For patients with an elevated platelet count who do not have the V617F mutation, it is important to exclude secondary causes of thrombocytosis, such as iron deficiency, infections, inflammatory conditions (especially rheumatoid arthritis, inflammatory bowel disease, and other autoimmune diseases) and hyposplenic states. Bone marrow examination in difficult cases may show clonal cytogenetic lesions or abnormalities of megakaryocyte morphology that are suggestive of ET.

Trephine histology has been suggested as a useful positive diagnostic criterion for diagnosing ET. It has been reported that patients can be divided into histologically distinct subgroups ('true ET' 'prefibrotic myelofibrosis', and early overt myelofibrosis) with different prognoses.[114] However, megakaryocyte morphology is notoriously difficult to assess in a reproducible manner and detailed studies of inter-observer variation are lacking. It is, therefore, not yet clear whether this sort of histological classification is robust enough to be applied widely outside specialized centers, and the inclusion of trephine biopsy histology in the WHO criteria is regarded by many as controversial.

MANAGEMENT OF ESSENTIAL THROMBOCYTHEMIA

Clinical trials

There have been only two prospective randomized studies of the treatment of patients with ET. In the first, 114 high-risk patients (age >60 years or prior thrombosis) were randomized to receive hydroxyurea or no cytoreductive agent.[114] During a median follow-up period of 27 months, patients on hydroxyurea developed significantly fewer thrombotic events. This was the first clear demonstration that cytoreductive therapy reduces thrombotic events in patients with ET.

The second randomized study was the Medical Research Council (MRC) primary thrombocythemia-1 (PT-1) trial,[20] in which high-risk patients (prior thrombosis, age >60 years or platelets >1000 × 10^9/l) were randomized to receive hydroxyurea plus aspirin or anagrelide plus aspirin. Compared to hydroxyurea plus aspirin, treatment with anagrelide plus aspirin was associated with increased rates of arterial

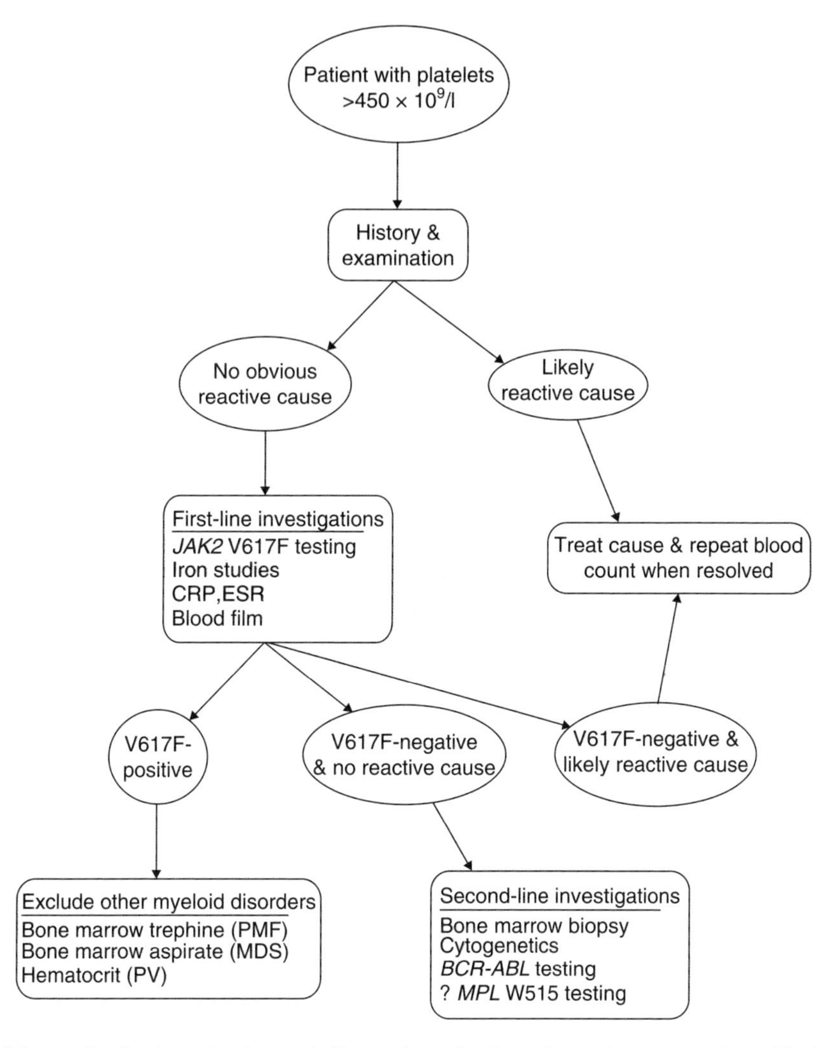

Figure 16.3 Schema for the investigation and diagnostic evaluation of a patient presenting with thrombocytosis. If initial history and examination do not reveal an obvious reactive cause, testing for *JAK2* V617F mutation, iron deficiency, and inflammatory markers should be performed. If the patient is V617F-positive, other myeloid disorders should be excluded, such as primary myelofibrosis (PMF), myelodysplasia (MDS), and polycythemia vera (PV). If the patient is V617F-negative and there is no obvious reactive cause, bone marrow biopsy and cytogenetics (including *BCR-ABL*) may provide supportive evidence. In difficult cases, testing for the *MPL* W515 mutations may be considered. If the patient is likely to have a reactive cause for the thrombocytosis, the blood count should be repeated 6–8 weeks after definitive correction of the secondary cause. CRP, C-reactive protein; ESR, erythrocyte sedimentation rate.

thrombosis, major hemorrhage, myelofibrotic transformation, and treatment withdrawal, but a decreased rate of venous thromboembolism. It is informative to compare these results with the other randomized study.[115] The actuarial rate of first thrombosis at 2 years was 4% for patients receiving hydroxyurea +/− aspirin in both studies, suggesting the two cohorts are broadly comparable. However, the rates of first thrombosis at 2 years were 8% and 26%

for patients receiving anagrelide plus aspirin (PT-1) or no cytoreductive therapy (Italian study), respectively. Notwithstanding the difficulties of such comparisons these data suggest that anagrelide plus aspirin provides partial protection against arterial thrombosis.

The results of the PT-1 trial suggest that hydroxyurea plus aspirin should remain first-line therapy for patients with ET at high risk of developing vascular events. For other patients at a lower risk of thrombosis, the situation is less clear. The decision whether to use a cytoreductive agent requires balancing two opposing risks, both of which are small: the risk of a thrombotic event and the risk of a significant drug-related side-effect. Unfortunately, the frequency of these two types of event is not clear from existing data. Some studies suggest that patients aged <60 years and with no prior thrombosis do not exhibit an increased frequency of thrombosis compared with controls.[116] However, the number of patients studied was small, the number of events very small, and the choice of an appropriate control population is difficult. Moreover, other studies have found that such patients do have a significant risk of thrombosis.[117]

Commonly used medications

Hydroxyurea

Hydroxyurea has emerged as first-line therapy for high-risk patients because of its efficacy, low cost, and rare acute toxicity. The main side-effects are leg ulcers, various other skin conditions (including photosensitivity and solar keratosis), and reversible bone marrow suppression. A common concern is whether hydroxyurea might be leukemogenic. There are now a number of studies which show that ET patients receiving hydroxyurea alone have a low incidence of acute myeloid leukemia myelodysplastic syndrome (3–4%)[118–120] and there are no data to show that this incidence is significantly different from that observed in untreated patients. Moreover, follow-up of patients receiving hydroxyurea for sickle cell disease over the past 10 years also suggests that its leukemogenic potential is very low.[121]

Anagrelide

Anagrelide is an imidazo quinazoline derivative originally developed as an inhibitor of platelet aggregation.[122] It was subsequently shown to lower the platelet count in a species-specific manner and at doses lower than that which inhibits platelet aggregation. It is a phosphodiesterase inhibitor and acts as a vasodilator and a positive inotrope. Acute side-effects include headaches, palpitations, and fluid retention.

Interferon

Interferon alfa is effective at reducing the platelet count below $600 \times 10^9/l$ in approximately 90% of patients with an average dose of 3 million international units per day. It is not known to be teratogenic or leukemogenic, does not cross the placenta and is often the treatment of choice during pregnancy.[123] However, the need for parenteral administration and its acute side-effects, particularly flu-like symptoms, are significant problems and result in treatment withdrawal in a substantial proportion of patients.

Aspirin

The European Collaboration on Low-dose Aspirin in Polycythemia Vera (ECLAP) trial was a randomized comparison of aspirin with placebo in patients with PV.[124] The key finding was a significantly reduced risk of vascular events in patients randomized to receive aspirin,[124] without a significant increase in major hemorrhage rates. The similarities in pathobiology between PV and ET, together with the central role of platelets in the vascular complications of ET, strongly argue that low-dose aspirin should be prescribed in all ET patients without a contraindication.

Management recommendations

An outline of a risk-stratified approach to the management of ET is presented in Table 16.3.

Table 16.3 Risk-stratified management recommendations for patients with essential thrombocythemia

All patients
Manage reversible cardiovascular risk factors aggressively (e.g. smoking, hypertension, hypercholesterolemia, obesity)
High-risk patients (prior thrombosis, age >60 years or platelets >1500 × 10^9/l)
Low-dose aspirin (unless specific contraindication)
Hydroxyurea (to maintain platelet count in normal range)
If hydroxyurea contraindicated, failure or toxicity, anagrelide or interferon alfa are acceptable second-line agents
Intermediate-risk patients (age 40–60 years and no high-risk features)
Either enter into randomized trial (e.g. PT-1 intermediate-risk arm)
Or low-dose aspirin (consider cytoreduction if other cardiovascular risk factors present)
Low-risk patients (age <40 years and no high-risk features)
Low-dose aspirin

The MRC PT-1 trial demonstrates that hydroxyurea should be first-line therapy for most patients with high-risk disease.[20] Interferon alfa and anagrelide are both reasonable second-line agents. The combination of hydroxyurea and anagrelide can be useful as a way of minimizing side-effects associated with the two drugs. All patients should receive aspirin, unless specifically contraindicated.

There is a general consensus that patients at particularly low risk of thrombotic events (age <40 years, no high-risk features) should receive low-dose aspirin alone (or equivalent). For the remaining intermediate-risk patients (age 40–60 years, no high-risk features), there are no good data to guide management and it is not clear whether cytoreduction is beneficial. Where possible such patients should be entered into a randomized trial such as the ongoing intermediate-risk PT-1 randomization (hydroxyurea plus aspirin versus aspirin alone).

There are few data to guide the management of ET in pregnancy.[123] It seems reasonable for patients to receive low-dose aspirin, but the decision whether to lower the platelet count is more contentious and there are conflicting reports as to whether the established factors for thrombosis in non-pregnant patients can predict poor pregnancy outcome. In the absence of clear data, it seems advisable to limit the use of platelet-lowering agents to patients thought to be at high risk of thrombosis and particularly to patients with a history of previous thrombosis or fetal loss. Anagrelide and hydroxyurea should be avoided because of the possibility of teratogenic effects, although there have been reports of normal pregnancies despite exposure to hydroxyurea. Interferon alfa is generally regarded as the treatment of choice and should be combined with heparin in patients at particularly high risk, with treatment continuing for several weeks postpartum.

REFERENCES

1. Campbell PJ, Green AR. The myeloproliferative disorders. N Engl J Med 2006; 355: 2452–66.
2. Adamson JW, Fialkow PJ, Murphy S, Prchal JF, Steinmann L. Polycythemia vera: stem-cell and probable clonal origin of the disease. N Engl J Med 1976; 295: 913–16.
3. Fialkow PJ, Faguet GB, Jacobson RJ, Vaidya K, Murphy S. Evidence that essential thrombocythemia is a clonal disorder with origin in a multipotent stem cell. Blood 1981; 58: 916–19.
4. Campbell PJ, Green AR. Management of polycythemia vera and essential thrombocythemia. Hematology Am Soc Hematol Educ Program 2005: 201–8.
5. Dameshek W. Some speculations on the myeloproliferative syndromes. Blood 1951; 6: 372–5.
6. Baxter EJ, Scott LM, Campbell PJ et al. Acquired mutation of the tyrosine kinase JAK2 in human myeloproliferative disorders. Lancet 2005; 365: 1054–61.
7. James C, Ugo V, Le Couedic JP et al. A unique clonal JAK2 mutation leading to constitutive signalling causes polycythaemia vera. Nature 2005; 434: 1144–8.
8. Levine RL, Wadleigh M, Cools J et al. Activating mutation in the tyrosine kinase JAK2 in polycythemia vera, essential thrombocythemia, and myeloid metaplasia with myelofibrosis. Cancer Cell 2005; 7: 387–97.

9. Kralovics R, Passamonti F, Buser AS et al. A gain-of-function mutation of JAK2 in myeloproliferative disorders. N Engl J Med 2005; 352: 1779–90.
10. Zhao R, Xing S, Li Z et al. Identification of an acquired JAK2 mutation in polycythemia vera. J Biol Chem 2005; 280: 22788–92.
11. Marchioli R, Finazzi G, Landolfi R et al. Vascular and neoplastic risk in a large cohort of patients with polycythemia vera. J Clin Oncol 2005; 23: 2224–32.
12. Passamonti F, Rumi E, Pungolino E et al. Life expectancy and prognostic factors for survival in patients with polycythemia vera and essential thrombocythemia. Am J Med 2004; 117: 755–61.
13. Johansson P, Kutti J, Andreasson B et al. Trends in the incidence of chronic Philadelphia chromosome negative (Ph-) myeloproliferative disorders in the city of Goteborg, Sweden, during 1983–99. J Intern Med 2004; 256: 161–5.
14. Mesa RA, Silverstein MN, Jacobsen SJ, Wollan PC, Tefferi A. Population-based incidence and survival figures in essential thrombocythemia and agnogenic myeloid metaplasia: an Olmsted County Study, 1976–1995. Am J Hematol 1999; 61: 10–15.
15. McNally RJ, Rowland D, Roman E, Cartwright RA. Age and sex distributions of hematological malignancies in the U.K. Hematol Oncol 1997; 15: 173–89.
16. Chaiter Y, Brenner B, Aghai E, Tatarsky I. High incidence of myeloproliferative disorders in Ashkenazi Jews in northern Israel. Leuk Lymphoma 1992; 7: 251–5.
17. Berglund S, Zettervall O. Incidence of polycythemia vera in a defined population. Eur J Haematol 1992; 48: 20–6.
18. Najean Y, Mugnier P, Dresch C, Rain JD. Polycythaemia vera in young people: an analysis of 58 cases diagnosed before 40 years. Br J Haematol 1987; 67: 285–91.
19. Danish EH, Rasch CA, Harris JW. Polycythemia vera in childhood: case report and review of the literature. Am J Hematol 1980; 9: 421–8.
20. Harrison CN, Campbell PJ, Buck G et al. Hydroxyurea compared with anagrelide in high-risk essential thrombocythemia. N Engl J Med 2005; 353: 33–45.
21. Bellanne-Chantelot C, Chaumarel I, Labopin M et al. Genetic and clinical implications of the Val617Phe JAK2 mutation in 72 families with myeloproliferative disorders. Blood 2006; 108: 346–52.
22. Ghilardi N, Wiestner A, Kikuchi M, Ohsaka A, Skoda RC. Hereditary thrombocythaemia in a Japanese family is caused by a novel point mutation in the thrombopoietin gene. Br J Haematol 1999; 107: 310–16.
23. Caldwell GG, Kelley DB, Heath CW Jr, Zack M. Polycythemia vera among participants of a nuclear weapons test. JAMA 1984; 252: 662–4.
24. Sandberg EM, Wallace TA, Godeny MD, Vonderlinden D, Sayeski PP. Jak2 tyrosine kinase: a true jak of all trades? Cell Biochem Biophys 2004; 41: 207–32.
25. Kisseleva T, Bhattacharya S, Braunstein J, Schindler CW. Signaling through the JAK/STAT pathway, recent advances and future challenges. Gene 2002; 285: 1–24.
26. Neubauer H, Cumano A, Muller M et al. Jak2 deficiency defines an essential developmental checkpoint in definitive hematopoiesis. Cell 1998; 93: 397–409.
27. Parganas E, Wang D, Stravopodis D et al. Jak2 is essential for signaling through a variety of cytokine receptors. Cell 1998; 93: 385–95.
28. Huang LJ, Constantinescu SN, Lodish HF. The N-terminal domain of Janus kinase 2 is required for Golgi processing and cell surface expression of erythropoietin receptor. Mol Cell 2001; 8: 1327–38.
29. Remy I, Wilson IA, Michnick SW. Erythropoietin receptor activation by a ligand-induced conformation change. Science 1999; 283: 990–3.
30. Lu X, Gross AW, Lodish HF. Active conformation of the erythropoietin receptor: random and cysteine-scanning mutagenesis of the extracellular juxtamembrane and transmembrane domains. J Biol Chem 2006; 281: 7002–11.
31. Seubert N, Royer Y, Staerk J et al. Active and inactive orientations of the transmembrane and cytosolic domains of the erythropoietin receptor dimer. Mol Cell 2003; 12: 1239–50.
32. Witthuhn BA, Quelle FW, Silvennoinen O et al. JAK2 associates with the erythropoietin receptor and is tyrosine phosphorylated and activated following stimulation with erythropoietin. Cell 1993; 74: 227–36.
33. Levine RL, Belisle C, Wadleigh M et al. X-inactivation based clonality analysis and quantitative JAK2V617F assessment reveals a strong association between clonality and JAK2V617F in PV but not ET/MMM, and identifies a subset of JAK2V617F negative ET and MMM patients with clonal hematopoiesis. Blood 2006; 107: 4139–41.
34. Campbell PJ, Scott LM, Buck G et al. Definition of subtypes of essential thrombocythaemia and relation to polycythaemia vera based on JAK2 V617F mutation status: a prospective study. Lancet 2005; 366: 1945–53.
35. Wolanskyj AP, Lasho TL, Schwager SM et al. JAK2 mutation in essential thrombocythaemia: clinical associations and long-term prognostic relevance. Br J Haematol 2005; 131: 208–13.
36. Antonioli E, Guglielmelli P, Pancrazzi A et al. Clinical implications of the JAK2 V617F mutation in essential thrombocythemia. Leukemia 2005; 19: 1847–9.
37. Jones AV, Kreil S, Zoi K et al. Widespread occurrence of the JAK2 V617F mutation in chronic myeloproliferative disorders. Blood 2005; 106: 2162–8.

38. Campbell PJ, Griesshammer M, Dohner K et al. V617F mutation in JAK2 is associated with poorer survival in idiopathic myelofibrosis. Blood 2006; 107: 2098–100.
39. Tefferi A, Lasho TL, Schwager SM et al. The JAK2(V617F) tyrosine kinase mutation in myelofibrosis with myeloid metaplasia: lineage specificity and clinical correlates. Br J Haematol 2005; 131: 320–8.
40. Scott LM, Scott MA, Campbell PJ, Green AR. Progenitors homozygous for the V617F JAK2 mutation occur in most patients with polycythemia vera but not essential thrombocythemia. Blood 2006; 108: 2435–7.
41. Steensma DP, Dewald GW, Lasho TL et al. The JAK2 V617F activating tyrosine kinase mutation is an infrequent event in both 'atypical' myeloproliferative disorders and myelodysplastic syndromes. Blood 2005; 106: 1207–9.
42. Scott LM, Campbell PJ, Baxter EJ et al. The V617F JAK2 mutation is uncommon in cancers and in myeloid malignancies other than the classic myeloproliferative disorders. Blood 2005; 106: 2920–1.
43. Levine RL, Loriaux M, Huntly BJ et al. The JAK2V617F activating mutation occurs in chronic myelomonocytic leukemia and acute myeloid leukemia, but not in acute lymphoblastic leukemia or chronic lymphocytic leukemia. Blood 2005; 106: 3377–9.
44. Jelinek J, Oki Y, Gharibyan V et al. JAK2 mutation 1849G>T is rare in acute leukemias but can be found in CMML, Philadelphia chromosome-negative CML, and megakaryocytic leukemia. Blood 2005; 106: 3370–3.
45. Lee JW, Kim YG, Soung YH et al. The JAK2 V617F mutation in de novo acute myelogenous leukemias. Oncogene 2006; 25: 1434–6.
46. Frohling S, Lipka DB, Kayser S et al. Rare occurrence of the JAK2 V617F mutation in AML subtypes M5, M6, and M7. Blood 2006; 107: 1242–3.
47. Melzner I, Weniger MA, Menz CK, Moller P. Absence of the JAK2 V617F activating mutation in classical Hodgkin lymphoma and primary mediastinal B-cell lymphoma. Leukemia 2006; 20: 157–8.
48. Patel RK, Lea NC, Heneghan MA et al. Prevalence of the activating JAK2 tyrosine kinase mutation V617F in the Budd-Chiari syndrome. Gastroenterology 2006; 130: 2031–8.
49. Saharinen P, Takaluoma K, Silvennoinen O. Regulation of the Jak2 tyrosine kinase by its pseudokinase domain. Mol Cell Biol 2000; 20: 3387–95.
50. Ugo V, Marzac C, Teyssandier I et al. Multiple signaling pathways are involved in erythropoietin-independent differentiation of erythroid progenitors in polycythemia vera. Exp Hematol 2004; 32: 179–87.
51. Socolovsky M, Fallon AE, Wang S, Brugnara C, Lodish HF. Fetal anemia and apoptosis of red cell progenitors in Stat5a-/-5b-/- mice: a direct role for Stat5 in Bcl-X(L) induction. Cell 1999; 98: 181–91.
52. Myklebust JH, Blomhoff HK, Rusten LS, Stokke T, Smeland EB. Activation of phosphatidylinositol 3-kinase is important for erythropoietin-induced erythropoiesis from CD34(+) hematopoietic progenitor cells. Exp Hematol 2002; 30: 990–1000.
53. Pikman Y, Lee BH, Mercher T et al. MPLW515L is a novel somatic activating mutation in myelofibrosis with myeloid metaplasia. PLoS Med 2006; 3: e270.
54. Pardanani AD, Levine RL, Lasho T et al. MPL515 mutations in myeloproliferative and other myeloid disorders: a study of 1182 patients. Blood 2006; 108: 3472–6.
55. Staerk J, Lacout C, Sato T et al. An amphipathic motif at the transmembrane-cytoplasmic junction prevents autonomous activation of the thrombopoietin receptor. Blood 2006; 107: 1864–71.
56. Wernig G, Mercher T, Okabe R et al. Expression of Jak2V617F causes a polycythemia vera-like disease with associated myelofibrosis in a murine bone marrow transplant model. Blood 2006; 107: 4274–81.
57. Lacout C, Pisani DF, Tulliez M et al. JAK2V617F expression in murine hematopoietic cells leads to MPD mimicking human PV with secondary myelofibrosis. Blood 2006; 108: 1652–60.
58. Zaleskas VM, Krause DS, Lazarides K et al. Molecular pathogenesis of polycythemia induced in mice by JAK2 V617F. Blood 2005; 106: A116.
59. Bumm TGP, Elsea C, Wood LG et al. JAK2 V617F Mutation Induces a Myeloproliferative Disorder in Mice. Blood 2005; 106: A116.
60. Bench AJ, Nacheva EP, Champion KM, Green AR. Molecular genetics and cytogenetics of myeloproliferative disorders. Baillieres Clin Haematol 1998; 11: 819–48.
61. Kralovics R, Teo SS, Li S et al. Acquisition of the V617F mutation of JAK2 is a late genetic event in a subset of patients with myeloproliferative disorders. Blood 2006; 108: 1377–80.
62. Campbell PJ, Baxter EJ, Beer PA et al. Mutation of JAK2 in the myeloproliferative disorders: timing, clonality studies, cytogenetic associations and role in leukemic transformation. Blood 2006; 108: 3548–55.
63. Kralovics R, Teo SS, Buser AS et al. Altered gene expression in myeloproliferative disorders correlates with activation of signaling by the V617F mutation of Jak2. Blood 2005; 106: 3374–6.
64. Silva M, Richard C, Benito A et al. Expression of Bcl-x in erythroid precursors from patients with polycythemia vera. N Engl J Med 1998; 338: 564–71.
65. Kieslinger M, Woldman I, Moriggl R et al. Antiapoptotic activity of Stat5 required during terminal

stages of myeloid differentiation. Genes Dev 2000; 14: 232–44.

66. Socolovsky M, Nam H, Fleming MD et al. Ineffective erythropoiesis in Stat5a(−/−)5b(−/−) mice due to decreased survival of early erythroblasts. Blood 2001; 98: 3261–73.
67. Zeuner A, Pedini F, Signore M et al. Increased death receptor resistance and FLIPshort expression in polycythemia vera erythroid precursor cells. Blood 2006; 107: 3495–502.
68. Walz C, Crowley BJ, Hudon HE et al. Activated JAK2 with the V617F point mutation promotes G1/S-phase transition. J Biol Chem 2006; 281: 18177–83.
69. Goerttler PS, Kreutz C, Donauer J et al. Gene expression profiling in polycythaemia vera: overexpression of transcription factor NF-E2. Br J Haematol 2005; 129: 138–50.
70. Labbaye C, Valtieri M, Barberi T et al. Differential expression and functional role of GATA-2, NF-E2, and GATA-1 in normal adult hematopoiesis. J Clin Invest 1995; 95: 2346–58.
71. Sayer MS, Tilbrook PA, Spadaccini A et al. Ectopic expression of transcription factor NF-E2 alters the phenotype of erythroid and monoblastoid cells. J Biol Chem 2000; 275: 25292–8.
72. Lu X, Levine R, Tong W et al. Expression of a homodimeric type I cytokine receptor is required for JAK2V617F-mediated transformation. Proc Natl Acad Sci U S A 2005; 102: 18962–7.
73. Tefferi A, Fonseca R, Pereira DL, Hoagland HC. A long-term retrospective study of young women with essential thrombocythemia. Mayo Clin Proc 2001; 76: 22–8.
74. Rozman C, Giralt M, Feliu E, Rubio D, Cortes MT. Life expectancy of patients with chronic nonleukemic myeloproliferative disorders. Cancer 1991; 67: 2658–63.
75. Wolanskyj AP, Schwager SM, McClure RF, Larson DR, Tefferi A. Essential thrombocythemia beyond the first decade: life expectancy, long-term complication rates, and prognostic factors. Mayo Clin Proc 2006; 81: 159–66.
76. Michiels JJ, Abels J, Steketee J, van Vliet HH, Vuzevski VD. Erythromelalgia caused by platelet-mediated arteriolar inflammation and thrombosis in thrombocythemia. Ann Intern Med 1985; 102: 466–71.
77. Michiels JJ, Berneman Z, Schroyens W, van Urk H. Aspirin-responsive painful red, blue, black toe, or finger syndrome in polycythemia vera associated with thrombocythemia. Ann Hematol 2003; 82: 153–9.
78. Itin PH, Winkelmann RK. Cutaneous manifestations in patients with essential thrombocythemia. J Am Acad Dermatol 1991; 24: 59–63.
79. Michiels JJ, Koudstaal PJ, Mulder AH, van Vliet HH. Transient neurologic and ocular manifestations in primary thrombocythemia. Neurology 1993; 43: 1107–10.
80. Valla D, Casadevall N, Huisse MG et al. Etiology of portal vein thrombosis in adults. A prospective evaluation of primary myeloproliferative disorders. Gastroenterology 1988; 94: 1063–9.
81. Lamy T, Devillers A, Bernard M et al. Inapparent polycythemia vera: an unrecognized diagnosis. Am J Med 1997; 102: 14–20.
82. Cortelazzo S, Finazzi G, Ruggeri M et al. Hydroxyurea for patients with essential thrombocythemia and a high risk of thrombosis. N Engl J Med 1995; 332: 1132–6.
83. Bellucci S, Janvier M, Tobelem G et al. Essential thrombocythemias. Clinical evolutionary and biological data. Cancer 1986; 58: 2440–7.
84. Colombi M, Radaelli F, Zocchi L, Maiolo AT. Thrombotic and hemorrhagic complications in essential thrombocythemia. A retrospective study of 103 patients. Cancer 1991; 67: 2926–30.
85. Regev A, Stark P, Blickstein D, Lahav M. Thrombotic complications in essential thrombocythemia with relatively low platelet counts. Am J Hematol 1997; 56: 168–72.
86. Besses C, Cervantes F, Pereira A et al. Major vascular complications in essential thrombocythemia: a study of the predictive factors in a series of 148 patients. Leukemia 1999; 13: 150–4.
87. Elliott MA, Tefferi A. Thrombosis and haemorrhage in polycythaemia vera and essential thrombocythaemia. Br J Haematol 2005; 128: 275–90.
88. Fenaux P, Simon M, Caulier MT et al. Clinical course of essential thrombocythemia in 147 cases. Cancer 1990; 66: 549–56.
89. Bellucci S, Legrand C, Boval B, Drouet L, Caen J. Studies of platelet volume, chemistry and function in patients with essential thrombocythaemia treated with Anagrelide. Br J Haematol 1999; 104: 886–92.
90. Falanga A, Marchetti M, Vignoli A, Balducci D, Barbui T. Leukocyte-platelet interaction in patients with essential thrombocythemia and polycythemia vera. Exp Hematol 2005; 33: 523–30.
91. Budde U, van Genderen PJ. Acquired von Willebrand disease in patients with high platelet counts. Semin Thromb Hemost 1997; 23: 425–31.
92. Budde U, Scharf RE, Franke P et al. Elevated platelet count as a cause of abnormal von Willebrand factor multimer distribution in plasma. Blood 1993; 82: 1749–57.
93. Buss DH, Stuart JJ, Lipscomb GE. The incidence of thrombotic and hemorrhagic disorders in association with extreme thrombocytosis: an analysis of 129 cases. Am J Hematol 1985; 20: 365–72.
94. Spivak JL. Polycythemia vera: myths, mechanisms, and management. Blood 2002; 100: 4272–90.
95. Bain BJ, Clark DM, Lampert IA, Wilkins BS. Bone Marrow Pathology, 3rd edn. London: Blackwell Publishing, 2001.
96. Barosi G, Ambrosetti A, Finelli C et al. The Italian Consensus Conference on Diagnostic Criteria for

Myelofibrosis with Myeloid Metaplasia. Br J Haematol 1999; 104: 730–7.

97. Najean Y, Rain JD. Treatment of polycythemia vera: the use of hydroxyurea and pipobroman in 292 patients under the age of 65 years. Blood 1997; 90: 3370–7.
98. Najean Y, Rain JD. Treatment of polycythemia vera: use of 32P alone or in combination with maintenance therapy using hydroxyurea in 461 patients greater than 65 years of age. The French Polycythemia Study Group. Blood 1997; 89: 2319–27.
99. Tatarsky I, Sharon R. Management of polycythemia vera with hydroxyurea. Semin Hematol 1997; 34: 24–8.
100. Cervantes F, Alvarez-Larran A, Talarn C et al. Myelofibrosis with myeloid metaplasia following essential thrombocythaemia: actuarial probability, presenting characteristics and evolution in a series of 195 patients. Br J Haematol 2002; 118: 786–90.
101. Najean Y, Dresch C, Rain JD. The very-long-term course of polycythaemia: a complement to the previously published data of the Polycythaemia Vera Study Group. Br J Haematol 1994; 86: 233–5.
102. Passamonti F, Malabarba L, Orlandi E et al. Polycythemia vera in young patients: a study on the long-term risk of thrombosis, myelofibrosis and leukemia. Haematologica 2003; 88: 13–18.
103. Kiladjian JJ, Gardin C, Renoux M, Bruno F, Bernard JF. Long-term outcomes of polycythemia vera patients treated with pipobroman as initial therapy. Hematol J 2003; 4: 198–207.
104. Najean Y, Deschamps A, Dresch C et al. Acute leukemia and myelodysplasia in polycythemia vera. A clinical study with long-term follow-up. Cancer 1988; 61: 89–95.
105. Finazzi G, Caruso V, Marchioli R et al. Acute leukemia in polycythemia vera: an analysis of 1638 patients enrolled in a prospective observational study. Blood 2005; 105: 2664–70.
106. Dupriez B, Morel P, Demory JL et al. Prognostic factors in agnogenic myeloid metaplasia: a report on 195 cases with a new scoring system. Blood 1996; 88: 1013–18.
107. Berk PD, Goldberg JD, Donovan PB et al. Therapeutic recommendations in polycythemia vera based on Polycythemia Vera Study Group protocols. Semin Hematol 1986; 23: 132–43.
108. Fruchtman SM, Mack K, Kaplan ME et al. From efficacy to safety: a Polycythemia Vera Study group report on hydroxyurea in patients with polycythemia vera. Semin Hematol 1997; 34: 17–23.
109. Sterkers Y, Preudhomme C, Lai JL et al. Acute myeloid leukemia and myelodysplastic syndromes following essential thrombocythemia treated with hydroxyurea: high proportion of cases with 17p deletion. Blood 1998; 91: 616–22.
110. Donovan PB, Landaw SA, Dresch C et al. Resistance to therapy of acute leukemia developing in the course of polycythemia vera. Nouv Rev Fr Hematol 1981; 23: 187–92.
111. Cheung B, Radia D, Pantelidis P et al. The presence of the JAK2 V617F mutation is associated with a higher haemoglobin and increased risk of thrombosis in essential thrombocythaemia. Br J Haematol 2006; 132: 244–5.
112. Scott LM, Scott MA, Campbell PJ, Green AR. Progenitors homozygous for the V617F mutation occur in most patients with polycythemia vera, but not essential thrombocythemia. Blood 2006; 108: 2435–7.
113. Campbell PJ, Scott LM, Baxter EJ et al. Methods for the detection of the JAK2 V617F mutation in human myeloproliferative disorders. Methods Mol Med 2006; 125: 253–64.
114. Thiele J, Kvasnicka HM, Zankovich R, Diehl V. Relevance of bone marrow features in the differential diagnosis between essential thrombocythemia and early stage idiopathic myelofibrosis. Haematologica 2000; 85: 1126–34.
115. Cortelazzo S, Finazzi G, Ruggeri M et al. Hydroxyurea for patients with essential thrombocythemia and a high risk of thrombosis. N Engl J Med 1995; 332: 1132–6.
116. Ruggeri M, Finazzi G, Tosetto A et al. No treatment for low-risk thrombocythaemia: results from a prospective study. Br J Haematol 1998; 103: 772–7.
117. Pearson TC, Bareford D, Craig J et al. The management of ‘low-risk’ and ‘intermediate-risk’ patients with primary thrombocythaemia. MPD (UK) Study Group. Br J Haematol 1999; 106: 833–4.
118. Sterkers Y, Preudhomme C, Lai JL et al. Acute myeloid leukemia and myelodysplastic syndromes following essential thrombocythemia treated with hydroxyurea: high proportion of cases with 17p deletion. Blood 1998; 91: 616–22.
119. Finazzi G, Ruggeri M, Rodeghiero F, Barbui T. Second malignancies in patients with essential thrombocythaemia treated with busulphan and hydroxyurea: long-term follow-up of a randomized clinical trial. Br J Haematol 2000; 110: 577–83.
120. Finazzi G, Caruso V, Marchioli R et al. Acute leukemia in polycythemia vera: an analysis of 1638 patients enrolled in a prospective observational study. Blood 2005; 105: 2664–70.
121. Hanft VN, Fruchtman SR, Pickens CV et al. Acquired DNA mutations associated with in vivo hydroxyurea exposure. Blood 2000; 95: 3589–93.
122. Spivak JL, Barosi G, Tognoni G et al. Chronic myeloproliferative disorders. Hematology Am Soc Hematol Educ Program 2003: 200–24.
123. Harrison C. Pregnancy and its management in the Philadelphia negative myeloproliferative diseases. Br J Haematol 2005; 129: 293–306.
124. Landolfi R, Marchioli R, Kutti J et al. Efficacy and safety of low-dose aspirin in polycythemia vera. N Engl J Med 2004; 350: 114–24.

Transplant options for patients with *BCR-ABL*-negative chronic myeloproliferative disorders

17

Nicolaus Kröger

INTRODUCTION

The chronic myeloproliferative disorders include chronic myeloid leukemia (CML), essential thrombocythemia (ET), polycythemia vera (PV), and idiopathic myelofibrosis (IMF). Each disorder is a clonal hematological malignancy originating at the pluripotent hematopoietic stem cell level. These clonal hematopoietic disorders are characterized by proliferation of one or more of the myeloid (granulocytic, erythroid, and megakaryocytic) lineages. While in ET and PV, a relative normal blood production exists, this proliferation results in an increased number of granulocytes, red blood cells, and/or platelets. In contrast, advanced IMF is associated with ineffective hematopoiesis leading to cytopenia. Both ET and PV are usually associated with a prolonged clinical course, and with appropriate treatment, patients often survive for >15 years.[1,2] In contrast, IMF has a more serious prognosis with a median survival of approximately 5 years.[3,4] IMF is characterized by cytopenia, megakaryocytic hyperplasia, splenomegaly, extramedullary hematopoiesis, and a leukoerythroblastic blood picture. The bone marrow histology shows fibrosis and increased angiogenesis. A number of agents, including erythropoietin, thalidomide, lenalidomide, hydroxyurea, melphalan, and busulfan, have been used to correct cytopenia or reduce splenomegaly. However, no drug has been shown to alter the natural course of the disease. The recent discovery of mutation of the Janus kinase 2 (JAK2)[5] and the thrombopoietin-receptor (MPL)[6] has resulted in activity towards development of inhibitors, which might be used as non-toxic specific agents for treatment of BCR-ABL-negative myeloproliferative disorders. Currently allogeneic stem cell transplantation is the only curative treatment approach in IMF.

AUTOLOGOUS STEM CELL TRANSPLANTATION

Few studies have investigated autologous stem cell transplantation after high-dose chemotherapy in patients with myelofibrosis.[7–9] In a pilot study, 21 patients received peripheral blood stem cell transplantation after myeloablative conditioning with busulfan (16 mg/kg body mass). The median time of leukocyte and platelet engraftment was 21 days; however, some patients had delayed engraftment of up to 96 days for leukocyte recovery, and more than 200 days for platelet recovery. Three patients died from non-relapse causes. Erythroid response without transfusion for >8 weeks was seen in ten out of 17 patients, and symptomatic splenomegaly improved in seven out of ten patients.[8] In a small series of three patients who received autologous stem cell transplantation after conditioning with treosulfan (42 g/m^2 body surface), a prolonged leukocyte reconstitution of 28–38 days was seen, and a significant reduction of spleen size was noted.[7] Overall, autologous stem cell transplantation is a potential treatment approach that can relieve disease-related symptoms such as splenomegaly, but the curative potential is very unlikely.

ALLOGENEIC STEM CELL TRANSPLANTATION AFTER STANDARD MYELOABLATIVE CONDITIONING

Despite the increased use of allogeneic stem cell transplantation in treatment of hematological malignancies, major concerns regarding performing this treatment approach in patients with IMF come from bone marrow histopathology which is distorted by fibrosis and might lead to a higher risk for engraftment failure. The first small reports and case reports in the early 1990s, however, suggested that engraftment is feasible and regression of bone marrow fibrosis was noted.[10,11] Furthermore, in relapsed patients after allografting, a graft versus myelofibrosis effect could be demonstrated by donor-lymphocyte infusions.[12,13] Larger retrospective studies including > 50 patients with myelofibrosis were reported by Guardiola *et al.* in a combined analysis of European and American centers,[14] and from Deeg *et al.* reporting the results of the Fred Hutchinson Cancer Research Center (FHCRC) in Seattle.[15] The latter study was recently updated and included 95 patients.[16] In the retrospective European–American study, Guardiola *et al.*[14] reported on 55 patients with myelofibrosis, who underwent conventional allogeneic stem cell transplantation. The median time from diagnosis to transplantation was 21 months (range 2–266 months). Most of the patients received conditioning regimens including total-body irradiation (TBI). Matched-related donors were used in the majority of the patients (n = 49). According to the Lille risk score, 76% had intermediate- or high-risk disease. Splenectomy prior transplantation was done in 27 patients. Graft failure occurred in 9% of the patients, and non-relapse mortality at 1 year was 27%. The 5-year overall and disease-free survival was 47% and 39%, respectively. Patients with low risk according to the Lille score had better overall survival than patients with intermediate- or high-risk disease (85% versus 45–30%). In a multivariate analysis, hemoglobin <10 g/dl, abnormal karyotype, high-risk disease according to the Lille score, and presence of osteosclerosis had an adverse impact on survival.

The Seattle group recently updated its results of allogeneic stem cell transplantation in patients with Philadelphia chromosome-negative myeloproliferative diseases.[16] The study included 104 patients, and standard myeloablative conditioning was used in 95 patients. Most patients had myelofibrosis (n = 62), advanced ET (n = 18), or PV (n = 12). The median age was 49 years (range 18–70 years), and stem cell donors were related (n = 59), syngeneic (n = 3), or unrelated (n = 45). The conditioning regimens mainly consisted of TBI plus cyclophosphamide, or busulfan plus cyclophosphamide. Non-relapse mortality at 5 years was 34%. The overall survival at 7 years was 61%. Improved survival in a multivariate analysis was seen for patients conditioned with targeting busulfan/cyclophosphamide regimen, for younger patients, for patients with a low co-morbidity score, and for patients with high platelet count at transplantation.

The results of both of these studies and of other studies of standard allografting are listed in Table 17.1.[14–22]

Taken together the results of the published studies on conventional allogeneic stem cell transplantation show the median age of the patients was between 38 and 54 years and significantly lower than the median age of about 60 years for patients with myelofibrosis at time of diagnosis. The long-term survival in the larger studies was 47% and 61%, respectively,[14,16] indicating the curative potential of standard myeloablative allograft. However, the non-relapse mortality at 1 year ranged from 20 to 48% (Table 17.1). One of the most significant prognostic factors for impaired survival was increasing age of the patient. In the European–American study, patients of <45 years of age experienced 62% survival, whereas patients >45 years had a survival of only 14%. In one study, stem cell transplantation from an unrelated donor was associated with worse outcome, while other studies did not show differences between related and unrelated stem cell transplantation.[15,16,23] Other factors for improved survival in multivariate

Table 17.1 Allogeneic stem cell transplantation after standard myeloablative conditioning

Author	*No. of patients*	*Median age (range)*	*Non-relapse mortality at 1 year (%)*	*Overall survival (%)*
Singhal *et al.*[17]	3	38 years (45–75)	33	66 (at 1 year)
Anderson *et al.*[18*]	13	38 years (18–49)	23	77 (at 2 years)
Deeg *et al.*[15*]	56	43 years (10–66)	20	58 (at 3 years)
Kerbauy *et al.*[16*†]	104	49 years (18–70)	34 (at 5 years)	61 (at 7 years)
Guardiola *et al.*[14]	55	42 years (4–53)	27	47 (at 5 years)
Daly *et al.*[19]	25	49 years (46–50)	48	41 (at 2 years)
Mittal *et al.*[20]	5	54 years (46–58)	40	60 (at 1 year)
Ditschkowski *et al.*[21]	20	45 years (22–57)	45	39 (at 3 years)
Przepiorka *et al.*[22]	5	43 years (34–51)	20	60 (at 2 years)

*Report from the same institution, therefore some patients were reported more than once.
†Including nine patients with non-myeloablative conditioning.

Table 17.2 Prognostic factors for better overall survival after myeloablative allograft

Conditioning regimen	*Reference*
Target busulfan/cyclophosphamide regimen versus others	15, 16
Younger age	14, 16
High platelet count	16
Low co-morbidity index	16
Low risk according to the Dupriez score	14, 15
Normal karyotype	14, 15
Hemoglobin >10 g/dl	14
No osteosclerosis	14

analysis were conditioning with targeting busulfan regimen,[15,16] high platelet count and low co-morbidity index,[16] low risk according to the Dupriez score,[14,15] normal karyotype,[14,15] hemoglobin >10 g/dl,[14] and non-osteosclerosis[14] (see Table 17.2).[24–29]

ALLOGENEIC STEM CELL TRANSPLANTATION AFTER DOSE-REDUCED CONDITIONING

Allogeneic stem cell transplantation after standard myeloablative conditioning chemotherapy has been shown to be a curative treatment approach in patients with myelofibrosis. The major limitation of this approach is that it can only be performed in younger patients with good performance status. The introduction of so called 'non-myeloablative', or 'dose-reduced', or 'toxicity-reduced' conditioning regimens is based on the concept of shifting the eradication of tumor cells from high-dose chemotherapy to the immunologically mediated graft versus tumor effect. The potential advantages are less treatment-related morbidity and mortality, and a broader application also in elderly patients. Evidence for an immunologically mediated graft versus myelofibrosis effect comes from reports on relapsed patients after allogeneic stem cell transplantation who show a remarkable reduction of bone marrow fibrosis after donor-lymphocyte infusion.[12,13] The feasibility of dose-reduced conditioning in patients with myelofibrosis has first been reported in small series of case reports.[26,27,30,31] In the two largest studies published so far[24,25] patients up to their 7th decade of age were included. In the German study,[25] 21 patients with a median age of 53 years (range 32–63 years) were included. The conditioning regimen consisted of busulfan (10 mg/kg), fludarabine (180 mg/m^2), and anti-thymocyte globulin (ATG, Fresenius) (30 mg/kg for related and 60 mg/kg for unrelated donors), followed by stem cell transplantation from related ($n = 8$) or unrelated ($n = 13$) donors. No primary graft failure was observed, and leukocyte and platelet engraftment were seen after a median of 16 days and 23 days, respectively. Complete donor chimerism was seen in 95% of the patients at day +100. Acute graft versus host disease grade II–IV and grade III/IV was observed in 48% and 19% of the patients, respectively. Chronic graft versus host disease occurred in 55% of patients. Non-relapse mortality was 16% at 1 year. After a median follow-up of 22 months (range 4–59 months), the 3-year estimated overall and disease-free survival was 84%. The second study from the Myelofibrosis Consortium also included 21 patients with a median age of 54 years (range 27–68 years). Different conditioning regimens were used, including melphalan plus fludarabine, cyclophosphamide plus fludarabine, thiotepa plus fludarabine, and TBI (2 Gy) in combination with fludarabine. All patients were intermediate or high risk according to the Lille score. One graft failure was observed. More than 95% donor chimerism was seen in 18 patients. Non-relapse mortality was 10%, and overall 2-year survival was 87%. Table 17.2 shows other published results including three or more patients. The most commonly used regimens were busulfan/fludarabine based, and melphalan/fludarabine based. In comparison to the reported myeloablative transplantations (Table 17.3), the median age of patients was >10 years older at 51–58 years. The non-relapse mortality was lower than 20%, and overall survival after a relatively short follow-up was between 84% and 100%. In a small study including nine patients, the non-relapse mortality was 40%,[29] and the overall survival was only 56% at 1 year. A retrospective comparison between conventional and reduced-intensity conditioning regimens was performed in 26 patients from the Swedish Group for Myeloproliferative Disorders.[28] Despite the fact that in the reduced-intensity group ($n = 10$), the median age was 14 years older than in the myeloablative group ($n = 17$), the non-relapse mortality was lower in the reduced-intensity conditioning regimen group than in the myeloablative group (10% versus 30%). Even if the follow-up of these studies is rather short, they demonstrate that reduced conditioning is effective and feasible with acceptable toxicity even in older patients.

ROLE OF SPLENECTOMY PRIOR TO TRANSPLANTATION

The role of pretransplant splenectomy is still controversial. A major concern regarding splenectomy and allogeneic stem cell transplantation is the risk of graft failure or delayed engraftment. Indeed, some reports have shown faster engraftment of splenectomized patients.[14,32] An analysis of 26 splenectomized patients showed less need for red blood cell or platelet transfusion in patients who underwent

Table 17.3 Allogeneic stem cell transplantation after reduced-intensity conditioning

Author	*No. of patients*	*Conditioning regimen*	*Median age (years)*	*Non-relapse mortality at 1 year (%)*	*Overall survival (%)*
Rondelli *et al.*[24]	21	Various	54	10	85 (at 2.5 years)
Kröger *et al.*[25]	21	Bu (10 mg/kg)/Flu	53	16	84 (at 3 years)
Hessling *et al.*[26*]	3	Bu (10 mg/kg)/Flu	51	0	100 (at 1 year)
Devine *et al.*[27]	4	Melph/Flu	56	0	100 (at 1 year)
Merup *et al.*[28]	10	Bu/Flu; Melph/Cyclo/Flu	58	10	90 (at 1 year)
Snyder *et al.*[29]	9	Flu/Melph; 2 Gy TBI/Flu	54	40	56 (at 1 year)

Bu, busulfan; Flu, fludarabine; Melph, melphalan; Cyclo, Cyclophosphamide; TBI, total-body irradiation.
[*]Patients were also reported with a longer follow-up in Kröger *et al.*

splenectomy prior to transplantation, but the 3-year probability of survival did not differ significantly in comparison to non-splenectomized patients (73% versus 64%).[33] Given the high risk of surgery-related morbidity and mortality, which exceeds 9%, as well as the increased risk of leukemia, removal of the spleen prior to allogeneic stem cell transplantation is currently not recommended.[33,34]

THE ROLE OF *JAK2* MUTATION IN THE TRANSPLANT SETTING

Recently, the *JAK2*-V617F mutation has been found to be present in 35–50% of patients with myelofibrosis.[35,36] Based thereon, methods such as real-time polymerase chain reaction (PCR) or pyrosequencing of blood granulocytes allow monitoring of treatment response on the molecular level.[35–39] The prognostic impact of *JAK2* mutation after allogeneic stem cell transplantation remains to be determined. A small series of 30 patients did not show any difference in outcome after allografting regarding the *JAK2* mutation status.[40] *JAK2* mutation screening with highly sensitive PCR might add helpful information regarding the depth of remission after allografting. The criteria for complete remission recently proposed by the International Working Group for myelofibrosis research and treatment (IWG-MRT) include disappearance of disease-related syndromes, peripheral blood levels of hemoglobin of ≥11 g/dl and platelet counts of ≥100 × 10^9/l.[41] After allogeneic stem cell transplantation these parameters are often influenced by graft versus host disease, infections, or poor graft function, and they cannot be used as valid remission criteria. On the other hand, normal blood counts and disappearance of disease-related syndromes do not exclude residual disease using highly sensitive PCR for *JAK2* mutation. After 22 allogeneic stem cell transplantation procedures in 21 JAK2-positive patients with myelofibrosis, 78% became PCR negative. In 15 out of 17 patients (88%), JAK2 remained negative after a median follow-up of 20 months. JAK2 negativity was achieved after a median of 89 days post-allograft (range 19–750 days). A significant inverse correlation was seen for JAK2 positivity and donor-cell chimerism (r −0.91, p <0.001). Four out of five patients who never achieved JAK2 negativity during the entire follow-up fulfilled all criteria for complete remission recently proposed by the International Working Group, suggesting a major role for JAK2 measurement to determine depth of remission. In one case, residual JAK2-positive cells were successfully eliminated by donor-lymphocyte infusion.[42]

BONE MARROW FIBROSIS REGRESSION

The interactions between cytokine release, myeloid stoma, and other bone marrow cells are only partially understood. Megakaryocytes are suggested to play a major role as a source of cytokine release.[43–45] Furthermore, pathological interaction between megakaryocytes and neutrophils (emperipolesis) contributes to abnormal cytokine release.[46] It seems reasonable that replacement of an abnormal clonal hematopoietic cell population by allogeneic stem cell transplantation would eliminate the stimulus for abnormal cytokine release. Indeed, several reports of allogeneic stem cell transplantation after standard conditioning for myelofibrosis reported a reversal of bone marrow fibrosis between 6 and 12 months after transplantation.[45,46] More recently, bone marrow fibrosis regression after dose-reduced allograft was investigated in 24 patients, who underwent allografting with either fibrosis grade 2 (MF-2) (n = 13) or fibrosis grade 3 (MF-3) (n = 11). After transplantation, a complete (MF-0) or nearly complete (MF-1) regression of bone marrow fibrosis was seen in 59% of patients at day +100, in 90% at day +180, and in 100% at day +360. No correlation between occurrence of acute graft versus host disease, and fibrosis regression on day +180 was seen.[47] More recently, monitoring of regression of myelofibrosis and osteosclerosis following hematopoietic stem cell

Table 17.4 Risk assessment in myelofibrosis

	No. of adverse prognostic factors	*Risk group*	*Median survival (months)*
'Lille' ('Dupriez') score[4]			
Adverse prognostic factors			
Hb < 10 g/dl			
WBC <4 or >30 × 10^9/l			
	0	Low	93
	1	Intermediate	26
	2	High	13
'Cervantes' score[3]			
Adverse prognostic factors			
Hb <10 g/dl			
Presence of constitutional symptoms (fever, night sweats, weight loss)			
Circulating blasts ≥1%			
	0–1	Low	176
	2–3	High	33
'Dingli' score[49]			
Adverse prognostic factors			
Hb <10 g/dl			
Platelet <100 × 10^9/l			
WBC <4 or >30 × 10^9/l			
	0	Low	155
	1	Intermediate	69
	≥2	High	23.5

Hb, hemoglobin; WBC, white blood count.

transplantation by magnetic resonance imaging (MRI) of the lumbar spine, pelvis, and femora has been reported to assess the pattern and extent of fibrosis.[48]

RISK ASSESSMENT AND ALLOGENEIC STEM CELL TRANSPLANTATION

Since allogeneic stem cell transplantation is increasingly used as a curative treatment option even in older patients, the still observed morbidity and mortality should be carefully balanced with the patients' life expectancy in order to offer optimal management. Several risk scores for myelofibrosis have been developed. The most widely used risk assessment model is the Lille (or 'Dupriez') score,[4] which distinguishes low, intermediate and high risk according to the hemoglobin (<10 g/dl) and white blood count (<4 × 10^9/l or >30 × 10^9/l) with overall survival of 93, 26, and 13 months, respectively. Another scoring system (Cervantes score)[3] includes hemoglobin (<10 g/dl), circulating blasts, and constitutional symptoms, and it distinguishes low risk (none to one adverse factor: median survival 176 months), and high risk (two to three adverse factors: median survival 33 months). More recently, a third risk-assessment score for transplantation-eligible patients was introduced,[49] which includes hemoglobin (<10 g/dl), white blood count ($<4 \times 10^9$/l or $> 30 \times 10^9$/l), and platelet count ($<100 \times 10^9$/l). Each event was given a score of 1, and patients with score 0 had a median survival of 155 months, while patients with a score of 1 had a median survival of 69 months, and those patients with a score of ≥2 had a median survival of 23.5 months. Table 17.4 shows the different risk models. This risk assessment model might help to select patients for allogeneic stem cell transplantation. However, other prognostic factors for decision-making such as age, comorbidities, or cytogenetic abnormalities[50] are not included in any of the models.

REFERENCES

1. Chim CS, Kwong YL, Lie AK et al. Long-term outcome of 231 patients with essential thrombocythemia: prognostic factors for thrombosis, bleeding, myelofibrosis, and leukemia. Arch Intern Med 2005; 165: 2651–8.
2. Wolanskyj AP, Schwager SM, McClure RF et al. Essential thrombocythemia beyond the first decade: life expectancy, long-term complication rates, and prognostic factors. Mayo Clin Proc 2006; 81: 159–66.
3. Cervantes F, Barosi G, Demory JL et al. Myelofibrosis with myeloid metaplasia in young individuals: disease characteristics, prognostic factors and identification of risk groups. Br J Haematol 1998; 102: 684–90.
4. Dupriez B, Morel P, Demory JL et al. Prognostic factors in agnogenic myeloid metaplasia: a report on 195 cases with a new scoring system. Blood 1996; 88: 1013–18.
5. James C, Ugo V, Le Couedic JP et al. A unique clonal JAK2 mutation leading to constitutive signalling causes polycythaemia vera. Nature 2005; 434: 1144–8.
6. Pardanani AD, Levine RL, Lasho T et al. MPL515 mutations in myeloproliferative and other myeloid disorders: a study of 1182 patients. Blood 2006; 108: 3472–6.
7. Fruehauf S, Buss EC, Topaly J et al. Myeloablative conditioning in myelofibrosis using i.v. treosulfan and autologous peripheral blood progenitor cell transplantation with high doses of CD34+ cells results in hematologic responses. Follow-up of three patients. Haematologica 2005; 90: ECR08.
8. Anderson JE, Tefferi A, Craig F et al. Myeloablation and autologous peripheral blood stem cell rescue results in hematologic and clinical responses in patients with myeloid metaplasia with myelofibrosis. Blood 2001; 98: 586–93.
9. Ngirabacu MC, Ravoet C, Dargent JL et al. Long term follow-up of autologous peripheral blood stem cell transplantation in the treatment of a patient with acute panmyelosis with myelofibrosis. Haematologica 2006; 91: ECR53.
10. Dokal I, Jones L, Deenmamode M et al. Allogeneic bone marrow transplantation for primary myelofibrosis. Br J Haematol 1989; 71: 158–60.
11. Creemers GJ, Lowenberg B, Hagenbeek A. Allogeneic bone marrow transplantation for primary myelofibrosis. Br J Haematol 1992; 82: 772–3.
12. Byrne JL, Beshti H, Clark D et al. Induction of remission after donor leucocyte infusion for the treatment of relapsed chronic idiopathic myelofibrosis following allogeneic transplantation: evidence for a 'graft vs. myelofibrosis' effect. Br J Haematol 2000; 108: 430–3.
13. Cervantes F, Rovira M, Urbano-Ispizua A et al. Complete remission of idiopathic myelofibrosis following donor lymphocyte infusion after failure of allogeneic transplantation: demonstration of a graft-versus-myelofibrosis effect. Bone Marrow Transplant 2000; 26: 697–9.
14. Guardiola P, Anderson JE, Bandini G et al. Allogeneic stem cell transplantation for agnogenic myeloid metaplasia: a European Group for Blood and Marrow Transplantation, Societe Francaise de Greffe de Moelle, Gruppo Italiano per il Trapianto del Midollo Osseo, and Fred Hutchinson Cancer Research Center Collaborative Study. Blood 1999; 93: 2831–8.
15. Deeg HJ, Gooley TA, Flowers ME et al. Allogeneic hematopoietic stem cell transplantation for myelofibrosis. Blood 2003; 102: 3912–18.
16. Kerbauy DM, Gooley TA, Sale GE et al. Hematopoietic cell transplantation as curative therapy for idiopathic myelofibrosis, advanced polycythemia vera, and essential thrombocythemia. Biol Blood Marrow Transplant 2007; 13: 355–65.
17. Singhal S, Powles R, Treleaven J et al. Allogeneic bone marrow transplantation for primary myelofibrosis. Bone Marrow Transplant 1995; 16: 743–6.
18. Anderson JE, Sale G, Appelbaum FR et al. Allogeneic marrow transplantation for primary myelofibrosis and myelofibrosis secondary to polycythaemia vera or essential thrombocytosis. Br J Haematol 1997; 98: 1010–16.
19. Daly A, Song K, Nevill T et al. Stem cell transplantation for myelofibrosis: a report from two Canadian centers. Bone Marrow Transplant 2003; 32: 35–40.
20. Mittal P, Saliba RM, Giralt SA et al. Allogeneic transplantation: a therapeutic option for myelofibrosis, chronic myelomonocytic leukemia and Philadelphia-negative/BCR-ABL-negative chronic myelogenous leukemia. Bone Marrow Transplant 2004; 33: 1005–9.
21. Ditschkowski M, Beelen DW, Trenschel R et al. Outcome of allogeneic stem cell transplantation

in patients with myelofibrosis. Bone Marrow Transplant 2004; 34: 807–13.

22. Przepiorka D, Giralt S, Khouri I et al. Allogeneic marrow transplantation for myeloproliferative disorders other than chronic myelogenous leukemia: review of forty cases. Am J Hematol 1998; 57: 24–8.
23. Guardiola P, Anderson JE, Gluckman E. Myelofibrosis with myeloid metaplasia. [Letter]. N Engl J Med 2000; 343: 659.
24. Rondelli D, Barosi G, Bacigalupo A et al. Myeloproliferative Diseases-Research Consortium. Allogeneic hematopoietic stem-cell transplantation with reduced-intensity conditioning in intermediate- or high-risk patients with myelofibrosis with myeloid metaplasia. Blood 2005; 105: 4115–19.
25. Kröger N, Zabelina T, Schieder H et al. Pilot study of reduced-intensity conditioning followed by allogeneic stem cell transplantation from related and unrelated donors in patients with myelofibrosis. Br J Haematol 2005; 128: 690–7.
26. Hessling J, Kröger N, Werner M et al. Dose-reduced conditioning regimen followed by allogeneic stem cell transplantation in patients with myelofibrosis with myeloid metaplasia. Br J Haematol 2002; 119: 769–72.
27. Devine SM, Hoffman R, Verma A et al. Allogeneic blood cell transplantation following reduced-intensity conditioning is effective therapy for older patients with myelofibrosis with myeloid metaplasia. Blood 2002; 99: 2255–8.
28. Merup M, Lazarevic V, Nahi H et al. Swedish Group for Myeloproliferative Disorders. Different outcome of allogeneic transplantation in myelofibrosis using conventional or reduced-intensity conditioning regimens. Br J Haematol 2006; 135: 367–73.
29. Snyder DS, Palmer J, Stein AS et al. Allogeneic hematopoietic cell transplantation following reduced intensity conditioning for treatment of myelofibrosis. Biol Blood Marrow Transplant 2006; 12: 1161–8.
30. Greyz N, Miller WE, Andrey J et al. Long-term remission of myelofibrosis following nonmyeloablative allogeneic peripheral blood progenitor cell transplantation in older age: the Scripps Clinic experience. Bone Marrow Transplant 2004; 34: 273–4.
31. Tanner ML, Hoh CK, Bashey A et al. FLAG chemotherapy followed by allogeneic stem cell transplant using nonmyeloablative conditioning induces regression of myelofibrosis with myeloid metaplasia. Bone Marrow Transplant 2003; 32: 581–5.
32. Li Z, Deeg HJ. Pros and cons of splenectomy in patients with myelofibrosis undergoing stem cell transplantation. Leukemia 2001; 15: 465–7.
33. Tefferi A, Mesa RA, Nagorney DM et al. Splenectomy in myelofibrosis with myeloid metaplasia: a single-institution experience with 223 patients. Blood 2000; 95: 2226–33.
34. Barosi G, Ambrosetti A, Centra A et al. Splenectomy and risk of blast transformation in myelofibrosis with myeloid metaplasia. Italian Cooperative Study Group on Myeloid with Myeloid Metaplasia. Blood 1998; 91: 3630–6.
35. Baxter EJ, Scott LM, Campbell PJ et al. Cancer Genome Project. Acquired mutation of the tyrosine kinase JAK2 in human myeloproliferative disorders. Lancet 2005; 365: 1054–61.
36. Levine RL, Wadleigh M, Cools J et al. Activating mutation in the tyrosine kinase JAK2 in polycythemia vera, essential thrombocythemia, and myeloid metaplasia with myelofibrosis. Cancer Cell 2005; 7: 387–97.
37. James C, Ugo V, Le Couedic JP et al. A unique clonal JAK2 mutation leading to constitutive signalling causes polycythaemia vera. Nature 2005; 434: 1144–8.
38. Jones AV, Silver RT, Waghorn K et al. Minimal molecular response in polycythemia vera patients treated with imatinib or interferon alpha. Blood 2006; 107: 3339–41.
39. Kralovics R, Passamonti F, Buser AS et al. A gain-of-function mutation of JAK2 in myeloproliferative disorders. N Engl J Med 2005; 352: 1779–90.
40. Ditschkowski M, Elmaagacli AH, Trenschel R et al. No influence of V617F mutation in JAK2 on outcome after allogeneic hematopoietic stem cell transplantation (HSCT) for myelofibrosis. Biol Blood Marrow Transplant 2006; 12: 1350–1.
41. Tefferi A, Barosi G, Mesa RA et al. International Working Group (IWG) consensus criteria for treatment response in myelofibrosis with myeloid metaplasia: On behalf of the IWG for myelofibrosis research and treatment (IWG-MRT). Blood 2006; 108: 1497–503.
42. Kröger N, Badbaran A, Holler E et al. Monitoring of the JAK2-V617F mutation by highly sensitive quantitative real-time PCR after allogeneic stem cell transplantation in patients with myelofibrosis. Blood 2007; 109: 1316–21.
43. Thiele J, Kvasnicka HM, Fischer R et al. Clinicopathological impact of the interaction between megakaryocytes and myeloid stroma in chronic myeloproliferative disorders: a concise update. Leuk Lymphoma 1997; 24: 463–81.
44. Wang JC, Chang TH, Goldberg A et al. Quantitative analysis of growth factor production in the mechanism of fibrosis in agnogenic myeloid metaplasia. Exp Hematol 2006; 34: 1617–23.
45. Katoh O, Kimura A, Itoh T et al. Platelet derived growth factor messenger RNA is increased in bone marrow megakaryocytes in patients with myeloproliferative disorders. Am J Hematol 1990; 35: 145–50.
46. Centurione L, Di Baldassarre A, Zingariello M et al. Increased and pathologic emperipolesis of neutrophils within megakaryocytes associated with marrow

fibrosis in GATA-1(low) mice. Blood 2004; 104: 3573–80.

47. Kröger N, Thiele J, Zander A et al. Rapid regression of bone marrow fibrosis after dose-reduced allogeneic stem cell transplantation in patients with myelofibrosis. Blood 2006; 108: 374, abstract.
48. Sale GE, Deeg HJ, Porter BA. Regression of myelofibrosis and osteosclerosis following hematopoietic cell transplantation assessed by magnetic resonance imaging and histologic grading. Biol Blood Marrow Transplant 2006; 12: 1285–94.
49. Dingli D, Schwager SM, Mesa RA et al. Prognosis in transplant-eligible patients with agnogenic myeloid metaplasia: a simple CBC-based scoring system. Cancer 2006; 106: 623–30.
50. Tefferi A, Dingli D, Li CY et al. Prognostic diversity among cytogenetic abnormalities in myelofibrosis with myeloid metaplasia. Cancer 2005; 104: 1656–60.

Non-transplant therapeutic strategies for patients with *BCR-ABL*-negative chronic myeloproliferative disorders

18

Jürg Schwaller, Radek Skoda

INTRODUCTION

Before activated kinases were discovered as the causative events in *BCR-ABL*-negative myeloproliferative disorders (MPD), patients with MPD were treated primarily with the intention to relieve symptoms and/or to prevent complications.[1–3] As discussed in the previous chapters, cytoreduction by hydroxyurea was shown to be beneficial in preventing thrombotic complications in patients with essential thrombocythemia (ET) who were considered to be 'high-risk' (age >60 years and/or previous thrombosis).[4] The Primary Thrombocythemia-1 (PT-1) study[5] showed that hydroxyurea plus aspirin was more effective in reducing thrombotic complications than anagrelide plus aspirin in high-risk ET patients. These differences were pronounced for arterial thromboses, but not for venous thromboses, where patients on anagrelide plus aspirin fared better.[5] The European Collaboration on Low-Dose Aspirin in Polycythemia Vera (ECLAP) study[6] recently provided a rational basis for the use of low-dose aspirin in the prevention thrombotic of complications in MPD and dissipated the fears of increasing morbidity and mortality from hemorrhagic events linked to the use of aspirin in these patients. These studies are currently the pillars for evidence-based therapeutic decisions. Although the latter results were obtained by studying patients with polycythemia vera (PV), it is now common practice to give aspirin also to patients with ET and during the cellular phase of primary myelofibrosis (PMF).[3] Interferon alfa (IFNα) showed promise as an alternative drug that could replace hydroxyurea in the management of MPD, but the high rate of unwanted side-effects limits its potential for long-term applications.[2,3] Thus, the therapeutic options in MPD are limited and new drugs are in demand. Particularly in young patients with ET or PV we are faced with difficult decisions, for which no data from controlled studies are available. The uncertainty concerning potential leukemogenic effects of hydroxyurea[7–9] weighs even more heavily in young patients with MPD, since the therapy once initiated is usually continued life-long. In advanced stages of PMF, allogeneic stem cell transplantation has been shown to be effective in some cases.[10,11] Whether reduced intensity conditioning regimens or standard conditioning should be used and the criteria for identifying patients who will benefit most from this form of therapy are currently the subject of further studies. The discovery of activating mutations in the Janus kinase 2 (*JAK2*) gene that can be found in the majority of patients with PV, ET, and PMF,[12–15] and the involvement of other kinases, such as platelet-derived growth factor receptor (PDGFR) and fibroblast growth factor receptor (FGFR) in rare forms of MPD, raised the hope that kinase inhibitors may soon become first-line therapy in MPD patients. Here, we primarily discuss the prospects of inhibitors of JAK2 and related downstream signaling molecules. The vast majority of patients with MPD carry a G>T transversion in exon 14 of *JAK2* that changes a valine in position 617 to a phenylalanine (*JAK2* V617F).[12–15] Recently, mutations in exon 12 of the *JAK2* gene have been found in PV patients who are negative for *JAK2* V617F.[16] These exon 12 mutations alter various nucleotide positions in the vicinity of codon 539 and frequently also involve deletions of 1–3 codons. Most of the patients studied had mutations at slightly different positions in exon 12, in sharp contrast to the uniform pattern of *JAK2* V617F. In cell lines, the exon 12 mutations led to stronger activation of the JAK2 activity than the *JAK2* V617F mutation. Recently, mutations in position 515 of MPL gene that change the wild-type tryptophane to leucine (W515L) or lysine (W515K) have been found in 1% of patients with ET and 5% of patients with PMF.[17,18] These mutations render MPL signaling independent of ligand binding, but JAK2 activity is required to transmit the signals. Thus, inhibitors of JAK2 can be expected to be effective both in patients with activating *JAK2* mutations and with activating *MPL* mutations.

IMATINIB IN *BCR-ABL*-NEGATIVE MYELOPROLIFERATIVE DISORDERS

Encouraged by the success of treating chronic myelogenous leukemia (CML) with small molecule tyrosine kinase inhibitors, several groups had tested the therapeutic potential of imatinib mesylate for *BCR-ABL*-negative MPD before the discovery of the *JAK2* mutations. Silver and colleagues observed that treatment of PV patients with 400–800 mg/day imatinib was able to reduce phlebotomy requirements.[19] The impaired autonomous *in vitro* growth of erythroid colonies from a significant fraction of PV patients by imatinib led to the suggestion that a 'yet unidentified kinase' might be involved in the pathogenesis of PV.[20] However, it remained unclear whether the observed *in vitro* growth reduction was indeed the consequence of imatinib effects on erythroid progenitors or on cells from the monocytic lineage.[21] Imatinib is highly efficient in blocking ABL, PDGFR and c-KIT, but the JAK2 kinase was never demonstrated to be a major target.[22] Interestingly, cells from MPD patients including PV have been demonstrated to frequently overexpress c-KIT.[23] Furthermore, potentially activating mutations in c-KIT have been described in seven out of 20 PV patients.[24] However, as no single clones have been analyzed it remains unclear whether activating mutations in c-KIT and JAK2 coexist in the same cells in PV patients. Although rare activating mutations or overexpression of c-KIT might explain the imatinib sensitivity of some patients, it is nevertheless surprising that the MPD phenotype caused by expression of the murine *JAK2* V617F in a mouse model of MPD has been found to be sensitive to systemic treatment with imatinib.[25] Similarly, murine FDPC1 cells transfected with *JAK2*-V617F were inhibited by imatinib.[26] Despite the interesting molecular interactions between JAK2 and c-KIT or possibly other imatinib sensitive kinases, only a minority of PV patients benefited from treatment with imatinib alone and no molecular remissions have been observed.[26,27]

TARGETING ACTIVATED JAK2 PROTEINS

In screening for small molecules that are able to inhibit the growth of blasts from patients with acute lymphoblastic leukemia (ALL) a tyrphostin compound (dihydroxy-N-benzylcinnnamide, AG-490) was identified that could block JAK2 kinase activity.[28] Selective anti-tumor activity was demonstrated in tissue culture as well as by treatment of severe combined immune deficiency (SCID) mice after xenotransplantation of human leukemic blasts. In addition, AG-490 showed cytotoxic effects against human myeloma cells with constitutive activation of an interleukin-6/JAK2 signaling pathway.[29] However, despite its efficacy, because of non-favorable pharmacokinetics, AG-490 never entered clinical trials. Although newer experimental data question the selectivity of AG-490 for JAK2, the compound is still often used to block JAK2 activity *in vitro*.[30] Interestingly, a murine MPD model induced by retroviral expression of *JAK2* V617F was sensitive to AG-490 therapy.[25] In addition, aberrant erythroid differentiation *in vitro* of human hematopoietic stem cells from *JAK2* V617F-positive PV patients was inhibited but not completely eliminated by AG-490.[31]

The identification of activating *JAK2* mutations in a large proportion of MPD patients has initiated an active search for small molecules able to selectively block activated JAK2 kinase. A milestone for the design of small molecular JAK2 inhibitors was reached by determining the crystallographic structure of the JAK2 kinase domain bound to the putative JAK2 inhibitor 'compound 6' (CMP6).[32] *In vitro*, CMP6 (also known as pyridone 6 or simply 'JAK2 inhibitor') is able to block all four JAK kinases at a nanomolar concentration.[33] CMP6 impairs growth and survival of the human HEL leukemia cell line that carries a homozygous *JAK2* V17F mutation. CMP6 also showed inhibitory activity against murine 32D hematopoietic cells stably transformed by expression of the constitutively active human thrombopoietin receptor (*MPL* W515L) or Ba/F3 cells stably expressing the *JAK2* V617F mutation.[17,25]

A new orally applicable piperazine-phenylaminopyrimidine compound (TG-1209,) was demonstrated to block several protein tyrosine kinases including JAK2 at a nanomolar concentration. TG-1209 impairs growth of murine Ba/F3 cells stably transformed by expression of *JAK2* V617F or *MPL* W515L at a median concentration of 200 nM. In addition, TG-1209 blocks *JAK2* V617F or *MPL* W515L induced signaling in human cells as shown in colony forming assays *in vitro* and in xenotransplantation experiments *in vivo*.[34] Phase I clinical trials are currently under way (TG-101348).

An increasing number of putative small molecular JAK2 inhibitors are undergoing preclinical evaluation as shown in several presentations at the recent meetings of the American Association for Cancer Research (AACR) and the European Hematology Association (EHA). Gourley and co-workers from SuperGen Inc. presented a series of small molecule JAK2 inhibitors (JAK2–14) with cellular antiproliferative activity at a nanomolar concentration range.[35] Further modification of these lead compounds might be necessary to begin a clinical trial. Another small molecule with selective JAK2 inhibitory activity was presented from InCyte Inc. This 'InCyte JAK2 inhibitor' showed JAK2 blocking activity at concentrations in the nanomolar range without affecting BCR-ABL. Oral application of this compound in a mouse model of *JAK2* V617F-induced myeloproliferation resulted in a significant decrease of the myeloid cell mass as assessed by a reduction of the spleen weight.[36] TG-1209, JAK2–14 as well as the 'InCyte JAK2 inhibitor' are ATP-competitive kinase inhibitors. In contrast, LS-104 (LymphoSign, Ontario) is a substrate-competitive small molecular JAK2 inhibitor. LS-104 is able to block JAK2 cellular signaling at a micromolar concentration range. Interestingly in combination with an ATP-competitive JAK2 inhibitor, LS-104 demonstrated a strong additive effect on cells expressing the *JAK2* V617F mutation.[37] Another lead molecule, the JAK2 inhibitory compound (SB1518), has been recently announced undergoing preclinical testing (S*Bio Ltd, Singapore) (information retrieved from www.biomedicine.org). In silico docking analysis has led to the identification of a hexabromocyclohexane compound that was able to block cellular JAK2 activity at a micromolar concentration.[38] Screening a library of close to 2000 compounds for candidates that modify cellular Stat3 activity in cancer cells has led to the identification of SD-1008, a small molecule able to inhibit SRC and JAK2 activity in ovarian cancer cells.[39] There are also studies, which propose that emodin, a compound extracted from the root of *Rheum palmatum* used in traditional Chinese medicine, exerts its anti-tumor activity by inhibiting JAK2.[40] All these studies suggest that JAK2 inhibitors might be soon available to undergo first clinical trials. Furthermore, these reports suggest that activated JAK2 kinases can be successfully targeted by small molecular inhibitors.

These studies also raise the question whether it will be possible to generate compounds that selectively target distinct mutations of JAK2. High-throughput screening approaches using large libraries could allow the identification of small molecules that inhibit mutated but not wild-type JAK2.[41] Using this approach it was demonstrated that the compound VX-680 with well-known activity against aurora kinases also interacts specifically and inhibits the T315I *BCR-ABL* mutant at a nanomolar concentration.[42] Although second generation ABL inhibitors such as dasatinib or nilotinib are able to block many or the resistance-associated *BCR-ABL* mutations, *BCR-ABL* T315I remains a major challenge to overcome. First studies demonstrate that the aurora kinase inhibitor VX-680 (renamed to MK-0456) has some clinical activity also against *BCR-ABL* T315I.[43] Interestingly, MK-0456 interacts and inhibits also JAK2 *in vitro*, but it is currently not known whether this compound is also able to block oncogenic JAK2 activity *in vivo*.[43] In addition, another compound initially developed as an inhibitor for aurora kinases, AT9283 not only interacts and inhibits *BCR-ABL*-T315I, but efficiently targets mutant JAK2 activity.[44] The prospect of developing V617F-specific pseudokinase inhibitors will depend on the precise mechanism, of how the pseudokinase domain alters the function of the kinase domain. Elucidation of the three-dimensional structure of the entire JAK2 protein in the presence and absence of the *JAK2* V617F mutation may be necessary to allow design of selective pseudokinase inhibitors.

It will be interesting to see whether other aurora kinase inhibitors that are currently in preclinical tests or entering phase I clinical trials are also capable of targeting activated JAK2 kinases. Large-scale and high-throughput screens have demonstrated that most small molecules can interact with more than one kinase, which might add to the clinical efficacy of a given compound. Several *in vitro* studies have revealed that an increasing number of previously known compounds such as erlotinib (epidermal growth factor receptor inhibitor), GO-6976 (FLT3 inhibitor), LFM-A13 (BTK inhibitor) or AT9283 (aurora kinase inhibitor) are also able to interact and block JAK2 activity.[45–47] Interestingly, lestaurtinib (also known as CEP701, Cephalon Inc.), a known FLT3 inhibitor currently undergoing clinical trials for acute myeloid leukemia (AML) carrying activating *FLT3* mutations, also inhibits wild-type as well as mutant JAK2 V617F at nanomolar concentrations, which makes it a good candidate for clinical trials for MPD patients.[48]

TARGETING COMPONENTS DOWNSTREAM OF JAK2

Although the precise mechanism of IFNα action in MPD is unknown, some patients with MPD respond well to IFNα treatment and in rare cases molecular remissions have been observed, with *JAK2* V617F decreasing below the detection limit of DNA based allele-specific PCR (i.e. <0.5% of chromosomes) (reference 49 and our own unpublished results). Unfortunately, the frequent side-effects limit the usefulness of IFNα for long-term therapy in most MPD patients. Are there any alternative ways to block oncogenic JAK2 activity to overcome the current limitations of small molecule JAK2 inhibitors? Constitutively active JAK2 leads to phosphorylation of signal transducers and activators of transcription (STAT) proteins that enter the nucleus and act as transcription factors regulating a large number of target genes including cyclins, *PIM1* kinase, or *BCL-XL* (Figure 18.1). Among the target genes that are directly regulated by STAT5 is a group of endogenous STAT inhibitors, the ‘cytokine-induced SRC-homology-2 protein’ (CIS) and ‘suppressors of cytokine signaling’ (SOCS). While CIS interferes with activated upstream tyrosine kinase receptors, SOCS proteins interact with activated JAK2, STAT3, and STAT5. This negative feedback mechanism serves to ‘fine tune’ the cellular JAK/STAT activity. Downregulation of *SOCS* mRNA expression (owing to aberrant tumor cell promoter methylation) results in constitutive activation of the JAK/STAT5 signal transduction cascade. This principle has led to the suggestion that one could block aberrant JAK2 activity through small peptides (‘SOCS mimetics’) that mimic endogenous SOCS activity.[50]

Several studies have demonstrated that constitutive activation of STAT3 and STAT5 is a hallmark of chronic MPD induced by deregulated protein tyrosine kinase activity.[51] In contrast to kinases, selective inhibition of a transcription factor by small molecules is a much more difficult task. Although there is evidence that such an approach might soon be possible, as recently demonstrated by blocking aberrant BCL6 activity in high-grade lymphoma cells by disrupting critical protein–protein interactions by small molecules, to date no such success has been achieved for oncogenic STAT proteins.[52] Several natural compounds

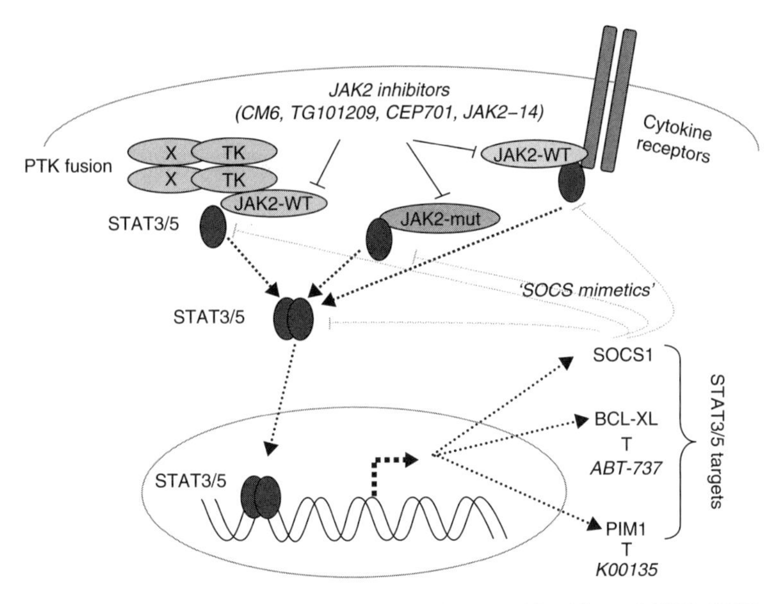

Figure 18.1 Therapeutic strategies to target oncogenic JAK2 kinase activity. Mutated JAK2 (JAK2-mut), or wild-type JAK2 (JAK2-WT) acting downstream of an oncogenic protein tyrosine kinase (PTK) or several cytokine receptors both lead to constitutive activation of the signal transducer and activators of transcription STAT3 and STAT5. Deregulated STAT activation results in upregulation of targets supporting cell proliferation and survival. Currently available small molecule JAK2 inhibitors, such as compound6 (CMP6), CEP701 or TG101209, block JAK2-WT as well as mutated JAK2. JAK2-induced cell survival might also indirectly be targeted by small molecules blocking STAT downstream targets such as BCL-XL (ABT-737) and PIM1 (K00135), or by peptides mimicking endogenous STAT inhibitors (SOCS mimetics). TK, tyrosine kinase.

seem to be able to functionally interfere with STAT proteins, although with a limited specificity.[53] However, these molecules could now act as lead compounds to develop small molecules that block critical protein–protein or protein–DNA interactions to abrogate constitutive STAT activity. To circumvent these limitations an increasing number of small molecules have been recently identified that are able to block critical downstream targets of STAT5 such as PIM1 or BCL-XL, both deregulated in MPD. *PIM1* and *PIM2* encode serine/threonine kinases that are upregulated in hematopoietic cells transformed by tyrosine kinase fusion genes involving *ABL*, *PDGFR*, or activating *JAK2* or *FLT3* mutations.[54–56] Using a structural approach, we have recently identified a group of imidazo[1,2-b]pyridazines as PIM kinase inhibitors with antileukemic activity.[57] Further optimization of these lead compounds might yield targeted therapeutics for hematological and solid malignancies with aberrant PTK activity. The pro-survival protein BCL-XL is a major target of oncogenic STAT activity. Overexpression of BCL-XL is associated with progression, poor prognosis, and resistance to chemotherapy in several human cancers. Several proteomimetics (such as ABT-737) have recently been identified to block the BCL-XL/BCL2-BH3 binding and were used as anticancer agents to overcome apoptosis resistance.[58] ABT-737 was shown to overcome resistance to imatinib or FLT3 inhibitors in chronic myeloid leukemia (CML) and acute myeloid leukemia (AML) cells, respectively.[59,60] However, in cells with high BCL2 phosphorylation and high levels of expression of *MCL1*, another pro-survival relative and STAT3 target, ABT-737 was inactive. Several strategies have been proposed to block BCL2 phosphorylation and to reduce *MCL1* expression to restore sensitivity to ABT-737.[61–63] ABT-737 seems to enhance the efficacy of combined chemotherapeutics that are used for the treatment of ALL.[64] Whether ABT-737 will find a place in the therapeutic regimen for MPD remains to be determined.

OUTLOOK

The availability of small molecular inhibitors of activated JAK2 and critical downstream mediators raises the hopes that new effective treatments for patients with MPD can be found that will not only reduce the number of cells derived from the MPD clone, but may induce lasting molecular remissions or in the best case cure the disease. The mechanism of how *JAK2* V617F increases the kinase activity will need to be resolved and may open ways to specifically target the mutated form of JAK2. Mice deficient for *JAK2* die during embryogenesis owing to lack of definitive erythropoiesis and the signaling by the EPO receptor, MPL and in part also the G-CSF receptor is dependent on JAK2.[65,66] Therefore, it is to be expected that a complete block of JAK2 activity will result in anemia, thrombocytopenia, and neutropenia. Another potential pitfall for JAK2 inhibitors could be cross-reactivity with other family members, in particular JAK3, potentially causing severe combined immunodeficiency.[67–69] Given these theoretical limitations, the phase I–II trials with FLT3 and aurora kinase inhibitors that also suppress JAK2 activity so far have shown surprisingly few side-effects. How effective will inhibition of JAK2 be in patients with MPD? Studies on familial MPD and analysis of clonality suggest that *JAK2* V617F may be preceded by mutation(s) in as yet unknown gene(s).[70–72] However, patients negative for *JAK2* mutations at diagnosis remain negative during follow-up[73] Thus, the phenotypic manifestation of MPD appears to be linked to the presence of *JAK2* V617F or other mutations. Nevertheless, a pre-JAK2 mutation in a progenitor or stem cell remains a possibility, as shown in some patients with deletions of chromosome 20q.[72] Surprisingly, patients with *JAK2* V617F-positive MPD when they transformed to secondary AML displayed leukemic blasts that frequently had no detectable *JAK2* mutation.[74,75] These data are compatible with the presence of a pre-*JAK2* mutation in a progenitor or stem cell as the common clonal origin for MPD and AML, although *de novo* AML also remains a possibility in these cases. Whether JAK2 inhibitors will have any impact (positive or negative) on leukemic transformation remains at present purely speculative. With the new JAK2 inhibitors in sight, the question is, who will profit most from such drugs? The generally mild clinical manifestations in ET and most cases of PV will make it necessary to find a good balance between the desired reduction of the cell mass and the complications and potential side-effects of such compounds. The new compounds could be effective in patients with myelofibrosis, where current drug therapies are ineffective. Ultimately, combinations of drugs may be able to induce lasting remissions or potentially cure MPD.

REFERENCES

1. Spivak JL. Polycythemia vera: myths, mechanisms, and management. Blood 2002; 100: 4272–90.
2. Silver RT. Treatment of polycythemia vera. Semin Thromb Hemost 2006; 32: 437–42.
3. Finazzi G, Barbui T. How I treat patients with polycythemia vera. Blood 2007; 109: 5104–11.
4. Cortelazzo S, Finazzi G, Ruggeri M et al. Hydroxyurea for patients with essential thrombocythemia and a high risk of thrombosis. N Engl J Med 1995; 332: 1132–6.
5. Harrison CN, Campbell PJ, Buck G et al. Hydroxyurea compared with anagrelide in high-risk essential thrombocythemia. N Engl J Med 2005; 353: 33–45.
6. Landolfi R, Marchioli R, Kutti J et al. Efficacy and safety of low-dose aspirin in polycythemia vera. N Engl J Med 2004; 350: 114–24.
7. Tefferi A. Is hydroxyurea leukemogenic in essential thrombocythemia? [letter]. Blood 1998; 92: 1459–60; discussion 1460–1.
8. Kiladjian JJ, Rain JD, Bernard JF et al. Long-term incidence of hematological evolution in three French prospective studies of hydroxyurea and pipobroman in polycythemia vera and essential thrombocythemia. Semin Thromb Hemost 2006; 32: 417–21.
9. Barbui T, Finazzi G. Therapy for polycythemia vera and essential thrombocythemia is driven by the cardiovascular risk. Semin Thromb Hemost 2007; 33: 321–9.
10. Barosi G, Hoffman R. Idiopathic myelofibrosis. Semin Hematol 2005; 42: 248–58.
11. Cervantes F, Barosi G. Myelofibrosis with myeloid metaplasia: diagnosis, prognostic factors, and staging. Semin Oncol 2005; 32: 395–402.
12. James C, Ugo V, Le Couedic JP et al. A unique clonal JAK2 mutation leading to constitutive signalling causes polycythaemia vera. Nature 2005; 434: 1144–8.

13. Baxter EJ, Scott LM, Campbell PJ et al. Acquired mutation of the tyrosine kinase JAK2 in human myeloproliferative disorders. Lancet 2005; 365: 1054–61.
14. Levine RL, Wadleigh M, Cools J et al. Activating mutation in the tyrosine kinase JAK2 in polycythemia vera, essential thrombocythemia, and myeloid metaplasia with myelofibrosis. Cancer Cell 2005; 7: 387–97.
15. Kralovics R, Passamonti F, Buser AS et al. A gain-of-function mutation of JAK2 in myeloproliferative disorders. N Engl J Med 2005; 352: 1779–90.
16. Scott LM, Tong W, Levine RL et al. JAK2 exon 12 mutations in polycythemia vera and idiopathic erythrocytosis. N Engl J Med 2007; 356: 459–68.
17. Pikman Y, Lee BH, Mercher T et al. MPLW515L is a novel somatic activating mutation in myelofibrosis with myeloid metaplasia. PLoS Med 2006; 3: e270.
18. Pardanani AD, Levine RL, Lasho T et al. MPL515 mutations in myeloproliferative and other myeloid disorders: a study of 1182 patients. Blood 2006; 108: 3472–6.
19. Silver RT. Imatinib mesylate [Gleevec(TM)] reduces phlebotomy requirements in polycythemia vera. Leukemia 2003; 17: 1186–7.
20. Oehler L, Jaeger E, Eser A et al. Imatinib mesylate inhibits autonomous erythropoiesis in patients with polycythemia vera in vitro. Blood 2003; 102: 2240–2.
21. Spivak JL, Silver RT. Imatinib mesylate in polycythemia vera. Blood 2004; 103: 3241; author reply 3241–2.
22. Druker BJ, Tamura S, Buchdunger E et al. Effects of a selective inhibitor of the Abl tyrosine kinase on the growth of Bcr-Abl positive cells. Nat Med 1996; 2: 561–6.
23. Siitonen T, Savolainen ER, Koistinen P. Expression of the c-kit proto-oncogene in myeloproliferative disorders and myelodysplastic syndromes. Leukemia 1994; 8: 631–7.
24. Fontalba A, Real PJ, Fernandez-Luna JL et al. Identification of c-Kit gene mutations in patients with polycythemia vera. Leuk Res 2006; 30: 1325–6.
25. Zaleskas VM, Krause DS, Lazarides K et al. Molecular Pathogenesis and Therapy of Polycythemia Induced in Mice by JAK2 V617F. PLoS ONE 2006; 1: e18.
26. Gaikwad A, Verstovsek S, Yoon D et al. Imatinib effect on growth and signal transduction in polycythemia vera. Exp Hematol 2007; 35: 931–8.
27. Jones AV, Silver RT, Waghorn K et al. Minimal molecular response in polycythemia vera patients treated with imatinib or interferon alpha. Blood 2006; 107: 3339–41.
28. Meydan N, Grunberger T, Dadi H et al. Inhibition of acute lymphoblastic leukaemia by a Jak-2 inhibitor. Nature 1996; 379: 645–8.
29. Levitzki A. Tyrosine kinases as targets for cancer therapy. Eur J Cancer 2002; 38(Suppl 5): S11–18.
30. Luo C, Laaja P. Inhibitors of JAKs/STATs and the kinases: a possible new cluster of drugs. Drug Discov Today 2004; 9: 268–75.
31. Jamieson CH, Gotlib J, Durocher JA et al. The JAK2 V617F mutation occurs in hematopoietic stem cells in polycythemia vera and predisposes toward erythroid differentiation. Proc Natl Acad Sci U S A 2006; 103: 6224–9.
32. Lucet IS, Fantino E, Styles M et al. The structural basis of Janus kinase 2 inhibition by a potent and specific pan-Janus kinase inhibitor. Blood 2006; 107: 176–83.
33. Thompson JE, Cubbon RM, Cummings RT et al. Photochemical preparation of a pyridone containing tetracycle: a Jak protein kinase inhibitor. Bioorg Med Chem Lett 2002; 12: 1219–23.
34. Pardanani A, Hood J, Lasho T et al. TG101209, a small molecule JAK2-selective kinase inhibitor potently inhibits myeloproliferative disorder-associated JAK2V617F and MPLW515L/K mutations. Leukemia 2007; 21: 1658–68.
35. Gourley E, Liu X-H, Grand C, Vankayalapati H, Bearss D. Discovery and characterization of small molecule inhibitors for JAK2. Proceedings of the 98th Annual Meeting of the American Association for Cancer Research, Los Angeles, 2007.
36. Fridman S, Li J, Liu P et al. Discovery and preclinical development of selective JAK inhibitors of the treatment of hematological malignancies. Haematologica 2007; S1: 117.
37. Lipka DB, Hoffmann L, Kasper S et al. LS104 is a novel substrate inhibitor of mutant JAK2 kinase and acts synergistically with ATP-binding-site kinase inhibitors in JAK2 V617F positive cells. Haematologica 2007; S1: 113.
38. Sandberg EM, Ma X, He K et al. Identification of 1,2,3,4,5,6-hexabromocyclohexane as a small molecule inhibitor of jak2 tyrosine kinase autophosphorylation [correction of autophosphorylation]. J Med Chem 2005; 48: 2526–33.
39. Duan Z, Bradner J, Greenberg E et al. SD-1008 a novel JAK2 inhibitor, increases chemotherapy sensitivity in human ovarian cancer cells. Mol Pharmacol 2007; 72: 1137–45.
40. Muto A, Hori M, Sasaki Y et al. Emodin has a cytotoxic activity against human multiple myeloma as a Janus-activated kinase 2 inhibitor. Mol Cancer Ther 2007; 6: 987–94.
41. Fabian MA, Biggs WH 3rd, Treiber DK et al. A small molecule-kinase interaction map for clinical kinase inhibitors. Nat Biotechnol 2005; 23: 329–36.
42. Carter TA, Wodicka LM, Shah NP et al. Inhibition of drug-resistant mutants of ABL, KIT, and EGF receptor kinases. Proc Natl Acad Sci U S A 2005; 102: 11011–16.
43. Giles FJ, Cortes J, Jones D et al. MK-0457, a novel kinase inhibitor, is active in patients with chronic myeloid leukemia or acute lymphocytic leukemia with the T315I BCR-ABL mutation. Blood 2007; 109: 500–2.

44. Lyons J, Curry J, Mallet K et al. JAK2 and T315I Abl activity of clinical candidate, AT9283. Proceedings of the 98th Annual Meeting of the American Association for Cancer Research, Los Angeles, 2007.
45. Li Z, Xu M, Xing S et al. Erlotinib effectively inhibits JAK2V617F activity and polycythemia vera cell growth. J Biol Chem 2007; 282: 3428–32.
46. Grandage VL, Everington T, Linch DC, Khwaja A. Go6976 is a potent inhibitor of the JAK 2 and FLT3 tyrosine kinases with significant activity in primary acute myeloid leukaemia cells. Br J Haematol 2006; 135: 303–16.
47. van den Akker E, van Dijk TB, Schmidt U et al. The Btk inhibitor LFM-A13 is a potent inhibitor of Jak2 kinase activity. Biol Chem 2004; 385: 409–13.
48. Carroll M. Signal transduction in myeloproliferative diseases and AML. FASEB Summer Research Conferences: hematopoietic malignancies. Vermont: Vermont Academy, 2007.
49. Kiladjian JJ, Cassinat B, Turlure P et al. High molecular response rate of polycythemia vera patients treated with pegylated interferon alpha-2a. Blood 2006; 108: 2037–40.
50. Flowers LO, Johnson HM, Mujtaba MG et al. Characterization of a peptide inhibitor of Janus kinase 2 that mimics suppressor of cytokine signaling 1 function. J Immunol 2004; 172: 7510–18.
51. Schwaller J, Parganas E, Wang D et al. Stat5 is essential for the myelo- and lymphoproliferative disease induced by TEL/JAK2. Mol Cell 2000; 6: 693–704.
52. Melnick A. Targetting transcriptional repression in B-cell lymphomas. FASEB Summer Research Conferences: hematopoietic malignancies. Vermont: Vermont Academy, 2007.
53. Sun J, Blaskovich MA, Jove R et al. Cucurbitacin Q: a selective STAT3 activation inhibitor with potent antitumor activity. Oncogene 2005; 24: 3236–45.
54. Adam M, Pogacic V, Bendit M et al. Targeting PIM kinases impairs survival of hematopoietic cells transformed by kinase inhibitor-sensitive and kinase inhibitor-resistant forms of Fms-like tyrosine kinase 3 and BCR/ABL. Cancer Res 2006; 66: 3828–35.
55. Goerttler PS, Kreutz C, Donauer J et al. Gene expression profiling in polycythaemia vera: overexpression of transcription factor NF-E2. Br J Haematol 2005; 129: 138–50.
56. Schwemmers S, Will B, Waller CF et al. JAK2(V617F)-negative ET patients do not display constitutively active JAK/STAT signaling. Exp Hematol 2007; 35: 1695–703.
57. Pogacic V, Bullock AN, Fedorov O et al. Structural analysis identifies imidazo[1,2-b]pyridazines as PIM kinase inhibitors with in vitro antileukemic activity. Cancer Res 2007; 67: 6916–24.
58. Oltersdorf T, Elmore SW, Shoemaker AR et al. An inhibitor of Bcl-2 family proteins induces regression of solid tumours. Nature 2005; 435: 677–81.
59. Kuroda J, Puthalakath H, Cragg MS et al. Bim and Bad mediate imatinib-induced killing of Bcr/Abl+ leukemic cells, and resistance due to their loss is overcome by a BH3 mimetic. Proc Natl Acad Sci U S A 2006; 103: 14907–12.
60. Kohl TM, Hellinger C, Ahmed F et al. BH3 mimetic ABT-737 neutralizes resistance to FLT3 inhibitor treatment mediated by FLT3-independent expression of BCL2 in primary AML blasts. Leukemia 2007; 21: 1763–72.
61. van Delft MF, Wei AH, Mason KD et al. The BH3 mimetic ABT-737 targets selective Bcl-2 proteins and efficiently induces apoptosis via Bak/Bax if Mcl-1 is neutralized. Cancer Cell 2006; 10: 389–99.
62. Konopleva M, Contractor R, Tsao T et al. Mechanisms of apoptosis sensitivity and resistance to the BH3 mimetic ABT-737 in acute myeloid leukemia. Cancer Cell 2006; 10: 375–88.
63. Chen S, Dai Y, Harada H, Dent P, Grant S. Mcl-1 down-regulation potentiates ABT-737 lethality by cooperatively inducing Bak activation and Bax translocation. Cancer Res 2007; 67: 782–91.
64. Kang MH, Kang YH, Szymanska B et al. Activity of vincristine, L-ASP, and dexamethasone against acute lymphoblastic leukemia is enhanced by the BH3-mimetic ABT-737 in vitro and in vivo. Blood 2007; 110: 2057–66.
65. Neubauer H, Cumano A, Muller M et al. Jak2 deficiency defines an essential developmental checkpoint in definitive hematopoiesis. Cell 1998; 93: 397–409.
66. Parganas E, Wang D, Stravopodis D et al. Jak2 is essential for signaling through a variety of cytokine receptors. Cell 1998; 93: 385–95.
67. Nosaka T, van DJ, Tripp RA et al. Defective lymphoid development in mice lacking Jak3. Science 1995; 270: 800–2.
68. Russell SM, Tayebi N, Nakajima H et al. Mutation of Jak3 in a patient with SCID: Essential role of Jak3 in lymphoid development. Science 1995; 270: 797–800.
69. Yamaoka K, Saharinen P, Pesu M et al. The Janus kinases (Jaks). Genome Biol 2004; 5: 253.
70. Bellanne-Chantelot C, Chaumarel I, Labopin M et al. Genetic and clinical implications of the Val617Phe JAK2 mutation in 72 families with myeloproliferative disorders. Blood 2006; 108: 346–52.
71. Levine RL, Belisle C, Wadleigh M et al. X-inactivation-based clonality analysis and quantitative JAK2V617F assessment reveal a strong association between clonality and JAK2V617F in PV but not ET/MMM, and identifies a subset of JAK2V617F-negative ET and MMM patients with clonal hematopoiesis. Blood 2006; 107: 4139–41.
72. Kralovics R, Teo SS, Li S et al. Acquisition of the V617F mutation of JAK2 is a late genetic event in a subset of patients with myeloproliferative disorders. Blood 2006; 108: 1377–80.

73. Barosi G, Bergamaschi G, Marchetti M et al. JAK2 V617F mutational status predicts progression to large splenomegaly and leukemic transformation in primary myelofibrosis. Blood 2007; 110: 4030–6.
74. Campbell PJ, Baxter EJ, Beer PA et al. Mutation of JAK2 in the myeloproliferative disorders: timing, clonality studies, cytogenetic associations, and role in leukemic transformation. Blood 2006; 108: 3548–55.
75. Theocharides A, Boissinot M, Girodon F et al. Leukemic blasts in transformed JAK2-V617F-positive myeloproliferative disorders are frequently negative for the JAK2-V617F mutation. Blood 2007; 110: 375–9.

Index